Your *Clinics* subscription

SO-BYD-710

You can now access the FULL TEXT of this publication online at no additional cost! Activate your online subscription today and receive...

- Full text of all issues from 2002 to the present
- Photographs, tables, illustrations, and references
- Comprehensive search capabilities
- Links to MEDLINE and Elsevier journals

Activate Your Online Access Today!

Plus, you can also sign up for E-alerts of upcoming issues or articles that interest you, and take advantage of exclusive access to bonus features!

To activate your individual online subscription:

1. Visit our website at **www.TheClinics.com**.

2. Click on "Register" at the top of the page, and follow the instructions.

3. To activate your account, you will need your subscriber account number, which you can find on your mailing label (note: the number of digits in your subscriber account number varies from six to ten digits). See the sample below where the subscriber account number has been circled.

This is your subscriber account number

```
***************************************3-DIGIT 001
FEB00   J0167   C7   123456-89   10/00   Q: 1

J.H. DOE, MD
531 MAIN ST
CENTER CITY, NY  10001-001
```

4. That's it! Your online access to the most trusted source for clinical reviews is now available.

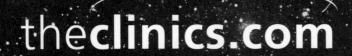

theclinics.com

ELSEVIER

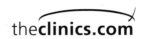
theclinics.com

PHYSICAL MEDICINE AND REHABILITATION CLINICS OF NORTH AMERICA

Aging with a Disability

GUEST EDITOR
Adrian Cristian, MD

CONSULTING EDITOR
George H. Kraft, MD, MS

February 2005 • Volume 16 • Number 1

SAUNDERS

An Imprint of Elsevier, Inc.
PHILADELPHIA   LONDON   TORONTO   MONTREAL   SYDNEY   TOKYO

W.B. SAUNDERS COMPANY
A Division of Elsevier Inc.

The Curtis Center • Independence Square West • Philadelphia, Pennsylvania 19106

http://www.theclinics.com

PHYSICAL MEDICINE AND REHABILITATION   Volume 16, Number 1
CLINICS OF NORTH AMERICA   ISSN 1047-9651
February 2005
Editor: Molly Jay

The ideas and opinions expressed in *Physical Medicine and Rehabilitation Clinics of North America* do not necessarily reflect those of the Publisher. The Publisher does not assume any responsibility for any injury and/or damage to persons or property arising out of or related to any use of the material contained in this periodical. The reader is advised to check the appropriate medical literature and the product information currently provided by the manufacturer of each drug to be administered to verify the dosage, the method and duration of administration, or contraindications. It is the responsibility of the treating physician or other health care professional, relying on independent experience and knowledge of the patient, to determine drug dosages and the best treatment for the patient. Mention of any product in this issue should not be construed as endorsement by the contributors, editors, or the Publisher of the product or manufacturers' claims.

Physical Medicine and Rehabilitation Clinics of North America (ISSN 1047-9651) is published quarterly by W.B. Saunders Company, Corporate and Editorial Offices: The Curtis Center, Independence Square West, Philadelphia, PA 19106-3399. Accounting and Circulation Offices: 6277 Sea Harbor Drive, Orlando, FL 32887-4800. Periodicals postage paid at Orlando, FL 32862, and additional mailing offices. Subscription price per year is $155.00 (US individuals), $238.00 (US institutions), $78.00 (US students), $188.00 (Canadian individuals), $305.00 (Canadian institutions), $108.00 (Canadian students), $215.00 (foreign individuals), $305.00 (foreign institutions), and $108.00 (foreign students). Foreign air speed delivery is included in all *Clinics* subscription prices. All prices are subject to change without notice. POSTMASTER: Send address changes to *Physical Medicine and Rehabilitation Clinics of North America*, W.B. Saunders Company, Periodicals Fulfillment, Orlando, FL 32887-4800. **Customer Service: 1-800-654-2452 (US). From outside of the US, call 1-407-345-4000.**

Physical Medicine and Rehabilitation Clinics of North America is indexed in *Excerpta Medica, Index Medicus, Cinahl,* and *Cumulative Index to Nursing and Allied Health Literature.*

Printed in the United States of America.

CONSULTING EDITOR

GEORGE H. KRAFT, MD, MS, Professor, Department of Rehabilitation Medicine; Adjunct Professor of Neurology; Director, Electrodiagnostic Medicine, Multiple Sclerosis Clinical Center; and Co-Director, Muscular Dystrophy Clinic, The University of Washington, Seattle, Washington

GUEST EDITOR

ADRIAN CRISTIAN, MD, Assistant Professor, Department of Rehabilitation Medicine, Mount Sinai School of Medicine, New York; Chief, Department of Rehabilitation Medicine, Bronx Veterans Affairs Medical Center, Bronx, New York

CONTRIBUTORS

MOHAMED S. AHMED, MD, Instructor, Department of Rehabilitation Medicine, Mount Sinai School of Medicine, New York; and Physiatrist, Department of Rehabilitation Medicine, Bronx Veterans Affairs Medical Center, Bronx, New York

DOUGLAS ALLEN, DO, Resident Physician, St. Vincent's Hospital, New York, New York

MATTHEW N. BARTELS, MD, MPH, Assistant Professor of Clinical Rehabilitation Medicine, Department of Rehabilitation Medicine, Columbia College of Physicians and Surgeons, Columbia University, New York, New York

JAISHREE CAPOOR, MD, Instructor, Department of Rehabilitation Medicine, The Mount Sinai School of Medicine, New York, New York

ADRIAN CRISTIAN, MD, Assistant Professor, Department of Rehabilitation Medicine, Mount Sinai School of Medicine, New York; Chief, Department of Rehabilitation Medicine, Bronx Veterans Affairs Medical Center, Bronx, New York

DANE B. COOK, PhD, Assistant Professor, Department of Radiology, University of Medicine and Dentistry of New Jersey-New Jersey Medical School, Newark; and Health Science Specialist, War-Related Illness and Injury Study Center, Department of Veteran Affairs, East Orange, New Jersey

CATHY M. CRUISE, MD, Clinical Assistant Professor, Department of Rehabilitation Medicine, Rusk Institute of Rehabilitation, New York University School of Medicine; and Physical Medicine and Rehabilitation Programs, Veterans Integrated Service Network #3, New York, New York

THOMAS W. FINDLEY, MD, PhD, Director of Research, War-Related Illness and Injury Study Center; Co-Director, Center for Healthcare Knowledge Management and Professor of Informatics, Department of Veteran Affairs, East Orange; and School of Health Related Professions, University of Medicine and Dentistry of New Jersey, Newark, New Jersey

STEVEN R. FLANAGAN, MD, Assistant Professor, Department of Rehabilitation Medicine, Mount Sinai School of Medicine, New York, New York

RICHARD A. FRIEDEN, MD, Assistant Professor, Department of Rehabilitation Medicine, The Mount Sinai School of Medicine, New York, New York

WAYNE A. GORDON, PhD, Professor, Department of Rehabilitation Medicine, Mount Sinai School of Medicine, New York, New York

MARY R. HIBBARD, PhD, Professor, Department of Rehabilitation Medicine, Mount Sinai School of Medicine, New York, New York

LILYANN JEU, PharmD, Clinical Pharmacy Specialist, Pharmacy Service, Bronx Veterans Affairs Medical Center, Bronx, New York

BRYAN J. KEMP, PhD, Director, Rehabilitation Research and Training Center on Aging with a Disability, Rancho Los Amigos National Rehabilitation Center, Downey; and Professor of Medicine and Psychology, University of California at Irvine, Irvine, California

ISAAC J. KREIZMAN, MD, Assistant Professor, Department of Rehabilitation Medicine, SUNY-Health Science Center of Brooklyn; and Director of Plain and Rehabilitation Services (PARS), Brooklyn, New York

JOSEPH M. LANE, MD, Attending Orthopedist, Department of Orthopedic Surgery, Hospital for Special Surgery; and Professor, Department of Orthopedic Surgery, The New York-Presbyterian Hospital, Weill Medical College of Cornell University, New York, New York

MATTHEW H.M. LEE, MD, Howard A. Rusk Professor and Chair, Department of Rehabilitation Medicine, Rusk Institute of Rehabilitation, New York University School of Medicine, New York, New York

JULIE T. LIN, MD, Assistant Attending Physiatrist, Department of Physiatry, Hospital for Special Surgery; and Clinical Instructor, Department of Rehabilitation Medicine, The New York-Presbyterian Hospital, Weill Medical College of Cornell University, New York, New York

BRITTANY MATSUMURA, MD, Chief Resident, Mount Sinai Medical Center, New York, New York

JOHN MORES, MS, Exercise Physiologist, War-Related Illness and Injury Study Center, Department of Veteran Affairs, East Orange, New Jersey

MICHELLE NISENBAUM, MD, Chief Resident, Department of Rehabilitation Medicine, Mount Sinai School of Medicine, New York, New York

ELLEN OLSON, Associate Professor, Department of Geriatrics and Adult Development, Mount Sinai School of Medicine; Chief, Extended Care, Mount Sinai School of Medicine, Bronx, New York

AKIKO OMURA, MD, Chief Resident, Department of Rehabilitation Medicine, Columbia College of Physicians and Surgeons, Columbia University, New York, New York

ASHOK POLURI, MD, Post-Doctoral Research Fellow, Exercise Physiology, War-Related Illness and Injury Study Center, Department of Veteran Affairs, East Orange, New Jersey

JAMES H. RIMMER, PhD, Professor, Department of Disability and Human Development, University of Illinois at Chicago, Chicago, Illinois

ADAM B. STEIN, MD, Associate Professor, Department of Rehabilitation Medicine, The Mount Sinai School of Medicine, New York, New York

MICHELLE STERN, MD, Assistant Clinical Professor, Department of Physical Medicine and Rehabilitation, Columbia University, College of Physicians and Surgeons, New York, New York

JODI THOMAS, MD, Instructor, Department of Rehabilitation Medicine, Mount Sinai School of Medicine, New York; Physiatrist, Bronx Veterans Affairs Medical Center, Bronx, New York

DAVID ULLMAN, Esq, New York State Bar Association, Section on Trustees & Estates, Albany, New York; American Trial Lawyers Association, Washington, DC

CELESTE D. ZAFFUTO-SFORZA, DO, Instructor, Department of Rehabilitation Medicine, Mount Sinai School of Medicine, New York; and Physician-in-Charge, Pediatric Rehabilitation, Elmhurst Hospital Center, Elmhurst, New York

MICHAEL E. ZULLER, Esq, New York, New York

CONTENTS

> Many people with disabilities from early in life (eg, cerebral palsy, spinal cord injury, and polio) are beginning to live into middle and late life. Recent evidence indicates that these individuals often do not age in a typical manner. A large proportion of these people develop new medical, functional, and support problems by the time they reach their late 40s and early 50s. This article reviews many of those changes and points to some ways to help intervene. Changes in rehabilitation education and programs need to begin to incorporate these recent findings.

> Changes in muscles and joints associated with aging can have a profound effect on the functionality of elderly and physically disabled persons. This article provides an overview of the current knowledge about how muscles and joints age and describes possible interventions.

FORTHCOMING ISSUES

RECENT ISSUES

VISIT OUR WEB SITE

The Clinics are now available online!
Access your subscription at <u>www.theclinics.com</u>

ELSEVIER
SAUNDERS

Phys Med Rehabil Clin N Am
16 (2005) xiii–xv

PHYSICAL MEDICINE
AND REHABILITATION
CLINICS OF
NORTH AMERICA

Foreword

Aging with a Disability

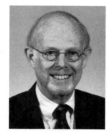

George H. Kraft, MD, MS
Consulting Editor

"[The best way to ensure a long, productive life is to] have a chronic disease and take care of it."

—Oliver Wendell Holmes, MD

Dr. Oliver Wendell Holmes had it right. This sensitive nineteenth-century physician–poet was aware of how continuous and attentive medical care could ward off accumulating maladies in persons who have chronic disease. However, the physician had to be attentive to them. This issue of the *Physical Medicine and Rehabilitation Clinics of North America* does just that—it details what the physician caring for patients who have chronic disabilities can do to give the best care possible to such persons.

I first became familiar with the problems of aging with a disability in the 1970s through the research of my colleagues Roberta Trieschmann, PhD, and Wilbert Fordyce, PhD [1]. Problems associated with the aging process may be amplified in individuals who have disabilities, or unrelated medical issues may develop and be overlooked, as they are inaccurately attributed to the primary disability.

Because I have focused my practice on the management of multiple sclerosis (MS), I have encountered this time and time again. Patients who have MS typically have a long course, in which they develop disease progression and worsening of neurologic symptoms. It is not uncommon for patients to complain of new symptoms but attribute them to their MS—such is their familiarity of living with the disease. Therefore, it is incumbent upon the practitioner to be ever vigilant and to tease out new neurologic disorders from the MS. The new disorders may be treatable or, at the least, must be

1047-9651/05/$ - see front matter © 2004 Elsevier Inc. All rights reserved.
doi:10.1016/j.pmr.2004.09.001

identified as separate entities so as to not confuse them with MS progression. It is not uncommon to see carpal tunnel syndrome as an offending new disorder—important to identify, because it is so successfully treated. Another example: I recently saw an MS patient who developed brachial neuritis—also important to identify so that it may be managed properly and so that it is not confused with MS [2].

Thus, those of us practicing chronic disease management need to be sensitive to both anticipated and unanticipated complications that may develop over time as the patient ages, and we need to work to prevent them [3]. This is a very important topic, and I am grateful to Dr. Adrian Cristian for taking on the task of organizing this issue. He has brought together a group of experts to share their areas of special interests on this theme. In large measure, the authors are colleagues of Dr. Cristian, coming from medical schools in the greater New York area. As such, these articles form a coherent text that discusses four overall themes:

The first theme—physical activity (Dr. Rimmer), aging muscles and joints (Dr. Ahmed), and falls (Drs. Lin and Lane)—covers the management of generic problems of the disabled elderly. The second theme discusses the management of two common symptoms: pain (Drs. Cristian, Thomas, Nisenbaum, and Jeuon) and fatigue (Drs. Poluri, Mores, Cook, Findley, and Cristian). The third theme deals with the problems of specific diseases: traumatic brain injury (Drs. Flanagan, Hibbard, and Gordon), cardiac (Dr. Kreitzman), cerebral palsy (Dr. Zaffuto-Sforza), amputations (Dr. Frieden), polio (Drs. Bartels and Omura), multiple sclerosis (Dr. Stern), and terminal diseases (Drs. Olson and Cristian). The last theme reviews practical applications: required knowledge for both provider and consumer (Dr. Kemp), legal aspects (Messrs. Ullman and Zuller), and service delivery (Drs. Cruise and Lee).

This is an ambitious and important issue. It contains practical guides and applications, such as the "pearls" in the article on falls, the practical tables in the article on pain, and the "boxes" in the article on fatigue. This issue belongs on the shelf of every physician who treats chronic disease. I am sure that the effort that has gone into it will be appreciated. My thanks again to Dr. Cristian and his coauthors for this fine issue of the *Physical Medicine and Rehabilitation Clinics of North America*.

George H. Kraft, MD, MS
Department of Rehabilitation Medicine
University of Washington School of Medicine
1959 NE Pacific Street, Box 356490
Seattle, WA 98195-6490, USA

E-mail address: ghkraft@u.washington.edu

References

[1] Trieschmann RB. Aging with a disability. New York: Demos; 1986.
[2] Walker M, Zunt JR, Kraft GH. Brachial neuropathy after immunosupression and stem cell transplantation for multiple sclerosis: a case report. Mult Scler (in press).
[3] Kraft GH. Rehabilitation principles for patients with multiple sclerosis. J Spinal Cord Med 1998;21:117–20.

PHYSICAL MEDICINE
AND REHABILITATION
CLINICS OF
NORTH AMERICA

Phys Med Rehabil Clin N Am
16 (2005) xvii–xviii

Preface

Aging with a Disability

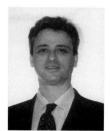

Adrian Cristian, MD
Guest Editor

Due to advances in modern medicine, millions of adults aging with disabilities are living longer lives. This increased lifespan is associated with an accelerated aging process due to the increased demands posed by the combination of normal aging changes superimposed on living with a disability. As a result, individuals with disabilities present at an earlier age with challenges not commonly encountered until much later in life by their nondisabled counterparts.

Although there are many diagnoses that lead to disability, common themes are emerging that connect many of them. Limited ambulation and wheelchair use is associated with a sedentary lifestyle. This predisposes to obesity, hypertension, diabetes, altered lipid profiles, and cardiovascular disease—often at a relatively young age. Common complaints expressed include pain, fatigue, and weakness. Pain is a major factor in the daily lives of people living with lower limb amputations, spinal cord injury, cerebral palsy, multiple sclerosis, and the late effects of polio. Overuse injuries of various organ systems are also common.

These complaints have a profound impact on the functionality of individuals living with these diseases. In addition, limited financial resources, transportation, access to medical specialists, and aging caregivers provide additional barriers to be overcome by this fragile population. At the end of life, ethical and legal challenges arise that affect patients, their families, and their physicians.

The goal of this issue is to provide clinicians with information on specific diagnoses and to lay a foundation on which future clinicians and researchers

doi:10.1016/j.pmr.2004.06.002

can build. Certain general topics that are pertinent to the care of the elderly patient (eg, falls) are also covered.

The contributors who have graciously devoted their time, energy, and knowledge for this endeavor are from a variety of health care settings across the United States. They care for patients in private, city, and federal facilities. An attempt was made to include the clinician's point of view and that of the ethicist and the lawyer because some issues straddle different fields.

Another goal of the issue was to identify some pressing research areas that contributors felt were needed to adequately provide care for this population in the future. Although the reader will find specific areas of inquiry in individual chapters, some common themes have emerged. The topic of aging with a disability desperately needs well-designed studies with adequate numbers of participants that reach statistical significance. There is a lack of long-term data on aging with some disabilities (traumatic brain injury), whereas others, although better described, lack adequately studied interventions. A grave concern is the potential impact of reduced reimbursement for rehabilitation services on patient care and their families.

I hope that the information provided in this text will teach present and future clinicians how to care for this delicate population, with the ultimate goal being their improved care and quality of life for many years to come.

I would like to thank the contributors, the staff at Elsevier, Dr. Kraft, and especially my family and my patients for their support and inspiration.

Adrian Cristian, MD
Department of Rehabilitation Medicine
Bronx Veterans Affairs Medical Center
130 West Kingsbridge Road
Bronx, NY 10468, USA

E-mail addresses: adrian.cristian@med.va.gov

ELSEVIER
SAUNDERS

Phys Med Rehabil Clin N Am
16 (2005) 1–18

PHYSICAL MEDICINE
AND REHABILITATION
CLINICS OF
NORTH AMERICA

What the rehabilitation professional and the consumer need to know

Bryan J. Kemp, PhD[a,b,*]

[a] *Rehabilitation Research and Training Center on Aging with a Disability,*
Rancho Los Amigos National Rehabilitation Center,
Downey, CA 90242, USA
[b] *Department of Medicine and Psychology, University of California at Irvine,*
Irvine, CA 92697, USA

The issue of aging of individuals with a disability is important to consumers, families, and practitioners. Because of improvements in medical care, rehabilitation, and technology, people with a disability have a good chance of living a nearly normal life expectancy. This means that people with a childhood-onset disability can expect to live into middle age and old age and that people with a mid-life onset can expect to live into later life. This has not always been the case. Until about 1960, people with cerebral palsy, spinal cord injury (SCI), Down syndrome, polio, and other impairments had a much shorter life expectancy. For example, in 1929, the general population had a life expectancy of about 55 years, but people with Down syndrome had a life expectancy of 10 years. In 1940, although the rest of the population enjoyed a life expectancy of about 60 years, a person with SCI could expect to live only 18 months after onset. Today, life expectancy for a person with SCI is about 85% of normal [1], and most people with Down syndrome and other major impairments can expect to live at least into their 60s.

Awareness of this increased life expectancy is new to nearly everyone; few people realize that it has changed as dramatically as it has. Even fewer people understand the consequences of it. For the person with a disability, it means that planning for the long run is important. This includes having

This work was supported by grants H133B980024 and H133B70011 from the National Institute on Disability and Rehabilitation Research, Office of Special Education and Rehabilitative Services, US Department of Education, Washington, DC.

* Rancho Los Amigos National Rehabilitation Center, RRTC on Aging with a Disability, 7601 E. Imperial Highway, 800 West Annex Downey, CA 90242.

E-mail address: bkemp@uci.edu

doi:10.1016/j.pmr.2004.06.009

a plan for obtaining ongoing primary health care, economic sufficiency, housing, and possibly eventual increased assistance from others. For parents of individuals with a developmental disability, it means that long-term planning is important because the children will probably outlive the parents (unlike earlier eras) and that support needs will fall on other family members, the formal support system, or on the individual with the disability. Rehabilitation practitioners can no longer be satisfied with helping the person to become as independent as possible; they must help the person stay independent in the community in the face of many challenges and changes that aging brings.

Most of what we know about aging with a disability has been discovered in the last 15 years. The theoretic understanding of what is happening to people as they age is unfolding, and the practical implications are just being incorporated into practice and training. This article covers the nature of aging and how and why people with disabilities seem to age differently. Some of the major health problems, the functional changes, the psychologic issues, and the social problems that need to be resolved are highlighted. The information comes from a variety of sources, including the Rehabilitation Research and Training Centers (RRTC) funded by the National Institute on Disability and Rehabilitation Research under the US Department of Education, Office of Special Education and Rehabilitation. These research centers have been tracking the nature of aging among people with a disability for about 20 years. In addition, individual investigators have been examining aging here and in a number of other countries.

Recent developments in aging with a disability

During the last several years, two overarching findings have emerged concerning aging with a disability. The first is that life expectancy has increased to about 80% to 90% of normal for people with even severe impairments. Most of this increase has occurred during the last 30 years, as opposed to the last 60 years for the rest of the population (Fig. 1) [1]. For the most part, many of the same factors that contributed to improvements in life expectancy for the general population (eg, improved public health, the advent of antibiotics, better primary care, improved surgery, and newer technology) have led to the improved life expectancy for people with disabilities. In addition, more interest in rehabilitation, better trauma care, increased funding for rehabilitation care and research, and the enactment of pro-disability legislation have added to the life expectancy of people with disabilities. The 30-year lag between people with and without disabilities in longevity means that it is a much newer occurrence for people with disability and one that most people are not aware of and do not understand.

The second most general finding is that this increased life expectancy is often accompanied by an increase in medical and functional problems at a relatively early age. It seems likely that many, if not a majority, of people

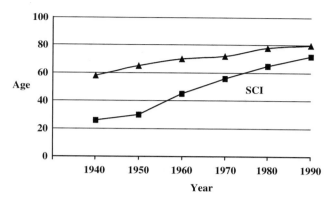

Fig. 1. Life expectancy of a 25-year-old person with and without SCI since 1940.

with a disability experience some form of premature aging changes in their health and in their functioning by the time they reach their 50s. This comes as a surprise to consumers and practitioners who expected that, after the hard work of rehabilitation and re-integration into life, the health of people with disabilities would remain stable. Many people with disabilities have been disappointed to find out about these mid-life changes first hand, and they want to know what to do about them. Many people with disabilities are searching for clinicians and services that can help them answer important questions about their health and about changes in function and independence. This article reviews some of the medical and functional changes that occur and offers ideas about why they seem to happen and what can be done about them. To understand what has been happening to people with a disability as they age, it is necessary to understand something about the nature of aging and to present a model for conceptualizing these age-related changes.

Aging is a natural and predictable component of life that begins almost as soon as the period of maturation and development ends, which typically is about 20 years of age. Aging changes can be viewed on a variety of levels, including subcellular, cellular, organ system, performance, psychologic, and social levels. Each level has its own measure of aging. At the cellular level aging is measured by cell death, at the organ level it is measured by the output of the organ, at the performance level it is measured by functional activities, and at the psychologic level it is measured by the ability to adapt.

The biologic changes that people go through as they age reflect gradual decreases in function at the cellular and organ system levels. Why we age and the mechanisms of aging are being better understood all the time, but we do not know all the answers. There are a number of theories about why we age, and these can be reviewed in major texts on gerontology [2]. Different kinds of aging—cellular, organ, functional, and psychologic—have different theories about them.

One of the more important theories for understanding what is happening to people with disabilities as they age is concerned with loss of function at the organ system level because this is often the underlying cause of the medical problems people with disabilities seem to be experiencing. This theory has been termed the "reserve capacity" theory of aging [3]. This theory holds that during normal maturation, each organ system gradually develops its capacity to carry out its functions. This development is usually accomplished by a combination of genetic and environmental influences. The cardiovascular system develops the capacity to circulate blood adequately as the tissue develops and as the demands for movement strengthen the tissue. The bones develop the ability to support weight, and the immune system develops the ability to resist disease. Capacity begins to develop before birth and reaches a peak at around 18 to 20 years of age. As part of its normal development, each organ system creates excess or reserve capacity over and above what is needed for basic survival. This excess capacity is supposed to protect us so that relatively minor injuries or illnesses do not turn out to be fatal, thus adding to our chances of survival. After reaching a peak at about 19 or 20 years of age, each of the organ systems begins to gradually lose some of that capacity. The loss is gradual and is not noticeable to the average person for many years. The rate of this decline in capacity has been the subject of much research. The Baltimore Longitudinal Studies of Aging [4] assessed several physical parameters of men of various ages over long periods of time and found that the rate of normal aging at the organ system level averaged about 1% per year across organ systems. The heart slowly loses its pumping ability, the kidneys slowly lose their filtering ability, and the bones slowly lose mineral content. This loss does not usually have much effect on daily functioning or much clinical significance because the excess capacity developed earlier in life keeps us above the minimum capacity needed for everyday life, which is generally about 40% to 50%. If capacity drops below that threshold, the person will be at risk for serious complications, such as an illness. At a rate of 1% per year, it takes between 50 and 60 years for the average person to go from his or her 100% peak capacity at age 20 to the 40% level at about the age of 75. This age is the beginning of the geriatric era. Fig. 2 depicts the course of normal aging at the organ system level.

Why people lose capacity in the organ systems is not completely known. Some of the prominent theories include genetics, the accumulation of toxic waste products within cells, loss of central regulatory mechanisms, wear and tear, and stress [2]. Perhaps each is true as it applies to a particular organ system. For example, the loss of cardiac contractility seems to be related to the accumulation of the effects of wear and tear, stress, and toxic products within the cells [3]. Cell death in the central nervous system seems to be caused by programmed death, small lesions, and abnormal toxins. Brain changes slowly lead to loss of some cognitive abilities, even in the absence of frank pathology (eg, Alzheimer disease).

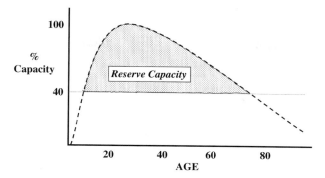

Fig. 2. Normal development and aging.

Loss of capacity in people with a disability: a model

What happens to people who have a disability? How do they age? How are the building of capacity and the loss of capacity affected by a disability? The answers to these questions depend in part on the kind of impairment, the age at which the impairment occurred, the effect of the impairment on activities that influence development and loss of capacity, and what organ system is studied. A person with SCI that occurred at age 23 ages in a way that is different from a person with cerebral palsy and different from a person who had SCI at age 50. These individuals each had a disability at different points of development and aging. The person with cerebral palsy may not reach the same absolute level of capacity in some organ systems and will therefore have less reserve capacity. As decline sets in, it may take less time before the 40% to 50% threshold is reached. The person with SCI at 50 years of age developed normal capacity but had been aging and losing reserve before the SCI. The SCI causes a rapid loss of capacity, thereby prematurely aging that person in terms of when that threshold is crossed. What can be discerned from the pattern of available literature in terms of how people with a disability are aging?

First, adults who have a disability after maturity seem to be aging from that point forward at a rate that is faster than normal when compared with nondisabled people. Instead of aging at a rate of 1% per year, the accumulating evidence (see below) suggests that the rate may be between 1.5% and 5% per year, depending upon the organ system. This means that a person who acquires a disability around 25 years of age reaches the 40% threshold capacity level in some organs around 55 to 60 years of age (95% remaining capacity at age 25 divided by 1.5% /year = 30 years to reach 50% capacity).

Second, the same absolute level of capacity may never be reached if the disability occurs before maturity and if the disability affects the activities needed for developing that organ's capacity. For example, a person with cerebral palsy may never reach the same level of bone mineral density

(BMD) as a nondisabled person if he or she lacked the ability to exercise or generate sufficient muscular force against the bones, which is essential to bone growth. These differences in aging are illustrated in Figs. 2 and 3. If the evidence holds, what could cause such accelerated aging? There are several possibilities, and each may play a role depending upon the organ system. One possibility is that there is more wear and tear in people with disabilities, particularly in the musculoskeletal system. This makes sense considering such commonly reported problems as joint injuries, carpal tunnel syndrome, fractures, and arthritis in people who have to use their shoulders to propel themselves, spend inordinate amounts of energy to be ambulatory, or put excess strain on their wrists to transfer. Wear and tear is more likely related to the duration of the impairment than to the age of the person. Thus, duration may be the key variable in some instances. Another possibility is that minute damage to organ systems may speed up aging in a particular organ. For example, repeated urinary tract infections may speed up aging in that system. Another possibility is that there is damage to central "pacemaker" systems, such as the immune system or the endocrine system, that affects end organs. There is evidence that multiple endocrine functions are disrupted in SCI, suggesting a central, "upstream" control mechanism.

If this model is correct, then three predictions can be made. (1) People with onset of disability after maturity should show declines in organ function that are steeper than nondisabled persons. (2) People with childhood or congenital disabilities should show less absolute levels of peak capacity in some organs. (3) Because organ system decline is happening sooner in people with a disability, people with a disability should show a higher number of secondary health problems by 50 or 60 years of age compared with their nondisabled peers.

It is difficult to estimate the size of the population of people aging with a disability who are having these kinds of problems due to semantic issues and the lack of sufficient information. The semantic difficulty arises because everyone over the age of 20 who has a disability is aging with it. Therefore,

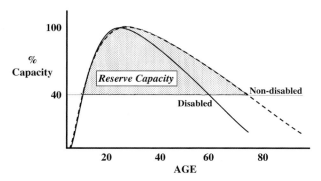

Fig. 3. Aging with and without disability.

this number equals all of the adults in the United States who have a disability, which is estimated at about 11% of the civilian population, or about 30,000,000 people [5]. However, that definition of disability is broad, including people who have any activity limitation. The problems discussed in this article apply to a subset of those persons—the ones with the most severe impairments. If the data are reduced to persons who have a severe disability in the sense that they cannot perform a major activity, then the number becomes about 6% of the population, or 15,500,000 people. If that number is further reduced to include only people who have a disability onset after the age of 20 but before age 60, then the estimate is about 2% to 3% of the population, or between 4,000,000 and 6,000,000 people. This is the estimated number of people at risk for developing later-life complications of disability.

Aging-related physical changes

By the time a person with a disability reaches 45 years of age, and often before then, many physical changes are well underway. Metabolic, orthopedic, cardiovascular, and respiratory changes have been documented in people aging with a disability. Most of the data that have been generated on physical changes are impairment specific, and there is a need for more information across impairments. A general principle that an earlier-than-expected loss of organ functioning exists is becoming clear. One caveat to this principle is that it is not always age that is the critical factor when comparing the difference between disabled and nondisabled individuals. Two other factors are also important. One is the duration of the impairment. Even though duration and age are highly correlated in many cases, duration may be the more important factor. The other is the historic era in which the impairment occurred, which can be significant because of changes in care, technology, and social policies. An older person received much different treatment when he was young than a young person receives today. Sophisticated research designs are needed to determine the contribution of each of these factors.

With these caveats in mind, it is still possible to discern aging differences between disabled and nondisabled individuals. Garland et al [6–8] assessed BMD in people who had SCI versus those who had no disability. Women without SCI showed a gradual decline in density until 55 years of age and then a more rapid loss of mineral after menopause. Women with SCI showed a linear loss of BMD that began immediately after the onset of the SCI and that continued throughout life at a rate of about 5% per year. The nondisabled women reached the threshold of having 40% remaining BMD about 70 years of age, but the women with SCI crossed that threshold at about 50 years of age. The deficit seems to be restricted to bones below the level of the injury because they have not found differences in the hip. Bach et al [9] studied respiratory changes in individuals with a history of polio. They measured vital capacity in adults of different ages and durations of polio who had no history of respiratory paralysis. They found that people with polio had a rate of loss of capacity that was about 1.9% per year compared with a rate of about 1% per year in the nondisabled population. Bauman and Spungen [10,11] assessed changes with age and duration in people with SCI in relation to growth hormones and body composition. The slope of loss in total body lean percentage was steeper (about 2.9% per year) in people with SCI than in nondisabled persons (about 1% per year) across a 60-year span. When they compared nondisabled people with people who had a SCI on free and total testosterone levels, they found that nondisabled men declined at rates of between 0.4% and 1.2%, respectively, but men with SCI declined at a rate of about 1.7% per year. In recent research from the RRTC (RRTC, unpublished data, 1998–2003), individuals of different ages and with various impairments received spirometry assessments. The nondisabled persons showed a normal slope of loss in vital capacity, but the group with a disability showed a slope that was twice as steep across ages. Recently, Linn et al [12] studied respiratory function in people with high-level SCI and found that it declined faster than in nondisabled persons but that the critical factor was duration, not age. Evidence has recently linked aging to a steeper decline in high-density cholesterol in people with disability than in persons without a disability [10]. Thus, evidence is accumulating of a steeper-than-normal loss of organ function for people who have a disability.

Evidence is being accumulated to support the prediction that if the person had a disability before maturity he or she may not reach the same peak level of organ capacity compared with nondisabled people. Henderson et al [13] studied bone density in people with cerebral palsy using DEXA scans. They found that nonambulatory individuals had lower peak bone density than their nondisabled counterparts at all ages. Mosqueda et al followed up on this study by assessing 50 people with cerebral palsy who averaged 34 years of age (L. Mosqueda, E. Fowler, S. Rao, unpublished data). In their sample, 82% had osteopenia or osteoporosis, even those who were only in their early 20s. Individuals with other impairments have low bone mass if they have lacked ambulation, such as people with a history of polio [14]. Several common clinical examples illustrate this principle. People with cystic fibrosis have been found not to develop the same respiratory capacity as nondisabled people, individuals with cerebral palsy or spina bifida do not have the same cardiovascular capacity as nondisabled people, and individuals with adolescent or childhood polio develop less respiratory capacity if the polio interfered with the ability to exercise. People with developmental mental retardation do not reach the same absolute level of brain development as their nondisabled peers [15].

One of the biggest differences between disabled and nondisabled people is in their rates of secondary heath problems. Bauman et al [16] studied glucose metabolism in middle-aged men with SCI compared with nondisabled men using a glucose tolerance test. The average age of the samples was the early

40s, and the duration of disability for those with SCI was about 18 years. In the control sample, 85% were considered normal as a result of the test, 9% were impaired to some degree, and 6% were diabetic. In the SCI sample, only 45% were normal, 31% were glucose intolerant, and 23% were diabetic. These rates of type II diabetes would not be expected in a nondisabled population until people were well into their 70s or 80s. Another study [17] found that more people with a history of post-polio syndrome had higher levels of total cholesterol than people with polio but no post-polio syndrome or nondisabled persons. They used laboratory samples to measure the number of people in each group who had total cholesterol levels above 240 and found that there was no statistical difference in the number of people with elevated cholesterol levels between the nondisabled people and the ones with a history of polio but no post-polio syndrome. However, the group that had post-polio syndrome had twice as many people with high cholesterol levels. The difference was 24% in the two former groups and 42% in the latter group. The authors speculated that the post-polio syndrome caused decreases in mobility, which contributed to the increased cholesterol levels. Similar results were obtained by Bauman et al [16], who studied individuals with SCI. Coyle et al [18] found that women with SCI had far more secondary health problems than women without disability.

Murphy et al [19] studied 101 persons with cerebral palsy who averaged 42 years of age. They found that more than 25% had had a fracture in the previous 5 years, 40% had new contractures, and more than 50% had new pain. People with developmental disabilities have higher rates of hypertension, incontinence, and swallowing difficulties [15]. People with SCI have much higher rates of fractures [6–8], heart disease, respiratory disorders, obesity, and diabetes [10] as do people with a history of polio [14,21]. The frequency of secondary and associated health problems in people with major physical impairments has been investigated by in studies by Seekins et al [22] and Campbell et al [23]. In the Seekins study, the investigators found that the participants reported an average of 13 new health problems per year, including such conditions as pressure sores, urinary tract infections, malnutrition, and depression. In the Campbell study, the investigators found equally high rates of health problems and functional problems such as pain, gait problems, weakness, and deconditioning. In the study done at the RRTC [47], the average person coming into the study had five secondary conditions. What causes the secondary conditions is open to debate, but they are likely due to organ system changes and a lack of adequate primary care to detect these problems earlier. For example, Murphy et al [19] found that in their sample of 101 people, 95% did not have a primary care physician. Similarly, Heller [15] found that people with developmental disabilities had access to primary care had fewer actual additional illnesses.

To demonstrate the magnitude of the problem that people with various impairments face in terms of the added risk and the added occurrence of

Table 1
Rates of secondary conditions of people with disability

Group	Problem	Mean age in study (y)	Percentage with problem	Reference
SCI	Osteoporosis	45	30%	Garland [6,7]
	Depression	48	42%	Krause et al [25]
	Diabetes	48	22%	Bauman and Spungen [16]
CP	Fracture	42	25%	Murphy et al [19]
	New Pain	42	30%	Murphy et al [19]
Down syndrome	Alzheimer's	50	40%	Sutton et al [24]
	Obesity	50	37%	Rubin et al [26]
Post-polio	Respiratory insufficiency	45	50%–60%	Halstead [21]

Abbreviations: SCI, spinal cord injury; CP, cerebral palsy.

additional health problems, Table 1 shows the rates of several major secondary health problems in studies of people with a primary impairment. For this table, data were collected to show the rate of these additional health problems in samples that averaged about 45 to 50 years of age.

Functional issues

Many people with disabilities experience changes in function and health as they age. Function refers to everything from mobility to employment. The first group to show new functional problems in large numbers was the post-polio population, whose report of new problems in the 1970s led to the defining of this post-polio syndrome [27]. It is estimated that up to 70% of people with a history of polio develop a syndrome of new weakness, pain, fatigue, and functional decline, the definition of post-polio syndrome [28]. These symptoms may occur in any sequence, but typically the process begins with new muscle weakness, and eventually fatigue and pain are present. The beginning is usually subtle. Often, it is only by taking a history that the person sees that there has been a slow progression of symptoms. As time passes, the person may notice that tasks become more difficult, that more rest is needed, or that he or she does not bounce back the way they used to. The fatigue factor becomes big because it is not necessarily activity related. Instead, people report that it is much like chronic fatigue syndrome in its severity and pervasiveness. More assistance from others or from equipment may be needed for certain activities. The loss of abilities usually is in a predictable pattern: social and recreational activities, work demands, instrumental activities of daily living (IADLs), and eventually some activities of daily living (ADLs).

It is not just people with polio who are reporting these problems. Recently, the RRTC on Aging With A Disability at Rancho Los Amigos reported in a study of over 600 people with various impairments that this combination of weakness, fatigue, and pain was a commonly expressed problem. It seems that this syndrome may be a general "post-impairment syndrome" because it is common across polio, SCI, cerebral palsy, arthritis, and other conditions that cause severe disability. Researchers at that Center labeled the symptoms of pain, fatigue, and weakness the "Functional Impairment Syndrome" because it occurs as a syndrome and because it usually marks the beginnings of change in function in major activities [29]. In studies at the RRTC, over a quarter of the persons with one of these impairments reported two or more of these problems.

Special attention has been paid to this problem by other investigators who attempted to identify who is most at risk of these problems and when they may be most likely to occur. Gerhart et al [30] investigated these problems in people living in England who had SCI of at least 20 years duration. They asked the subjects whether they had experienced a need for new assistance, and, if so, when it had occurred. They reported that approximately half the sample had reported new needs for assistance with ADLs or IADLs and that this occurred at an average age of 49 years for people with tetraplegia and age 54 for persons with paraplegia. The average duration of injury was a little over 20 years. Thompson and Yakura [29] reported that the age at which changes occurred averaged 45 years and that the average duration was 18 years. The difference between these two sets of figures is probably due to the fact that Thompson and Yakura assessed the age of onset of pain, fatigue, or weakness, whereas Gerhart et al [30] assessed the age at changes in needs for assistance. It is possible that the added years in the latter study represent how long it takes for the syndrome to evolve into needs for assistance with activities. Also, the former study showed differences between people with tetraplegia versus paraplegia, whereas the latter did not. This could be due to the nature of the outcome in each study. Pentland et al [31], Rintala et al [32], and Thompson [33] noted the increased likelihood of these problems with age or duration and the fact that it seems to take fewer years to start to experience these changes the later the onset in life of the SCI, as might be expected because those people would have less reserve capacity [33]. Murphy et al [19] found that about 40% of their sample of people with cerebral palsy had changes in mobility and other functional abilities that began as early as their mid-20s. A generalized principle seems to be emerging regarding changes in functional abilities and functional symptoms that applies to a variety of impairment groups, a principle first articulated by Gerhart et al [30]. That principle is the "20/40" rule. It means that functional issues are likely to begin to emerge by the time the person reaches 40 years of age or has 20 years duration of disability, whichever comes first. There is variation around this rule (it is 45/25 in some cases), but the principle seems applicable enough that it has become one of the teaching points in all of the professional and consumer training done by the RRTC on Aging With A Disability.

In a large sample of qualitative interviews at the RRTC, people reported similar ways of coping with these problems. First came the onset of some or all of the symptoms of pain, fatigue, and weakness, followed by a realization that some things have to change because of limited endurance and increasing pain or weakness. Most people reported that first they changed social activities or strenuous physical activities, such as sports. Then they started to rest more and started to reduce IADL demands. If they were working, they tried to maintain that role and eventually they possibly needed to cut back work activities or retire early. McNeal et al [34] studied changes in work patterns and needs for accommodation in people with polio, cerebral palsy, or SCI. They found that many people with disabilities needed additional job accommodations in the form of adjusted work schedules, new equipment, altered task techniques, or rest periods to keep working. Despite these adjustments, many people had to work part-time or retire by the time they reached their mid-50s.

Research efforts are underway to try to determine the causes of the pain, fatigue, and weakness in different impairment groups and to try to reduce these symptoms and maintain function. In many post-polio clinics, there is an emphasis on modifying life styles to maintain function, such as reducing activities and resting more [27]. Thompson [35] examined causes of fatigue in people with SCI and found that there was no single cause across individuals. Instead, there was a combination of medical, pharmacologic, psychologic, orthopedic, and functional issues that contributed to their fatigue. In many cases, no cause could be found. It seems that the method of treating these problems is three pronged: (1) a thorough evaluation to try to discover underlying conditions that can reverse the problem (eg, a medical cause for fatigue, an offending drug side effect, the presence of depression, or an inappropriate way of performing a task); (2) consideration of assistive devices and technology that could help the problem; and (3) changes in lifestyle to adjust to the diminished ability. As far as could be determined, there are no outcome data on the percentage of people who are assisted by each of these efforts.

Psychosocial considerations

At least three psychosocial issues are important in the context of aging with a disability. These are (1) how to maintain as high a quality of life as possible while adjusting to these age-related changes, (2) the problem of depression as people try to cope with these changes and losses, (3) and the issue of caregiving in the family context and in terms of service systems.

The concept of quality of life (QOL) can be approached objectively or subjectively. Objective QOL refers to empiric, observable entities that one can count, such as employment, income, marital status, home ownership, and educational level. These are important considerations in determining how well a person is doing in society compared with others. The other conceptualization of QOL is subjective: The level of QOL is whatever the person believes it is. Research on objective QOL began in the Eisenhower administration as a way to examine how the country as a whole was doing compared with earlier times. The research began to reveal the importance of subjective QOL at the individual level. One reason for this expanded interpretation was that there was often little correlation between objective indicators of QOL and subjective measures. A person with high income, a home, and a job could have low subjective QOL, and a person with no job, little income, and who did not own a home could have high subjective QOL. This is an important point when it comes to the issue of QOL in persons with a disability because the stereotype is that people with disabilities must have a lower QOL than people without a disability. This is not the case. Dijkers [36] and Fuhrer [37] did meta-analyses on life satisfaction and disability and concluded that there was little correlation between the two. Recently, Kemp [38] reported on QOL in people aging with a disability using a two-factor model of QOL. In his research, QOL was arranged on a continuum, from negative (or low) to positive (or high), with a neutral point in the middle. Kempe had about 1000 people with various impairments and people with no disability rate their overall QOL using a seven-point Likert-type scale. Although the group with no disability had somewhat higher QOL scores, there were some interesting findings in the group with disability. First, a large number of people with disabilities had high levels of QOL. Second, QOL in the group of people with disability was unrelated to the severity of the impairment or the degree of disability. For example, there were as many people with high QOL who had tetraplegia as had paraplegia. Finally, the factors that were most correlated with high QOL were engagement in social, recreational, family, and productive activities. As long as these could be accomplished, QOL was high. What happens to QOL as people with a disability age and undergo age-related changes in health and function? Does the disability affect their QOL?

Gerhart et al [30] examined this issue in a study of people with SCI who were at least 20 years post-onset. They found that people who had not undergone any significant changes in health and function rated their overall QOL (life satisfaction) as higher presently than it had been 20 years earlier. This is a common finding: People who have a disability rate their QOL higher as time passes [39]. However, for those who had a change in function, the time 20 years earlier was rated more satisfactory than the present. Therefore, it seems that the challenge of coping with age-related changes in health and functioning can have an impact on QOL. When Kemp correlated levels and changes in ADLs, IADLs, and community activities with ratings of QOL, it was only the latter that had a significant relationship. Thus, it seems reasonable to conclude that the critical factor is the ability to engage in these more social and meaningful activities as a factor in QOL. This is also consistent with the findings of McNeal et al [34], who found that people with disabilities would decrease their IADLs to preserve strength and stamina for employment, which they valued more highly.

The issue of coping with age-related changes in disability has an impact on the development of depression, arguably the most important psychologic problem among people with a disability. Rates of moderate and major depression are three to four times higher in people with a disability than in the nondisabled population [40]. The published rates for either level of depression among people who have a disability are from 20% to 55%, depending upon the nature of the impairment. For example, people with polio have been found to have a rate of about 24% [41], people with SCI have a rate of about 40% [41,42], and people with stroke have a rate of about 50% [43]. As in the case of QOL, depression is not strongly related to the severity of the impairment or to the degree of disability. For example, Krause et al [25] found that the rate was the same among people with tetraplegia or paraplegia. Depression is much more related to the person's ability to cope with changes and losses than it is with the disability. In this context, such factors as the number and type of life changes (stressors), the amount of emotional support received, the person's coping methods, and their view of the changes in terms of future impact are more important. Depression has devastating effects on a person who has a disability. It is highly correlated with increased health problems, decreased functioning, and a shorter life expectancy. For example, Morris [43] demonstrated that people with a stroke were half as likely to live 10 years if they were also depressed compared with if they were free of depression. In the research by Thompson [44] on changes in function in persons with SCI, twice as many people were depressed who had functional changes compared with those who did not have functional changes. Depression has not been found to be associated with age in groups of people with disability, although an onset of disability later in life is correlated with depression [25]. This finding seems to imply that living longer with a disability is not related to depression and goes with the finding that longer durations are associated with higher life satisfaction. It is possible that people who are depressed do not live as long and hence are not in the study sample as time goes by. Depression does seem to be treatable to a high degree in people who have a disability, and neither the disability nor the age of the person seem to matter in terms of who benefits from treatment. Treatment with antidepressant medication, especially selective serotonin reuptake inhibitors, is effective, and combining it with psychotherapy yields improvements rates similar to the nondisabled population [40].

The caregiving responsibilities of families and society are an issue for this population. Most people with a developmental disability outlive their primary source of support (ie, their parents), and many if not most people with a physical disability experience changes in function and health by 60 years of age that put extra responsibility, if not stress, on some member or members of the family of origin or the family of marriage. In the developmental disability population, the issue of long-term care and support of the person with the disability has been rated the number one issue worldwide [20]. This is easy to understand when one recognizes that the average life expectancy of the person with an intellectual developmental disability is about 60 years, meaning that the parents of this person are in their 80s if they are alive. It is not unusual for families to come to the clinic at the Medical Center of the University of California at Irvine where the "identified" patient is a person 54 years of age with an 82-year-old mother who has her own health problems. It is estimated that there are more than 500,000 people with a developmental disability who are living with a parent over the age of 65 in the United States [20,45], a number that is likely to increase by 25% in the next 30 years.

In the study by Thompson [33] concerning changes in function in people with SCI, data were collected on who was providing the extra help needed for assistance with IADL and ADL as the person with SCI sustains some of these changes. In the majority of the cases, it was the spouse who, because most people with SCI are men, was the wife. In other impairments it is likely to be either the wife or the husband. Next in terms of likelihood of providing help was a parent, a sibling, or a child. The extra responsibilities placed on the spouse are important because often these responsibilities come at a time when the spouse is busy with child rearing, employment, and caregiving responsibilities for parents or in-laws who are also aging. Aranda [46] found that family members were often stressed by these added responsibilities and had not expected that the person with the disability would need extra help as time went by. Their biggest concerns reported in that study were assisting with pain, fatigue, and emotional problems of the person with the disability, especially depression.

The systems of care that people aging with a disability need are nearly non-existent. There are few medical professionals knowledgeable about these age-related changes; there are few out-patient facilities where these persons can go to have their health status evaluated comprehensively; there are few therapists educated about the new functional problems people are facing; and there are few resources available for people who are aging with a disability to seek economic, technologic, or personal assistance help. One of the biggest needs in the field of physical medicine and rehabilitation in the next few years will be the development of comprehensive out-patient assessment clinics where people aging with a disability can go to have their health, functional, and psychosocial needs evaluated.

References

[1] Sasma GP, Patrick CH, Feussner JR. Long-term survival of veterans with traumatic spinal cord injury. Arch Neurol 1993;50:909–14.
[2] Birren J, Schaie W. The handbook of the psychology of aging. 5th edition. New York: Van Norstrand; 2001.
[3] Kane RL, Ouslander JG, Abrass IB. Essentials of clinical geriatrics. 4th edition. New York: McGraw-Hill; 1999.
[4] Shock NW, Gruelich RC, Andres R, Arenberg D, Costa PT Jr, Lakatte EG, et al. Normal human aging: the Baltimore Longitudinal Study of Aging. NIH publication no. 84–2450; Washington D.C.: US Department of Health and Human Services; 1984.

[5] Institute on Medicine. Committee on a National Agenda for Prevention of Disabilities. Disability in America: toward a national agenda for prevention. National Academy Press: Washington, DC; 1991.

[6] Garland DE, Maric Z, Adkins RH, Stewart CA, Yakura JS. Regional osteoporosis following incomplete spinal cord injury. Contemp Orthop 1994;28:134–9.

[7] Garland DE, Adkins RH, Rah A, Stewart CA. Bone loss with aging and the impact of SCI. Top Spinal Cord Inj Rehabil 2001;6:47–60.

[8] Garland DE, Adkins RH, Stewart CA, Ashford R, Vigil D. Regional osteoporosis in women who have a complete spinal cord injury. J Bone Joint Surg 2001;83A:1195–200.

[9] Bach JR, Alba AS. Pulmonary dysfunction and sleep disordered breathing as post-polio sequelae: evaluation and management. Orthopedics 2001;14:1329–37.

[10] Bauman WA, Spungen AM. Disorder of carbohydrate and lipid metabolism in veterans with paraplegia or quadriplegia: a model of premature aging. Metabolism 1994;43:749–56.

[11] Bauman WA, Spungen AM, Adkins RH, Kemp BJ. Metabolic and endocrine changes in persons aging with spinal cord injury. Assist Technol 1999;11:88–96.

[12] Linn WS, Adkins RH, Gong H Jr, Waters RH. Pulmonary function in chronic spinal cord injury: a cross-sectional survey of 222 southern California adult outpatients. Arch Phys Med Rehabil 2000;81:757–63.

[13] Henderson RC, Lark RK, Gurka MJ, Worley G, Fung E, Conaway M, et al. Bone density and metabolism in children and adolescents with moderate to severe cerebral palsy. Pediatrics 2002:110:e5.

[14] Silver JK. Keeping bones healthy and strong. In: Silver JK, editor. Post-polio syndrome: a guide for polio survivors and their families. New Haven: Yale University Press; 2001. p. 159–69.

[15] Heller T. Aging with developmental disabilities: emerging models for promoting health, independence, and quality of life. In: Kemp BJ, Mosqueda L, editors. Aging with a disability: what the clinician needs to know. Baltimore: The Johns Hopkins University Press; 2004. p. 213–33.

[16] Bauman WA, Adkins RH, Spungen AM, Waters RL. The effect of residual neurological deficit on oral glucose tolerance in persons with chronic spinal cord injury. Spinal Cord 1999; 37:765–71.

[17] Kemp BJ, Campbell ML. Health, functioning and psychosocial aspects of aging with disability: final report of the Rehabilitation Research and Training Center on Aging. Downey (CA): Los Amigos Research and Education Institute, Inc.; 1993.

[18] Coyle CP, Santiago MC, Shank JW, Ma GX, Boyd R. Secondary conditions and women with physical disabilities: a descriptive study. Arch Phys Med Rehabil 2000;81:1380–7.

[19] Murphy KP, Molnar GE, Lankasky K. Medical and functional status of adults with cerebral palsy. Dev Med Child Neurol 1995;37:1075–84.

[20] Adkins RH. Research and interpretation perspectives on aging related physical morbidity with spinal cord injury and brief review of systems. NeuroRehabilitation 2004;19:3–13.

[21] Halstead LS, Rossi C. New problems in old polio patients: results of a survey of 539 polio survivors. Orthopedics 1985;8:845–50.

[22] Seekins T, Clay J, Ravesloot C. A descriptive study of secondary conditions reported by a population of adults with physical disabilities, served by the three independent living centers in a rural state. J Rehabil 1994;60:47–51.

[23] Campbell M, Sheets D, Strong P. Secondary health conditions among middle-aged individuals with chronic physical disabilities: implications for unmet needs for services. Assist Technol 1999;11:105–22.

[24] Sutton E, Factor AR, Hawkins BA, Heller T, Seltzer GB. Older adults with developmental disabilities. Baltimore: Brookes Publishing; 1993.

[25] Krause JS, Kemp BJ, Coker JL. Depression after spinal cord injury: relation to gender, ethnicity, aging, and socioeconomic indicators. Arch Phys Med Rehabil 2000;81:1099–109.

[26] Rubin S, Rimmer J, Chicoine B, Braddock D, McGuire D. Overweight prevalence in persons with Down syndrome. Ment Retard 1998;36:175–81.

[27] Perry J. Aging with poliomyelitis. In: Kemp BJ, Mosqueda L, editors. Aging with a disability: what the clinician needs to know. Baltimore: The Johns Hopkins University Press; 2004. p. 175–95.

[28] Silver JK. Post-polio syndrome. In: Silver JK, editor. Post-polio syndrome: a guide for polio survivors and their families. New Haven (CT): Yale University Press; 2001. p. 12–20.

[29] Thompson L, Yakura J. Aging related functional changes in persons with spinal cord injury. Top Spinal Cord Inj Rehabil 2001;6:69–82.

[30] Gerhart KA, Bergstrom E, Charilifue SW, Menter RR, Whiteneck GG. Long-term spinal cord injury: functional changes over time. Arch Phys Med Rehabil 1993;74:1030–4.

[31] Pentland W, McColl MA, Rosenthal C. The effect of aging and duration of disability on long-term health outcomes following spinal cord injury. Paraplegia 1995;33:367–73.

[32] Rintala DH, Loubser PG, Castro J, Hart KA, Fuhrer MJ. Chronic pain in a community-based sample of men with spinal cord injury: prevalence, severity and relationship with impairment, disability, handicap and subjective well-being. Arch Phys Med Rehabil 1998;79: 604–14.

[33] Thompson L. Functional changes in persons aging with spinal cord injury. Assist Technol 1999;11:123–9.

[34] McNeil DR, Somerville NJ, Wilson DJ. Work problems and accommodations reported by persons who are postpolio or have a spinal cord injury. Assist Technol 1999;11: 137–157.

[35] Thompson L, Waters RL, Kemp BJ. Functional changes in longstanding spinal cord injury: the need for multi-disciplinary interventions. J Spinal Cord Med 2001;24:S6.

[36] Dijkers M. Quality of after spinal cord injury: a meta-analysis of the effect of disablement components. Spinal Cord 1997;35:829–40.

[37] Fuhrer MJ. The subjective well-being of people with spinal cord injury: relationships to impairment, disability and handicap. Top Spinal Cord Inj Rehabil 1996;1:56–71.

[38] Kemp BJ. Quality of life, coping, and depression. In: Kemp BJ, Mosqueda L, editors. Aging with a disability: what the clinician needs to know. Baltimore: The Johns Hopkins University Press; 2004. p. 48–67.

[39] Krause JS, Crewe NM. Chronologic age, time since injury, and time of measurement: effect on adjustment after spinal cord injury. Arch Phys Med Rehabil 1991;72:91–100.

[40] Kemp BJ, Kahan JS, Krause JS, Adkins RH, Nava G. Treatment of major depression among persons with SCI: changes in depressive symptoms, life satisfaction and community activities over six months. J Spinal Cord Med 2004;27:35–41.

[41] Kemp BJ, Krause JS. Depression and life satisfaction among people aging with a disability: a comparison of post-polio and spinal injured individuals. Disabil Rehabil 1999;21: 241–9.

[42] Fuhrer MJ, Rintala DH, Hart KA, Clearman R, Young ME. Depressive symptomatology in persons with spinal cord injury who reside in the community. Arch Phys Med Rehabil 1993; 74:255–60.

[43] Morris PL, Robinson RG, Andrzejewski P, Samuels J, Price TR. Association of depression with 10-year post-stroke mortality. Am J Psychiatry 1993;150:124–9.

[44] Thompson L, Kemp BJ, Waters RL. Aging with spinal cord injury: clinical implications from recent research findings. Presented at the American Spinal Injury Association. Long Beach (CA), May 17, 2001.

[45] Janicki MP, Dalton AJ, Henderson CM, Davidson PW. Mortality and morbidity among older adults with intellectual disability: health services considerations. Disabil Rehabil 1999; 21:284–94.

[46] Aranda MP, Clark LJ, Adams BM, Ettelson DM, Kemp BJ, Gunderson AS. Psycho-educational interventions for family caregivers of people aging with physical disabilities.

Presented at the Annual Meeting of the Gerontological Society of America. Chicago, November 15–18, 2001.

[47] Rehabilitation Research and Training Center on Aging with Disability. Variations in late onset complications, risk factors and health care needs for four groups of people aging with physical disabilities. Richmond (VA): Rehabilitation Research Training Center. Grant H133B30004; 1993.

ELSEVIER
SAUNDERS

Phys Med Rehabil Clin N Am
16 (2005) 19–39

PHYSICAL MEDICINE
AND REHABILITATION
CLINICS OF
NORTH AMERICA

Age-related changes in muscles and joints

Mohamed S. Ahmed, MD[a,b,*], Brittany Matsumura, MD[c], Adrian Cristian, MD[a,b]

[a]Department of Rehabilitation Medicine, Mount Sinai School of Medicine,
One Gustave L. Levy Place, 1190 5th Avenue, New York, NY 10029, USA
[b]Department of Rehabilitation Medicine, Bronx Veterans Affairs Medical Center,
130 West Kingsbridge Road, Bronx, NY 10468, USA
[c]Mount Sinai Medical Center, 1425 Madison Avenue, New York, NY 10029-6574, USA

As people get older, multiple factors play roles in their disability. The impact of the aging process on skeletal muscles and joints can have a profound effect on the functionality of an individual. This article discusses the changes seen in aging muscles and joints and describes possible treatment options to minimize them. The changes described are based on human and animal models. Many studies involving human subjects are limited by a small sample size.

Theories on aging

There are two common theories for aging: the "programmed theory" and the "damage theory." The programmed theory states that aging follows a genetic timetable. The damage theory states that aging may be due to the cumulative consequences of free radical reactions. The source of these toxic and inert substances can be outside the body or can be a by-product of cellular metabolism. Some of them can transform DNA into an inert state [1].

Structural and mechanical change in aging skeletal muscle

Skeletal muscles mainly consist of two types of muscle fibers: fast-twitch and slow-twitch. Fast-twitch muscles (type II) can generate power over short

* Corresponding author. Department of Rehabilitation Medicine, Bronx Veterans Affairs Medical Center, Room 3d-16 526/117 Bronx VAMC, 130 West Kingsbridge Road, Bronx, NY 10468.

E-mail address: mohamed.ahmed2@med.va.gov (M.S. Ahmed).

periods of time by using energy derived from anaerobic metabolism. Slow-twitch muscles (type I) derive their energy from aerobic metabolism, using more mitochondria, more myoglobin, and more capillaries per square inch. They are primarily involved in endurance-related activities.

In the geriatric population, skeletal muscle changes are related to aging, inactivity, underlying medical conditions, poor nutritional status, and hormonal changes. The human body contains over 400 skeletal muscles, which make up 30% to 40% of the total body weight. Multiple studies suggest that muscle mass decreases with aging. A recent study showed that the prevalence of low muscle mass increases with aging from 8.9% in the 76- to 80-year age group to 10.9% in 86- to 95-year age group [2].

In healthy young people, about 30% of the body weight is muscle, 20% is adipose tissue, and 10% is bone. By age 75, about 15% of body weight is muscle, representing a loss of half of the muscle mass with aging. Additionally, there is a doubling of adipose tissue to approximately 40% of body weight [3].

Age-related skeletal muscle changes vary among muscle groups and for different muscle fiber types and do not affect all muscles equally [4]. It has been reported that aging muscle shows a reduction in the number and total size of fast-twitch muscle fibers and a reduction in number of slow-twitch muscle fibers [5]. A study by Poggi et al [6] showed a predominance of type I fibers in aging muscles and suggested that this could be secondary to selective atrophy of type II fibers or a conversion of type II fibers to type I. In comparison to nonweight-bearing muscles, weight-bearing muscles with higher proportion of type IIb fibers showed marked atrophy [7].

There is a marked reduction in the total number of anterior horn cells with aging. This can be as much as 50% when compared with early adult life or middle age [8]. The loss of motor neurons contributes to the reduction of muscle mass by denervating the muscle fibers within the motor unit. Motor unit remodeling takes place in aging and is accompanied by a higher proportion of denervated muscle fibers [9,10]. Lewis et al [11] suggested that fast motor neurons may transform to slow motor neurons by a trophic chemical release from the slow-twitch muscle fibers [11].

Aging can significantly affect antioxidant activity and oxidative damage to skeletal muscles [12]. Pansarasa et al [13] have shown a reduction of superoxide dismutase activity in human muscles with aging. Animal models have reported lower glutathione peroxidase activity in the muscles of aging rats [14].

Satellite cells are specialized cells located in the basal membrane of muscle cells. They are necessary for the development of new muscle tissue and repair [15]. The number of satellite cells in skeletal muscle decreases with age; thus, the ability of muscle to regenerate after injury or overload decreases with aging [16]. The impaired propensity of satellite cells to proliferate and to produce myoblasts that are necessary for muscle regeneration in aging is secondary to insufficient Notch signaling [17].

There is a 50% reduction in oxidative capacity per volume of muscle in older adults when compared with younger adults. This is believed to be secondary to a reduction in mitochondrial content and to a lower oxidative capacity of mitochondria with age [18]. An aging-associated decreased content of mitochondrial coenzyme Q in skeletal muscles has been described [19]. Oxidant-induced mitochondrial DNA damage in aging muscles results in a decline in the content and rate of production of ATP. Animal models have shown that ATP content and production decrease by approximately 50% in skeletal muscles as a result of aging [20].

Tumor necrosis factor (TNF)-α is considered to be a contributing factor to aging-related loss of skeletal muscle mass [21]. Well-functioning older men and women show lower muscle mass and lower muscle strength when elevated plasma concentrations of interleukin-6 and TNF-α are present [22].

Inadequate dietary protein intake by elderly individuals has been associated with a loss of skeletal muscle mass. The recommended dietary protein allowance might not meet the protein requirement for the elderly persons [23]. Protein-calorie supplement in the aging population has shown to be helpful in gaining strength and muscle mass [24].

The rate of muscle protein synthesis is lower in older adults [25,26] secondary to a reduced synthesis of protein from amino acids [27,28] and leads to a loss of muscle mass. Reductions in myosin heavy chain and mitochondrial protein synthesis lead to a loss of muscle strength and poor aerobic exercise tolerance [26].

There has been little literature on the relationship between aging muscle changes and physical disabilities or disease states in humans. Electron microscopy of the muscles of diabetic rats has shown an abnormal arrangement of myofibrils along with mitochondrial swelling, with sparing of the neuromuscular junction and capillaries [29]. Chronic congestive heart failure causes significant change in skeletal muscle mitochondria and capillary distribution, which affects the oxidative capacity of working muscle [30]. Chronic renal failure affects the muscle energy metabolism by decreasing the mitochondrial enzymatic activity [31].

Elderly individuals whose mobility is restricted because of acute illness are at greater risk of deconditioning. Absolute bed rest can accelerate the loss of muscle mass and strength. The rate of loss can be 1.5% per day. Deconditioning seems to affect antigravity muscles to a greater extent [3].

There is growing evidence to indicate that age-related decline in the production and activity of hormones plays an important role in aging muscle. In healthy individuals, circulating levels of testosterone, estrone, estradiol, growth hormone (GH), insulin-like growth factor (IGF)-1, and IGF hormone binding protein-3 are significantly decreased with advancing age.

Age-related declines in testosterone in men have been observed cross-sectionally [32] and longitudinally [33]. A cross-sectional study of 403 elderly men showed a significant reduction of testosterone with aging. A correlation was noted between testosterone levels and muscle strength. Normal levels correlated with good muscle strength, whereas reduced levels correlated with decreased muscle strength [34]. Testosterone deficiency has been associated with a marked decrease in measures of whole body protein anabolism, decreased strength, decreased fat oxidation, and increased adiposity [35].

A correlation has been shown in healthy individuals over 60 years of age between a reduced lean body mass and an increase in adipose mass, with lower IGF-I [36]. In women, an additional 15% decline in muscle strength around menopause may be related to a reduction in estrogen [37].

A cross-sectional study comparing 21 adults with GH deficiency (GHD) and 29 non-GH-deficient adults showed that adults with GHD have increased body fat and a reduction of fat-free soft tissue mass [38].

Skelton et al [39] have shown that strength declines at a rate of about 1% to 2% per year between 65 and 89 years of age. By the seventh and eight decade of life, maximal voluntary contractile strength is decreased about 20% to 40% [40]. It has been suggested that change in muscle mass is a major determinant of age- and gender-related differences in skeletal muscle strength [41]. Much of the age-associated muscle atrophy and declining strength can be explained by motor unit remodeling. This is the process whereby there is selective denervation of muscle fibers and reinnervation by axonal sprouting from adjacent motor units.

Fast-twitch muscle fibers are associated with strength, whereas slow-twitch muscle fibers are associated with endurance. In aging, there is a greater proportional loss of fast-twitch muscle fibers compared with slow-twitch muscle fibers. This may explain the greater reduction in strength versus endurance with aging [42].

There is approximately a 3.5% annual loss in power generated by muscles for individuals between 65 and 89 years of age [39]. Normally, the greater the number of fast-twitch muscle fibers, the greater the force and power generated during a muscle contraction [43]. However, the force developed by the fast- and slow-twitch fibers (predominantly the fast-twitch fiber) declines with age [44]. The maximal isometric contraction force decreases 20% by the sixth decade and about 50% by the eighth decade [3]. Aging muscles show a lower muscle torque secondary to the small contractile muscle mass and increased coactivation of the antagonist muscles [45].

The speed of movement is greater in muscles with a higher percentage of fast-twitch fibers [46]. A slower contractile speed has been associated with aging secondary to a loss of fast-twitch muscle fibers, a predominance of slow-twitch muscle fibers, and a qualitative change in the contractile properties of skeletal muscles [47]. Age-related changes in the molecular dynamics of myosin can alter force production [48]. Decreased membrane permeability to calcium ions [49] and impaired calcium reuptake by the sarcoplasmic reticulum may be also responsible for the decreased muscle contractility with aging [50].

Other changes that have been reported include (1) a reduction in the elasticity of skeletal muscles secondary to an increased presence of fibrotic tissue, (2) an impaired healing of injured muscles [51], and (3) an increased fatigability believed to be associated with reduced motor unit firing rate [52].

The impact of changes in aging muscle in the elderly population

The changes described above can have a profound impact on aging individuals. The impaired muscle function can adversely affect elderly individuals' balance and ability to ambulate and perform activities of daily living. The reduced skeletal muscle mass has been associated with functional impairment and disability, particularly in older women [53]. The decreased muscle strength, decreased muscle mass, and poor standing balance can be associated with a higher risk for falls [54].

Management

This section presents various interventions, such as exercise, electrical stimulation, and hormonal treatments, that can potentially offset these changes.

Physical activity and exercise

It is important to encourage adults to remain as physically active as possible for as long as possible. It has been shown that the muscles of active individuals have a greater resistance to fatigue and have a greater strength when compared with sedentary individuals [55,56]. Clinicians should educate their older patients to maintain a lean body mass [57].

A regular exercise program has been shown to help in maintaining postural balance, muscle strength, and endurance in adults who exercised on a regular basis compared with those who do not [58]. Regular exercise has also been found to be helpful in preventing oxidative damage to muscles by increasing the resistance to oxidative stress [59]. An adequate warm-up period is essential to prevent injury and improve the elasticity of skeletal muscles [60].

Exercise should be goal oriented and performed on a regular basis. The exercise regimen should focus on an identified problem. For example, if the problem is with endurance, then an endurance-improving exercise program is advised. Although endurance training may reduce the extent of loss of strength [61], a strength-training program may be more appropriate for that problem.

The subject of benefit versus risk associated with a heavy-resistance strength exercise program is controversial. Some researchers found that a heavy-resistance strength training program causes muscle damage in an older population [62], whereas another study reported that heavy-resistance strength training can increase the number of satellite cells [63].

There is evidence to suggest that endurance and strength training programs help improve muscle strength and walking speed [64]. Endurance exercise in old animal models improves the visco-elastic properties of muscles [65]. Strengthening exercises have been shown to result in muscle hypertrophy [66].

Evans et al [67] showed that a high-intensity resistance training (above 60% of the one repetition maximum) exercise program can result in significant gains in strength and functional status in nursing home residents. It can also attenuate the age-related decline in force-generating capacity of muscles and can lead to muscle fiber hypertrophy [68]. Resistance exercise training has also been shown to improve protein synthesis and muscle strength [69]. Other benefits of resistance training include (1) an improved torque due to decreased antagonist muscle coactivation [70]; (2) improved oxidative capacity (31%), mitochondrial volume density (31%), and muscle size (10%) [71]; (3) increased muscle cell size, strength, contractile velocity, and power in slow- and fast-twitch muscle fibers [72]; (4) suppressed levels of muscle TNF-α [73]; (5) a partial reversal of the reduced Ca^{2+} re-uptake by the sarcoplasmic reticulum [50]; and (6) a positive effect on the synthesis rate of protein myosin heavy chain [74]. Even low-intensity resistance exercises with short rest period intervals can lead to muscle hypertrophy and improved strength [75].

Tai Chi Chuan

A Tai Chi Chuan program has been shown to improve knee extensors strength and endurance in the elderly population [76].

Electrical stimulation

Electrical stimulation can be useful as an initial therapeutic option for aging individuals with muscle weakness who have difficulty participating in a regular exercise program. Caggiano et al [77] showed that electrical stimulation on the quadriceps femoris muscle can improve muscle strength in aging individuals. McMiken et al [78] demonstrated a comparable benefit between cutaneous electrical stimulation and isometric exercise for quadriceps strengthening in the normal healthy population.

Gene therapy

Gene therapy may have a role in the strengthening of muscles. Scientists have developed a novel gene therapy treatment that blocks the age-related loss of muscle size and strength in mice. A recombinant adeno-associated virus directing overexpression of IGF-I was injected into muscle fibers and found to be associated with a 15% increase in muscle mass and a 27% increase in strength compared with uninjected muscles [79].

Antioxidant therapy

The antioxidant N-acetylcysteine has been shown to be effective in improving muscle strength and in reducing the plasma level of TNF-α [80].

Estrogen therapy

Controversy exists regarding the role of estrogen replacement therapy (ERT) in the management of sarcopenia. Some feel that oral estrogen therapy may accelerate the lean mass loss in postmenopausal women by reducing the concentration of bio-available free testosterone [81], whereas others feel that ERT does not protect against the muscle loss of aging [82].

A 16-week, double-blind, randomized trial of 40 postmenopausal women found a greater improvement in total lean body mass and a reduction of fat mass with estrogen-androgen therapy when compared with ERT alone [83]. Aloia et al [84] reported that hormone replacement therapy (HRT) was unable to prevent fat mass gain and loss of lean body mass in postmenopausal women. Sorensen et al [85] reported on 16 healthy postmenopausal women who showed that HRT (17β estradiol plus cyclic norethisterone acetate) had a reversal effect on menopause-related obesity and loss of lean body mass.

The route of ERT has different effects on the body composition of postmenopausal women. Oral estrogen resulted in an increased in fat mass and a decrease in lean mass compared with transdermal estrogen [86].

Dehydroepiandrosterone

Dehydroepiandrosterone (DHEA) is a precursor for estrogens and androgens. A prospective 6-month trial of oral DHEA replacement (50 mg/d) resulted in an increase in serum IGF-I, total serum testosterone concentrations, and fat-free mass. It decreased the fat mass [87], which suggests that increases in IGF-I or testosterone may play a role in mediating the effects of DHEA.

Testosterone

A randomized, double-blind study of 108 men over 65 years of age showed that treatment with testosterone significantly reduced fat mass and increased lean body mass [88]. Significant side effects associated with the use of testosterone can preclude its use. For example, testosterone has been associated with an elevation of prostate-specific antigen [89].

Growth hormone

Mixed results with the use of GH have been reported. Some studies have shown an improvement in lean body mass and a decrease in fat mass [90,91], whereas others did not [92,93].

A double-blind, placebo-controlled study of 1 year's duration on adults with acquired growth hormone deficiency (GHD) showed significant improvement in body composition with GH therapy. Daily subcutaneous injection of GH (2.0 IU/m², Norditropin) increased serum IGF-I 200% and lean body mass 5.7%. Fat mass was reduced by 21.5% [90]. Long-term (3 years) uninterrupted GH replacement treatment in the GHD adult showed improvement in isometric muscle strength and thigh muscle volume, which was maintained throughout the treatment period without significant side effects [94]. Blackman et al [91] reported on a 26-week randomized, double-blind, placebo-controlled, parallel-group trial conducted in healthy, ambulatory, community-dwelling men and women 65 to 88 years of age in the United States. GH with or without sex steroids was found to increase lean body mass and decrease fat mass [91].

Contrary to these studies, Whitehead et al [92] reported that a 6-month program with recombinant human growth hormone (rhGH) did not result in a significant change in muscle fibers of adults with GHD; however, the study was limited by a small sample size. Friedlander et al [93] reported that self-injection with IGF-I (15 µg/kg twice daily) by postmenopausal women over 60 years of age for 1 year did not show significant changes in lean body mass when compared with placebo, but this study size was also limited by a small sample size ($n = 16$) [93].

A comparison study between rhGH (0.025 mg/kg/d) and one of two doses of recombinant human insulin-like growth factor-I (rhIGF-I) (0.015 and 0.060 mg/kg) twice daily was performed on elderly women. All treatment groups showed a significant improvement in lean body mass. The lower IGF dose was better tolerated when compared with the higher dose of IGF and the GH dose [95]. It is believed that IGF-I increases satellite cell proliferation [96] and improves protein synthesis [97].

The synovial joint

The synovial joint has several key components that contribute to its overall structure and function. The capsule, ligaments, and tendons of the synovial joint are made up of fibrous connective tissue that provides stability and strength to the joint. Articular cartilage provides the articulating surfaces that participate in load bearing and distribution and lower the friction-bearing surface. Subchondral bone provides nutrients to the base of the cartilage. A layer of calcified cartilage separates the articular cartilage with the subchondral bone and is known as the "tide mark." The synovial membrane is responsible for the secretion and maintenance of synovial fluid that provides nutrition to articular cartilage and lubricates the joint space. Each of these components undergoes age-related changes that can lead to overall impairment of joint structure and function, making the joint more susceptible to age-related diseases and injury of the joint (Fig. 1). Muscles envelop the joint, providing movement and stability.

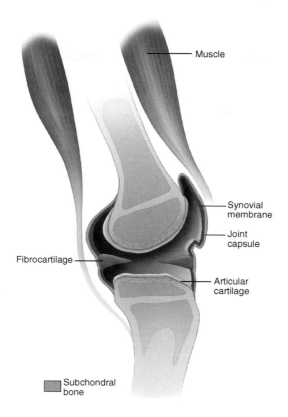

Fig. 1. Each of these components undergoes age-related changes that can lead to overall impairment of joint structure and function, making the joint more susceptible to age-related diseases and injury of the joint. Muscles envelop the joint, providing movement and stability.

Articular cartilage is made up of a matrix composed mainly of proteoglycans and collagens. Aggrecans are molecules consisting of multiple chondroitin sulfate and keratan sulfate chains covalently bound to a central protein core. Aggrecans are the basic structure that gives cartilage the qualities of compression stiffness, resiliency, and durability [98]. Multiple aggrecans create noncovalent associations with a hyaluronic filament to form large proteoglycan aggregates. Link proteins stabilize the associations between aggrecans and hyaluronan. The proteoglycan aggregates become enmeshed in a network of predominantly type II collagen, forming the cartilage matrix. It is the proteoglycans that bind to the majority of water within cartilage.

Age-related changes in articular cartilage

In the past, the degenerative changes of osteoarthritis were considered an inevitable consequence of aging; however, several studies have illustrated distinct differences between the effects of natural aging and the manifestations of osteoarthritis in joints. An alternative view has surfaced in which joint degeneration is not an inevitable consequence of aging; rather, the alterations in the aging joint make it more susceptible to degeneration. Age-related changes observed in articular cartilage, including those of a structural, compositional, and mechanical nature, have been shown to vary to from changes of degenerative diseases such as osteoarthritis [99–102].

With age, there is a noted decrease in keratan sulfate chains and aggrecan size. The mean number of aggrecans per aggregate decreases, leading to smaller proteoglycan aggregates [102,103]. Whether this is due to increased proteoglycan degradation, decreased proteoglycan synthesis, or a combination of both is not clear. Some studies suggest that with age, chondrocytes produce shorter aggrecans and more variable aggregates [101,104]. It has also been suggested that there is an age-related alteration in the small-link proteins that stabilize the association between aggrecans and hyaluronan [101,105,106]. The molecular changes within the articular cartilage matrix may play a role in the altered biomechanical properties of articular cartilage (eg, decreased tensile stiffness and strength) [102].

Collagen and other proteins within the matrix undergo non-enzymatic reactions with glucose to form advanced glycosylation end products (AGEs) that participate in collagen cross-linking. Studies have noted increased concentrations of pentosidine, a measure of AGEs, with age resulting in increases in collagen cross-linking [107]. Due to a prolonged half-life, collagen may be susceptible to the accumulation of AGEs [108]. Increased collagen cross-linking may be central to stiffening of the collagen network in cartilage.

Proteoglycan synthesis seems to decline with age. A study of age-related decreased proteoglycan synthesis suggested that accumulation of AGEs may correspond to declining proteoglycan synthesis [109]. The mechanism of how this may take place is not clear; hypotheses vary between a direct interference of AGEs with growth factor's ability to stimulate receptors and a more indirect effect. Altered proteoglycan synthesis and structure seen with aging may contribute to the finding of decreased water concentration in aging cartilage because proteoglycans bind water in cartilage [110].

Research has shown an increased prevalence of cartilage calcification with age [111,112]. The presence of calcium pyrophosphate dihydrate crystals has been found in the cartilage of elderly individuals. Transglutaminase is an enzyme that is involved in the biomineralization process. Age-related increases in transglutaminase activity may contribute to the finding of increased calcium pyrophosphate crystals found in older cartilage [113].

Structurally, aging articular cartilage tends to have increased superficial fibrillations, roughening of the surface, and erosions [114]. Thinning of the articular cartilage has been noted with age and is associated with a decline in cell numbers. Research findings have not concurred upon a specific amount of chondrocyte cell loss attributed to age [115,116].

Age-related changes in chondrocytes

Age-related decline in the mitotic and synthetic activity of articular cartilage chondrocytes has been a subject of investigation [117]. The ability of chondrocytes to proliferate seems to decrease with age. Research suggests that this is due to decreased responsiveness to growth factor stimulation and replicative senescence [118].

Telomeres are DNA sequences found at the ends of chromosomes. Telomeres play an important role in the replication and maintenance of normal chromosome function. The protective role of a telomere includes the prevention of enzymatic degradation of the chromosome. Over the cells' replicative cycle, incremental loss of telomere length to DNA damage may lead to telomere exhaustion [119]. Telomere erosion effects the ability of the cell to replicate and can lead to cell senescence, a state of arrest in the cell cycle [102,120]. Research findings are consistent with the accumulation of senescent chondrocytes in aging articular cartilage that is associated with telomere shortening [117]. Cell senescence impairs the ability of chondrocytes to maintain the articular cartilage.

In studies of chondrocytes in rat articular cartilage, researchers have found an age-related decline in chondrocyte responsiveness to the anabolic factor IGF-I [121–123]. IGF-I seems to have a central role in stimulating the chondrocyte synthesis of collagen and proteoglycans to maintain articular cartilage. It has been suggested that the alterations in chondrocyte responsiveness to this anabolic factor may be secondary to increased production of IGF-binding proteins [124]. Response to other growth factors, such as transforming growth factor-beta, is maintained; however, the ability of these anabolic factors to overcome the antianabolic effects of other mediators is decreased [125], The overall result is a decreased ability of chondrocytes to repair and maintain the cartilage matrix.

Oxidative damage may contribute to decreased chondrocyte responsiveness to growth factors. Studies have shown an age-related increase in oxidative damage by endogenous reactive oxygen species in various human tissues [126]. Mitochondria play a central role in the protection of the cell from the harmful effects of free radical derivatives. An age-associated decline in the activity level and number of mitochondria and alterations in the mitochondrial genome have been observed [127,128]. Such changes may lead to increased reactive oxygen species, furthering oxidative damage. Studies of articular cartilage found markers for oxidative damage present in nonarthritic elderly individuals. These markers were not found in normal cartilage samples from young adults [129]. Studies have suggested that mitochondrial degeneration is associated with in vitro articular cartilage chondrocyte senescence [102].

Age-related changes in subchondral bone and synovial membrane

It is unclear whether age-related changes in subchondral bone lead to cartilage matrix deterioration or if degeneration of cartilage leads to the subchondral bone findings. Studies using a monkey model have suggested that increased density of subchondral bone (also known as osteopetrosis) appears before articular cartilage changes [130]. This is consistent with a previous hypothesis that the sclerotic changes within the subchondral bone are due to the healing of microfractures. This leads to bone stiffening and increased shear forces upon the cartilage matrix. It is hypothesized that forces over time lead to cartilage matrix degeneration [131]. Recent research has suggested a modest decrease in the thickness of subchondral bone with aging [132]. Further evaluation of the aging changes of subchondral bone would be helpful in elucidating the effects subchondral bone has on cartilage and visa versa.

The cells lining the synovial membrane can be separated into two types: type A and type B. Type A cells are rich in lysosomes and play an important role in phagocytosis. Type B cells are primarily involved in synthesis, particularly of hyaluronan. Hyaluronan plays an important role in cell regulation and phenotypic expression. In the intercellular space of the synovial membrane, hyaluronan regulates the diffusion of proteins from the plasma to the synovial fluid. With age, there is an alteration in the hyaluronan structure that contributes to a breakdown of the hyaluronan barrier. As a result, formerly excluded components of the plasma are introduced into the synovial fluid [133].

The impact of age-related muscle and soft tissue changes on aging joints

Sarcopenia may play a significant role in promoting joint injury because the stabilizing function of muscles in joint biomechanics is compromised [134]. Animal studies using Botox to weaken joint muscle forces have shown that decreased muscle forces in knee extensor muscles are associated with degeneration of the knee despite normal joint stability [135]. It is unclear what direct effects sarcopenia may play in the development of degenerative arthritis, although it is hypothesized that decreased ability for the muscles to distribute joint load by controlling joint movement leads to increased susceptibility for joint damage [134].

Tendons, menisci, and the joint capsule make up the soft tissues surrounding a joint. Ligaments and tendons consist of collagen, which undergoes increased cross-linking with age. This occurs via a mechanism similar to those observed in cartilage involving AGEs. These alterations in structure lead to increases in collagen stiffness and reduced flexibility of these structures. This plays an important role in transmitting muscle power and providing joint stability [136]. Evidence suggests that an age-related decline in the tensile strength of ligament–bone complexes leads to a failure of these complexes at loads much lower than in younger populations [137,138].

The menisci participate in load bearing and stabilization of the joint during flexion-extension. They act as shock absorbers for the knee joint by distributing the loads of pressure across it. These fibrocartilaginous structures are made up collagen fibers and proteoglycans. An age-associated decrease in proteoglycan synthesis has been observed in the menisci [139]. Structural changes that occur with age within the menisci reduce its ability to transmit tensional stresses, which compromises their function [140].

Biomechanical changes in the aging joint

Muscle contractions play an important role in the stability of a joint. As muscles contract around the joint, the forces and loads are dissipated across the joint. Research studies in the elderly population have shown a decline of quadriceps strength with age [141,142]. Further studies of quadriceps strength in subjects with degenerative changes of osteoarthritis (OA) suggest that individuals with OA tend to have greater weakness in the quadriceps than age-matched control subjects without OA [143]. These findings imply that quadriceps weakness is associated with joint degeneration; however, no direct correlation has been shown.

Maintaining appropriate joint alignment is important to joint integrity. There seems to be a correlation between knee joint varus-valgus laxity and age. Evidence suggests that an increased degree of varus-valgus laxity correlates with a greater decline in the joint space [144,145].

Joint stiffness increases the joint's vulnerability to injury. This is probably due to the combination of age-related changes seen in articular cartilage, ligaments, and synovium. With age, tensile stiffness, fatigue resistance, and cartilage strength decline [146].

An age-associated decrease in joint proprioception has been noted in several studies, including in patients with osteoarthritis [147,148]. Proprioception plays an important role in maintaining the joint structure. Animal studies have shown that disruption of proprioceptive feedback from the mechanoreceptors of a joint leads to advanced and accelerated degenerative changes of the joint [149].

Aging joint in disability

There is a paucity of research evaluating the specific age-related joint alteration in adults with physical disabilities. The exception to this seems to be overuse injuries of the shoulder in wheelchair users. This is described elsewhere in this issue. Further investigation is warranted to describe aging joint changes in this population so that appropriate interventions can be developed, tested, and implemented.

Potential interventions to minimize age-related joint changes

Appropriate strength training can slow the progression of muscle loss associated with age. Improvements in muscle strength have been shown with resistance exercises in the elderly population and may prove beneficial in slowing the progression of age-associated muscle mass loss [150,151].

Studies comparing knee proprioception in active elderly and sedentary elderly participants suggest that regular exercise may attenuate the proprioceptive decline seen with aging [152,153]. Tai Chi has been shown to improve joint proprioception in the elderly population [153,154].

Summary

Aging muscle and joint changes can have a tremendous impact on the functionality of elderly people with and without disabilities. Studies in animal models have shown some potentially beneficial interventions (eg, gene therapy). Further research is needed to ascertain their benefits in humans.

A better understanding of mechanisms by which skeletal muscle and joint changes take place in a geriatric population will be helpful to find reasonable ways to prevent age-related change and improve disability. Although some agents have been reported to have significant positive effects, further studies are needed to determine long-term side effects. More information is needed with respect to the changes in muscles and joints in various disabilities.

References

[1] Lee HC, Wei YH. Mitochondrial alterations, cellular response to oxidative stress and defective degradation of proteins in aging. Biogerontology 2001;2:231–44.

[2] Gillette-Guyonnet S, Nourhashemi F, Andrieu S, Cantet C, Albarede JL, Vellas B, et al. Body composition in French women 75+ years of age: the EPIDOS study. Ageing Dev 2003;124:311–6.

[3] Beers MH, Berkow R, editors. Aging and the musculoskeletal system. In: The Merck Manual of Geriatrics. Whitehouse Station (NJ): Merck Research Laboratories; 2000.

[4] Nikolic M, Malnar-Dragojevic D, Bobinac D, Bajek S, Jerkovic R, Soic-Vranic T. Age-related skeletal muscle atrophy in humans: an immunohistochemical and morphometric study. Coll Antropol 2001;25:545–53.

[5] Kamel HK, Maas D, Duthie EH Jr. Role of hormones in the pathogenesis and management of sarcopenia. Drugs Aging 2002;19:865–77.

[6] Poggi P, Marchetti C, Scelsi R. Automatic morphometric analysis of skeletal muscle fibers in the aging man. Anat Rec 1987;217:30–4.

[7] Holloszy JO, Chen M, Cartee GD, Young JC. Skeletal muscle atrophy in old rats: differential changes in the three fiber types. Mech Ageing Dev 1991;60:199–213.

[8] Tomlinson BE, Irving D. The numbers of limb motor neurons in the human lumbosacral cord throughout life. J Neurol Sci 1977;34:213–9.

[9] Grimby G, Danneskiold-Samsoe B, Hvid K, Saltin B. Morphology and enzymatic capacity in arm and leg muscles in 78–81 year old men and women. Acta Physiol Scand 1982;115:125–34.

[10] Brooks SV, Faulkner JA. Skeletal muscle weakness in old age: underlying mechanisms. Med Sci Sports Exerc 1994;26:432–9.

[11] Lewis DM, Chamberlain S. Differences between contractions in vitro of slow and fast rat skeletal muscle persist after random reinnervation. J Physiol 1993;465:731–45.

[12] Mecocci P, Fano G, Fulle S, MacGarvey U, Shinobu L, Polidori MC, et al. Age-dependent increases in oxidative damage to DNA, lipids, and proteins in human skeletal muscle. Free Radic Biol Med 1999;26:303–8.

[13] Pansarasa O, Bertorelli L, Vecchiet J, Felzani G, Marzatico F. Age-dependent changes of antioxidant activities and markers of free radical damage in human skeletal muscle. Free Radic Biol Med 1999;27:617–22.

[14] Ji LL, Wu E, Thomas DP. Effect of exercise training on antioxidant and metabolic functions in senescent rat skeletal muscle. Gerontology 1991;37:317–25.

[15] Morgan JE, Partridge TA. Muscle satellite cells. Int J Biochem Cell Biol 2003;35: 1151–6.

[16] Renault V, Thornell LE, Eriksson PO, Butler-Browne G, Mouly V, Thorne LE. Regenerative potential of human skeletal muscle during aging. Aging Cell 2002;1:132–9.

[17] Conboy IM, Conboy MJ, Smythe GM, Rando TA. Notch-mediated restoration of regenerative potential to aged muscle. Science 2003;302:1575–7.

[18] Conley KE, Jubrias SA, Esselman PC. Oxidative capacity and ageing in human muscle. J Physiol 2000;526:203–10.

[19] Lass A, Kwong L, Sohal RS. Mitochondrial coenzyme Q content and aging. Biofactors 1999;9:199–205.

[20] Drew B, Phaneuf S, Dirks A, Selman C, Gredilla R, Lezza A, et al. Effects of aging and caloric restriction on mitochondrial energy production in gastrocnemius muscle and heart. Am J Physiol Regul Integr Comp Physiol 2003;284(2):R474–80.

[21] Pedersen M, Bruunsgaard H, Weis N, Hendel HW, Andreassen BU, Eldrup E, et al. Circulating levels of TNF-alpha and IL-6-relation to truncal fat mass and muscle mass in healthy elderly individuals and in patients with type-2 diabetes. Mech Ageing Dev 2003; 124:495–502.

[22] Visser M, Pahor M, Taaffe DR, Goodpaster BH, Simonsick EM, Newman AB, et al. Relationship of interleukin-6 and tumor necrosis factor-alpha with muscle mass and muscle strength in elderly men and women: the Health ABC Study. J Gerontol Med Sci 2002;57: M326–32.

[23] Campbell WW, Trappe TA, Wolfe RR, Evans WJ. The recommended dietary allowance for protein may not be adequate for older people to maintain skeletal muscle. J Gerontol Med Sci 2001;56A:M373–80.

[24] Evans WJ. Protein nutrition and resistance exercise. Can J Appl Physiol 2001;26(Suppl): S141–52.

[25] Nair KS. Age-related changes in muscle. Mayo Clin Proc 2000;75(Suppl):S14–8.

[26] Proctor DN, Balagopal P, Nair KS. Age-related sarcopenia in humans is associated with reduced synthetic rates of specific muscle proteins. J Nutr 1998;128(Suppl):351S–5S.

[27] Dorrens J, Rennie MJ. Effects of ageing and human whole body and muscle protein turnover. Scand J Med Sci Sports 2003;13:26–33.

[28] Farrell PA. Protein metabolism and age: influence of insulin and resistance exercise. Int J Sport Nutr Exerc Metab 2001;11(Suppl):S150–63.

[29] Ozaki K, Matsuura T, Narama I. Histochemical and morphometrical analysis of skeletal muscle in spontaneous diabetic WBN/Kob rat. Acta Neuropathol (Berl) 2001;102: 264–70.

[30] Drexler H, Riede U, Munzel T, Konig H, Funke E, Just H. Alterations of skeletal muscle in chronic heart failure. Circulation 1992;85:1751–9.

[31] Conjard A, Ferrier B, Martin M, Caillette A, Carrier H, Baverel G. Effects of chronic renal failure on enzymes of energy metabolism in individual human muscle fibers. J Am Soc Nephrol 1995;6:68–74.

[32] Gray A, Feldman HA, McKinlay JB, Longcope C. Age, disease, and changing sex hormone levels in middle-aged men: results of the Massachusetts Male Aging Study. J Clin Endocrinol Metab 1991;73:1016–25.

[33] Harman SM, Metter EJ, Tobin JD, Pearson J, Blackman MR. Longitudinal effects of aging on serum total and free testosterone levels in healthy men. Baltimore Longitudinal Study of Aging. J Clin Endocrinol Metab 2001;86:724–31.

[34] van den Beld AW, de Jong FH, Grobbee DE, Pols HA, Lamberts SW. Measures of bioavailable serum testosterone and estradiol and their relationships with muscle strength, bone density, and body composition in elderly men. J Clin Endocrinol Metab 2000;85: 3276–82.

[35] Mauras N, Hayes V, Welch S, Rini A, Helgeson K, Dokler M, et al. Testosterone deficiency in young men: marked alterations in whole body protein kinetics, strength, and adiposity. J Clin Endocrinol Metab 1998;83:1886–92.

[36] Rudman D, Feller AG, Nagraj HS, Gergans GA, Lalitha PY, Goldberg AF, et al. Effects of human growth hormone in men over 60 years old. N Engl J Med 1990;323:1–6.

[37] Phillips SK, Rook KM, Siddle NC, Bruce SA, Woledge RC. Muscle weakness in women occurs at an earlier age than in men, but strength is preserved by hormone replacement therapy. Clin Sci (Lond) 1993;84:95–8.

[38] Hoffman DM, O'Sullivan AJ, Freund J, Ho KK. Adults with growth hormone deficiency have abnormal body composition but normal energy metabolism. J Clin Endocrinol Metab 1995;80:72–7.

[39] Skelton DA, Greig CA, Davies JM, Young A. Strength, power and related functional ability of healthy people aged 65–89 years. Age Ageing 1994;23:371–7.

[40] Doherty TJ. Invited review: aging and sarcopenia. J Appl Physiol 2003;95:1717–27.

[41] Frontera WR, Hughes VA, Lutz KJ, Evans WJ. A cross-sectional study of muscle strength and mass in 45- to 78-yr-old men and women. J Appl Physiol 1991;71:644–50.

[42] Johnson T. Age-related differences in isometric and dynamic strength and endurance. Phys Ther 1982;62:985–9.

[43] Fitts RH, McDonald KS, Schluter JM. The determinants of skeletal muscle force and power: their adaptability with changes in activity pattern. J Biomech 1991;24(Suppl 1): 111–22.

[44] Gonzalez E, Messi ML, Delbono O. The specific force of single intact extensor digitorum longus and soleus mouse muscle fibers declines with aging. J Membr Biol 2000;178: 175–83.

[45] Macaluso A, Nimmo MA, Foster JE, Cockburn M, McMillan NC, De Vito G. Contractile muscle volume and agonist-antagonist coactivation account for differences in torque between young and older women. Muscle Nerve 2002;25:858–63.

[46] Thorstensson A, Grimby G, Karlsson J. Force-velocity relations and fiber composition in human knee extensor muscles. J Appl Physiol 1976;40:12–6.

[47] Larsson L, Li X, Frontera WR. Effects of aging on shortening velocity and myosin isoform composition in single human skeletal muscle cells. Am J Physiol 1997;272: C638–49.

[48] Lowe DA, Thomas DD, Thompson LV. Force generation, but not myosin ATPase activity, declines with age in rat muscle fibers. Am J Physiol Cell Physiol 2002;283:C187–92.

[49] Saito M, Kondo A, Gotoh M, Kato K. Age-related changes in the rat detrusor muscle: the contractile response to inorganic ions. J Urol 1991;146:891–4.

[50] Hunter SK, Thompson MW, Ruell PA, Harmer AR, Thom JM, Gwinn TH, et al. Human skeletal sarcoplasmic reticulum Ca2+ uptake and muscle function with aging and strength training. J Appl Physiol 1999;86:1858–65.

[51] Brooks SV, Faulkner JA. Contraction-induced injury: recovery of skeletal muscles in young and old mice. Am J Physiol 1990;258:C436–42.

[52] Merletti R, Farina D, Gazzoni M, Schieroni MP. Effect of age on muscle functions investigated with surface electromyography. Muscle Nerve 2002;25:65–76.

[53] Rantanen T, Guralnik JM, Leveille S, Izmirlian G, Hirsch R, Simonsick E, et al. Racial differences in muscle strength in disabled older women. J Gerontol Biol Sci 1998;53: B355–61.

[54] de Rekeneire N, Visser M, Peila R, Nevitt MC, Cauley JA, Tylavsky FA, et al. Is a fall just a fall: correlates of falling in healthy older persons. The Health, Aging and Body Composition Study. J Am Geriatr Soc 2003;51:841–6.

[55] Laforest S, St-Pierre DM, Cyr J, Gayton D. Effects of age and regular exercise on muscle strength and endurance. Eur J Appl Physiol Occup Physiol 1990;60:104–11.

[56] Rantanen T, Era P, Heikkinen E. Physical activity and the changes in maximal isometric strength in men and women from the age of 75 to 80 years. J Am Geriatr Soc 1997;45: 1439–45.

[57] Newman AB, Haggerty CL, Goodpaster B, Harris T, Kritchevsky S, Nevitt M, et al. Strength and muscle quality in a well-functioning cohort of older adults: the Health, Aging and Body Composition Study. Health Aging And Body Composition Research Group. J Am Geriatr Soc 2003;51:323–30.

[58] Liang MT, Cameron Chumlea WM. Balance and strength of elderly Chinese men and women. J Nutr Health Aging 1998;2:21–7.

[59] Radak Z, Taylor AW, Ohno H, Goto S. Adaptation to exercise-induced oxidative stress: from muscle to brain. Exerc Immunol Rev 2001;7:90–107.

[60] Safran MR, Garrett WE Jr, Seaber AV, Glisson RR, Ribbeck BM. The role of warmup in muscular injury prevention. Am J Sports Med 1988;16:123–9.

[61] Alway SE, Coggan AR, Sproul MS, Abduljalil AM, Robitaille PM. Muscle torque in young and older untrained and endurance-trained men. J Gerontol Biol Sci 1996;51: B195–201.

[62] Roth SM, Martel GF, Ivey FM, Lemmer JT, Metter EJ, Hurley BF, et al. High-volume, heavy-resistance strength training and muscle damage in young and older women. J Appl Physiol 2000;88:1112–8.

[63] Roth SM, Martel GF, Ivey FM, Lemmer JT, Tracy BL, Metter EJ, et al. Skeletal muscle satellite cell characteristics in young and older men and women after heavy resistance strength training. J Gerontol Biol Sci 2001;56A:B240–7.

[64] Sipila S, Multanen J, Kallinen M, Era P, Suominen H. Effects of strength and endurance training on isometric muscle strength and walking speed in elderly women. Acta Physiol Scand 1996;156:457–64.

[65] Gosselin LE, Adams C, Cotter TA, McCormick RJ, Thomas DP. Effect of exercise training on passive stiffness in locomotor skeletal muscle: role of extracellular matrix. J Appl Physiol 1998;85:1011–6.

[66] Frontera WR, Meredith CN, O'Reilly KP, Knuttgen HG, Evans WJ. Strength conditioning in older men: skeletal muscle hypertrophy and improved function. J Appl Physiol 1988;64:1038–44.

[67] Evans W. Functional and metabolic consequences of sarcopenia. J Nutr 1997;127(Suppl): 998S–1003S.

[68] Hopp JF. Effects of age and resistance training on skeletal muscle: a review. Phys Ther 1993;73:361–73.

[69] Yarasheski KE. Exercise, aging, and muscle protein metabolism. J Gerontol Med Sci 2003;58A:M918–22.

[70] Ferri A, Scaglioni G, Pousson M, Capodaglio P, Van Hoecke J, Narici MV. Strength and power changes of the human plantar flexors and knee extensors in response to resistance training in old age. Acta Physiol Scand 2003;177:69–78.

[71] Jubrias SA, Esselman PC, Price LB, Cress ME, Conley KE. Large energetic adaptations of elderly muscle to resistance and endurance training. J Appl Physiol 2001;90:1663–70.

[72] Trappe S, Williamson D, Godard M, Porter D, Rowden G, Costill D. Effect of resistance training on single muscle fiber contractile function in older men. J Appl Physiol 2000; 89:143–52.

[73] Greiwe JS, Cheng B, Rubin DC, Yarasheski KE, Semenkovich CF. Resistance exercise decreases skeletal muscle tumor necrosis factor alpha in frail elderly humans. FASEB J 2001;15:475–82.

[74] Balagopal P, Schimke JC, Ades P, Adey D, Nair KS. Age effect on transcript levels and synthesis rate of muscle MHC and response to resistance exercise. Am J Physiol Endocrinol Metab 2001;280:E203–8.

[75] Takarada Y, Ishii N. Effects of low-intensity resistance exercise with short interset rest period on muscular function in middle-aged women. J Strength Cond Res 2002;16:123–8.

[76] Lan C, Lai JS, Chen SY, Wong MK. Tai Chi Chuan to improve muscular strength and endurance in elderly individuals: a pilot study. Arch Phys Med Rehabil 2000;81:604–7.

[77] Caggiano E, Emrey T, Shirley S, Craik RL. Effects of electrical stimulation or voluntary contraction for strengthening the quadriceps femoris muscles in an aged male population. J Orthop Sports Phys Ther 1994;20:22–8.

[78] McMiken DF, Todd-Smith M, Thompson C. Strengthening of human quadriceps muscles by cutaneous electrical stimulation. Scand J Rehabil Med 1983;15:25–8.

[79] Barton-Davis ER, Shoturma DI, Musaro A, Rosenthal N, Sweeney HL. Viral mediated expression of insulin-like growth factor I blocks the aging-related loss of skeletal muscle function. Proc Natl Acad Sci USA 1998;95:15603–7.

[80] Hauer K, Hildebrandt W, Sehl Y, Edler L, Oster P, Droge W. Improvement in muscular performance and decrease in tumor necrosis factor level in old age after antioxidant treatment. J Mol Med 2003;81:118–25. Epub February 8, 2003.

[81] Gower BA, Nyman L. Associations among oral estrogen use, free testosterone concentration, and lean body mass among postmenopausal women. J Clin Endocrinol Metab 2000;85:4476–80.

[82] Kenny AM, Dawson L, Kleppinger A, Iannuzzi-Sucich M, Judge JO. Prevalence of sarcopenia and predictors of skeletal muscle mass in nonobese women who are long-term users of estrogen-replacement therapy. J Gerontol Med Sci 2003;58A:M436–40.

[83] Dobs AS, Nguyen T, Pace C, Roberts CP. Differential effects of oral estrogen versus oral estrogen-androgen replacement therapy on body composition in postmenopausal women. J Clin Endocrinol Metab 2002;87:1509–16.

[84] Aloia JF, Vaswani A, Russo L, Sheehan M, Flaster E. The influence of menopause and hormonal replacement therapy on body cell mass and body fat mass. Am J Obstet Gynecol 1995;172:896–900.

[85] Sorensen MB, Rosenfalck AM, Hojgaard L, Ottesen B. Obesity and sarcopenia after menopause are reversed by sex hormone replacement therapy. Obes Res 2001;9:622–6.

[86] O'Sullivan AJ, Crampton LJ, Freund J, Ho KK. The route of estrogen replacement therapy confers divergent effects on substrate oxidation and body composition in postmenopausal women. J Clin Invest 1998;102:1035–40.

[87] Villareal DT, Holloszy JO, Kohrt WM. Effects of DHEA replacement on bone mineral density and body composition in elderly women and men. Clin Endocrinol (Oxf) 2000; 53:561–8.

[88] Snyder PJ, Peachey H, Hannoush P, Berlin JA, Loh L, Lenrow DA, et al. Effect of testosterone treatment on body composition and muscle strength in men over 65 years of age. J Clin Endocrinol Metab 1999;84:2647–53.

[89] Tenover JS. Effects of testosterone supplementation in the aging male. J Clin Endocrinol Metab 1992;75:1092–8.

[90] Hansen TB, Vahl N, Jorgensen JO, Christiansen JS, Hagen C. Soft tissue changes in adults with acquired growth hormone deficiency during substitution treatment: a double-blind, randomized, placebo-controlled study after a year of treatment. Ugeskr Laeger 1997;159: 4394–9.

[91] Blackman MR, Sorkin JD, Munzer T, Bellantoni MF, Busby-Whitehead J, Stevens TE, et al. Growth hormone and sex steroid administration in healthy aged women and men: a randomized controlled trial. JAMA 2002;288:2282–92.

[92] Whitehead HM, Gilliland JS, Allen IV, Hadden DR. Growth hormone treatment in adults with growth hormone deficiency: effect on muscle fiber size and proportions. Acta Paediatr Scand 1989;356(Suppl):65–8, 73–4.

[93] Friedlander AL, Butterfield GE, Moynihan S, Grillo J, Pollack M, Holloway L, et al. One year of insulin-like growth factor I treatment does not affect bone density, body composition, or psychological measures in postmenopausal women. J Clin Endocrinol Metab 2001;86:1496–503.

[94] Jorgensen JO, Thuesen L, Muller J, Ovesen P, Skakkebaek NE, Christiansen JS. Three years of growth hormone treatment in growth hormone-deficient adults: near normalization of body composition and physical performance. Eur J Endocrinol 1994;130:224–8.

[95] Thompson JL, Butterfield GE, Marcus R, Hintz RL, Van Loan M, Ghiron L, et al. The effects of recombinant human insulin-like growth factor-I and growth hormone on body composition in elderly women. J Clin Endocrinol Metab 1995;80:1845–52.

[96] Chakravarthy MV, Davis BS, Booth FW. IGF-I restores satellite cell proliferative potential in immobilized old skeletal muscle. J Appl Physiol 2000;89:1365–79.

[97] Vary TC, Jefferson LS, Kimball SR. Role of eIF4E in stimulation of protein synthesis by IGF-I in perfused rat skeletal muscle. Am J Physiol Endocrinol Metab 2000;278: E58–64.

[98] Buckwalter JA, Rosenberg LC. Electron microscopic studies of cartilage proteoglycans: direct evidence for the variable length of chondroitin sulfate rich region of the proteoglycan subunit core protein. J Biol Chem 1982;257:9830–9.

[99] Roth V, Mow VC. The intrinsic tensile behavior of the matrix of bovine articular cartilage and its variation with age. J Bone Joint Surg 1980;62A:1102–17.

[100] Buckwalter JA, Woo SL-Y, Goldberg VM, Hadley EC, Booth F, Oegema TR, et al. Soft tissue aging and musculoskeletal function. J Bone Joint Surg 1993;75A:1533–48.

[101] Buckwalter JA, Roughley PJ, Rosenberg LC. Age-related changes in cartilage proteoglycans: quantitative electron microscopic studies. Microsc Res Tech 1994;28:398–408.

[102] Martin JA, Buckwalter JA. Aging, articular cartilage chondrocyte senescence and osteoarthritis. Biogerontology 2002;3:257–64.

[103] Wells T, Davidson C, Norgelin M, Bird JL, Bayliss MT, Dudhia J. Age-related changes in the composition, the molecular stoichiometry and the stability of proteoglycan aggregates extracted from human articular cartilage. Biochem J 2003;370:69–79.

[104] Buckwalter JA, Kuettner KE, Thonar EJ-M. Age-related changes in articular cartilage proteoglycans: electron microscopic studies. J Orthop Res 1985;3:251–7.

[105] Bolton MC, Dudhia J, Bayliss MT. Age-related changes in the synthesis of link protein and aggrecan in human articular cartilage: implications for aggregate stability. Biochem J 1999;337:77–82.

[106] Tang LH, Buckwalter JA, Rosenberg LC. The effect of link protein concentration on articular cartilage proteoglycan aggregation. J Orthop Res 1996;14:334–9.

[107] Bank RA, Bayliss MT, Lafeber FP, Maroudas A, Tekoppele JM. Ageing and zonal variation in post-translational modification of collagen in normal human articular cartilage: the age-related increase in non-enzymatic glycation affects biomechanical properties of cartilage. Biochem J 1998;330:345–51.

[108] Verzijl N, DeGroot J, Ben ZC, Brau-Benjzmin O, Maroudas A, Bank RA, et al. Crosslinking by advanced glycation end products increases the stiffness of the collagen network in human articular cartilage: a possible mechanism through which age is a risk factor for osteoarthritis. Arthritis Rheum 2002;46:114–23.

[109] DeGroot J, Verzijl N, Bank RA, Lafeber FP, Bijlsma JW, TeKoppele JM. Age-related decrease in proteoglycan synthesis of human articular chondrocytes: the role of nonenzymatic glycation. Arthritis Rheum 1999;42:1003–9.

[110] Grushko G, Schneiderman R, Maroudas A. Some biochemical and biophysical parameters for the study of the pathogenesis of osteoarthritis: a comparison between the processes of ageing and degeneration in human hip cartilage. Connective Tissue Res 1989;19:149–76.

[111] Felson DT, Anderson JJ, Naimark A, Kannel W, Mennan RF. The prevalence of chondrocalcinosis in the elderly and its association with knee osteoarthritis: the Framingham Study. J Rheumatol 1989;16:1241–5.

[112] Wilkins E, Dieppe P, Maddison P, Evison G. Osteoarthritis and articular chondrocalcinosis in the elderly. Ann Rheum Dis 1983;42:280–4.

[113] Rosenthal AK, Derfus BA, Henry LA. Transglutaminase activity in aging articular chondrocytes and articular cartilage vesicles. Arthritis Rheum 1997;40:966–70.

[114] Martin JA, Buckwalter JA. Articular cartilage aging and degeneration. Sports Med Arthroscopy Rev 1996;4:263.

[115] Aigner T, Hemmel M, Neureiter D, Gebhard PM, Zeiler G, Kirchner T, et al. Apoptotic cell death is not a widespread phenomenon in normal aging and osteoarthritis human articular knee cartilage: a study of proliferation, programmed cell death (apoptosis), and viability of chondrocytes in normal and osteoarthritic human knee cartilage. Arthritis Rheum 2001;44:1304–12.

[116] Vignon E, Arlot M, Patricot LM, Vignon G. The cell density of human femoral head cartilage. Clin Orthop 1976;121:303–8.

[117] Martin JA, Buckwalter JA. Telomere erosion and senescence in human articular cartilage chondrocytes. J Gerontol Biol Sci 2001;56A:B172–9.

[118] Guerne PA, Blance F, Kaelin A, Desgeorges A, Lotz M. Growth factor responsiveness in human articular chondrocytes in aging and development. Arthritis Rheum 1995;38: 960–8.

[119] Allsopp RC, Chang E, Kashefi-Aazam M, Rogaev EI, Piatyszek MA, Shay JW, et al. Telomere shortening is associated with cell division in vitro and in vivo. Exp Cell Res 1995;220:194–200.

[120] Allsopp RC, Vaziri H, Patterson C, Goldstein S, Younglai E, Futcher AB, et al. Telomere length predicts replicative capacity of human fibroblasts. Proc Natl Acad Sci USA 1992; 89:10114–8.

[121] Martin JA, Buckwalter JA. The role of chondrocyte-matrix interactions in maintaining and repairing articular cartilage. Biorheology 2000;37:129–40.

[122] Loeser RF, Shanker G, Carlson CS, Gardin JF, Shelton BJ, Sonntag WE. Reduction in the chondrocyte response to insulin-like growth factor I in aging and osteoarthritis: studies in a non-human primate model of naturally occurring disease. Arthritis Rheum 2000;43:2110–20.

[123] Messai H, Duchossoy Y, Khatib A, Panasyuk A, Mitrovic DR. Articular chondrocytes from aging rats respond poorly to insulin-like growth factor-I: an altered signaling pathway. Mech Ageing Dev 2000;115:21–37.

[124] Martin JA, Ellerbroek SM, Buckwalter JA. The age-related decline in chondrocyte response to insulin-like growth factor-I: the role of growth factor binding proteins. J Ortho Res 1997;15:491–8.

[125] Scharstuhl A, van Beuningen HM, Vitters EL, van der Kraan PM, van den Berg WB. Loss of transforming growth factor counteraction on interleukin 1 mediated effects in cartilage of old mice. Ann Rheum Dis 2002;61:1095–8.

[126] Finkel T, Holbrook NJ. Oxidants, oxidative stress and the biology of ageing. Nature 2000;408:239–47.

[127] Kopsidas GS, Kovalenko A, Kelso JM, Linnane AW. An age-associated correlation between cellular bioenergy decline and mt DNA rearrangements in human skeletal muscle. Mutat Res 1998;421:27–36.

[128] Lee CM, Weindrich R, Aiken JM. Age-related alterations of the mitochondrial genome. Free Rad Biol Med 1997;22:1259–69.

[129] Loeser RF, Carlson CS, Carlo MD, Cole A. Detection of nitrotyrosine in aging and osteoarthritic cartilage correlation of oxidative damage with the presence of interleukin-1 beta and with chondrocyte resistance to insulin -like growth factor 1. Arthritis Rheum 2002;46:2349–57.

[130] Carlson CS, Loeser RF, Purser CB, Gardin JF, Jerome CP. Osteoarthritis in cynomolgus macaques III: effects of age, gender and subchondral bone thickness on severity of the disease. J Bone Miner Res 1996;11:1209–17.
[131] Radin EL, Burr DB, Caterson B, Fyhrie D, Brown TD, Boyd RD. Mechanical determinants of osteoarthrosis. Semin Arthritis Rheum 1991;21:12–21.
[132] Yamada K, Healey R, Amiel D, Lotz M, Coutts R. Subchondral bone of the human knee joint in aging and osteoarthritis. Osteoarthritis Cartilage 2002;10:360–9.
[133] Hamerman D. Biology of the aging joint. Clin Geriatr Med 1998;14:417–33.
[134] Brandt KD. Putting some muscle into osteoarthritis. Ann Intern Med 1997;128:154–6.
[135] Herzog W, Longino D, Clark A. The role of muscles in joint adaptation and degeneration. Langenbecks Arch Surg 2003;388:305–15.
[136] Birch HL, Bailey JV, Bailey AJ, Goodship AE. Age-related changes to the molecular and cellular components of equine flexor tendons. Equine Vet J 1999;31:391–6.
[137] Noyes FR, Grood ES. The strength of the anterior cruciate ligament in humans and Rhesus monkeys. J Bone Joint Surg 1976;58:1074–82.
[138] Neumann P, Ekstrom LA, Keller TS, Perry L, Hansson TH. Aging, vertebral density and disc degeneration alter the tensile stress-strain characteristics of the human anterior longitudinal ligament. J Orthop Res 1994;12:103–12.
[139] McAlinden A, Dudhia J, Bolton MC, Lorenzo P, Heinegard D, Bayliss MT. Age-related changes in the synthesis and mRNA expression of decorin and aggrecan in human meniscus and articular cartilage. Osteoarthritis Cartilage 2001;9:33–41.
[140] Ghosh P, Taylor TK. The knee joint meniscus: a fibrocartilage of some distinction. Clin Orthop 1987;224:52–63.
[141] Hurley MV, Rees J, Newham DJ. Quadriceps function, proprioceptive acuity and functional performance in healthy young, middle-aged and elderly subjects. Age Ageing 1998;27:55–62.
[142] Stevens JE, Binder-Macleod S, Snyder-Mackler L. Characterization of the human quadriceps muscle in active elders. Arch Phys Med Rehabil 2001;82:973–8.
[143] Messier SP, Loeser RF, Hoover JL, Semble EL, Wise CM. Osteoarthritis of the knee effects on gait, strength and flexibility. Arch Phys Med Rehabil 1992;73:29–36.
[144] Sharma L, Lou C, Felson DT, Dunlop DD, Kirwan-Mellis G, Hayes KW, et al. Laxity in healthy and osteoarthritic knees. Arthritis Rheum 1999;42:861–70.
[145] Sharma L, Song J, Felson DT, Cahune S, Shamiyeh E, Dunlop DD. The role of knee alignment in disease progression and functional decline in knee osteoarthritis. JAMA 2001;286:792.
[146] Sherman C, Buckwalter JA, DiNubile NA. Decreased mobility in the elderly: the exercise antidote. Phys Sportsmed 1997;25:126.
[147] Pai YC, Rymer WZ, Chang RW, Sharma L. Effect of age and osteoarthritis on knee proprioception. Arthritis Rheum 1997;10:2260–5.
[148] Barrett DS, Cobb AG, Bentley G. Joint proprioception in normal, osteoarthritic and replaced knees. J Bone Joint Surg Br 1991;71:53–6.
[149] O'Connor BL, Brandt KD. Neurogenic factors in the etiopathogenesis of osteoarthritis. Rheum Dis Cln North Am 1993;19:581–605.
[150] Fiatarone MA, Marks EC, Ryan ND, Meredith CN, Lipsitz LA, Evans WJ. High-intensity strength training in nonagenarians: effect on skeletal muscle. JAMA 1990;263:3029–34.
[151] Brandon LJ, Boyette LW, Lloyd A, Gaasch DA. Resistive training and long-term function in older adults. J Aging Phys Act 2004;12:10–28.
[152] Petrella RJ, Lattanzio PJ, Nelson MG. Effect of age and activity on knee joint proprioception. Am J Phys Med Rehabil 1997;76:235–41.
[153] Tsang WW, Hui-Chan CW. Effects of exercise on joint sense and balance in elderly men: Tai Chi versus golf. Med Sci Sports Exerc 2004;36:658–67.
[154] Tsang WW, Hui-Chan CW. Effects of Tai Chi on joint proprioception and stability limits in elderly subjects. Med Sci Sports Exerc 2003;35:1962–71.

ELSEVIER
SAUNDERS

Phys Med Rehabil Clin N Am
16 (2005) 41–56

PHYSICAL MEDICINE
AND REHABILITATION
CLINICS OF
NORTH AMERICA

Exercise and physical activity in persons aging with a physical disability

James H. Rimmer, PhD

*Department of Disability and Human Development, University of Illinois at Chicago,
1640 West Roosevelt Rd., Chicago, IL 60608-6904, USA*

The life expectancy of older Americans is on the rise [1]. Persons 65 years of age and older make up the fastest growing portion of the United States population [2]. Among people with physical disabilities, life expectancy has also risen [3]. Hicks et al [4] reported that the life expectancy of persons with spinal cord injury (SCI) is approaching that of the general population.

Although medical advances have allowed persons with disabilities to live longer, quality of life issues related to health and well-being have become increasingly important [5,6]. Roller [7] and others [8,9] have noted that as persons with physical disabilities move into middle and later adulthood, there is an enormous physical and psychologic burden associated with having to manage various secondary health conditions associated with the primary disability in addition to managing the health effects associated with the aging process. This interaction between the natural aging process and the disability can create a demanding physical environment [10,11]. Tasks that might have been easily accomplished in younger adulthood, such as transferring from a wheelchair to an automobile, ascending a ramp, or walking with braces, can become major obstacles for individuals aging with a physical disability and often require greater assistance from friends, family members, and personal care assistants.

Health conditions that affect the general population (eg, arthritis, type 2 diabetes, and coronary heart disease) will become greater concerns among individuals aging with a disability [4–6]. The interaction between these health conditions and the associated and secondary conditions

This work was supported in part by the National Institute on Disability and Rehabilitation Research grant #H133E020715 and the Centers for Disease Control and Prevention, National Center on Birth Defects and Developmental Disabilities, Division of Human Development and Disability grant #U59CCU516732.

E-mail address: jrimmer@uic.edu

doi:10.1016/j.pmr.2004.06.013

accommodating various types of physical disabilities will impose greater demands on physical and psychologic functioning and could challenge the person's independence and ability to continue working, socializing, and maintaining routine daily activities [8,9].

As researchers and public policy makers explore ways to increase health and function among older populations, physical activity as an intervention strategy for older adults with disabilities is starting to receive more attention [12,13]. As a result of several landmark studies that have shown a graded, inverse relationship between physical activity/fitness and the incidence of morbidity and mortality, public health officials and federal agencies are recommending that all Americans, including persons with disabilities, engage in a minimum of 30 minutes a day of moderate aerobic exercise [14,15]. Despite strong endorsements from the CDC [16], the National Institutes of Health [17], the Surgeon General's Office [18], and the American College of Sports Medicine [17], most Americans do not obtain the recommended amount of physical activity that is necessary for maintaining health, and the level of inactivity among persons with disabilities is higher than the general population [19,20].

In some respects, addressing the physical activity needs in middle and older adults with disabilities has greater urgency than in the general population. A small reduction in strength or endurance could diminish a person's physical independence [21]. It has been suggested that part of the loss in function observed in many older adults with disabilities may be related to sedentary behavior and a reduction in physical fitness [22,23].

Impact of physical activity on health and function

The high incidence of secondary and associated conditions in persons aging with disabilities compounded by environmental barriers that make participating in physical activity difficult present a unique problem to health professionals. These secondary and associated conditions include chronic pain, fatigue, deconditioning, excessive/sudden weight gain, depression, spasticity, pressure ulcers, and impaired thermoregulation among others and lead to severe reductions in health and independence, causing further impairments and activity limitations [1,10,24].

Given the empirical evidence linking physical activity with functional status and overall health [25,26] and the fact that impaired health and functioning can impede participation in physical activity, one can postulate a downward cyclical pattern in health and functioning that results from prolonged physical inactivity. Fig. 1 illustrates this cyclical relationship between disability and physical inactivity. First, the onset of disability (left circle) often results in greater effort required to engage in physical activity (top circle), thereby causing persons with disabilities to remain sedentary (right circle). Physical inactivity over a prolonged period results

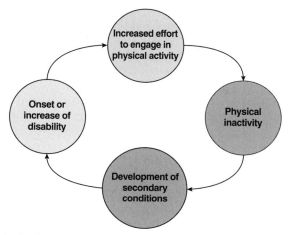

Fig. 1. Cyclical relationships between disability and physical inactivity.

in the development of secondary conditions and further functional loss (bottom circle), which results in greater effort to participate in physical activities.

There has been growing support for the use of physical activity for enhancing health and well-being among older populations. In a large-scale epidemiologic study evaluating the relationship between aerobic fitness and functional limitations in 3495 men and 1175 women, Huang et al [27] reported a strong association between low levels of aerobic fitness and a higher rate of functional limitations. The investigators also found that in subjects who were classified as having one or more chronic diseases, subjects who were more aerobically fit had a lower level of functional limitation (defined as the inability to carry out normal daily tasks and roles).

Binder et al [28] examined the relationship between peak Vo_2 and physical performance among older women between 75 and 94 years of age who were affected by chronic disease and functional limitations. They found that Vo_2 peak was an important independent predictor of task performance (eg, stair climbing and gait speed).

Lawrence and Jette [29] examined the causes of functional limitations in older adults and noted that lower extremity functional limitation, defined as the inability to walk 1 mile, was the single largest predictor of subsequent inability to perform instrumental activities of daily living (IADLs) (eg, shopping, housekeeping, and food preparation). They concluded that IADLs are strongly influenced by a person's physical activity level and, as a strategy for preventing further disablement, recommended that clinical trials focus on minimizing functional limitations through various interventions aimed at enhancing aerobic physical activity.

Stessman et al [30] examined the effects of exercise on the performance of activities of daily living (ADLs) and IADLs among older men and women. For nearly every task studied, subjects who reported exercising 4 days a week at age 70 were more likely to report ease in performance at age 77. After controlling for baseline levels (ease of performance of ADLs and IADLs, health, and psychosocial and demographic factors), ease of performance in at least three of four ADL tasks at age 77 was independently related to exercise at age 70 for women and men. Ease of independent function in at least four of five IADL tasks correlated to exercise for men but not for women. Ease in shopping correlated with physical activity for women and men.

Rimmer et al [31] reported in a population of stroke survivors that their low aerobic capacity has the potential to make it difficult to sustain various activities and IADLs (Fig. 2). Stroke participants had an average peak energy expenditure level of 3.77 METs (metabolic equivalents). Relative to this value, Fig. 2 shows the average estimated MET levels required for the performance of various ADLs. Performance of several activities, including sweeping, gardening, and climbing stairs, would result in an energy deficit, thereby limiting the ability of the individual to perform these activities over sustained periods.

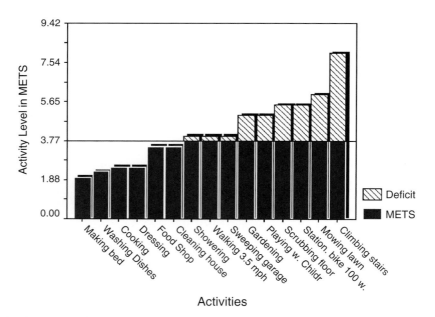

Fig. 2. MET levels of ADLs relative to maximum aerobic capacity of sample of stroke survivors.

Exercise guidelines for aging persons with physical disabilities

Regular physical activity has the potential to allow individuals aging with a physical disability to maintain their independence and to continue to enjoy life's pleasures. In addition, individuals with greater levels of physical fitness will be able to perform ADLs and IADLs with lower levels of energy expenditure and with a higher level of physical independence [32–36]. When planning physical activity programs for individuals with various types of physical disabilities, conditions associated with various impairments must be considered. Several of these are described below.

1. Certain physical disabilities are progressive in nature, and the potential for exacerbation is always present [37]. In cases where the individual has a progressive condition (eg, multiple sclerosis [MS], rheumatoid arthritis, postpolio syndrome, amyotrophic lateral sclerosis, Parkinson disease), it is important to monitor physical performance on a more regular basis to ensure that the activity is safe and effective for the individual. Progressive disorders often result in a gradual loss of muscle strength. When muscle soreness occurs in persons who have a progressive condition, it may be an indication that the overload or intensity of the exercise was too high. It is important to take the proper precautions to prevent pain, fatigue, or potential injury from overuse syndrome.
2. Persons with physical disabilities often exhibit asymmetrical weakness. Many individuals with cerebral palsy or stroke, for example, have hemiplegia, which results in significant differences in strength between the stronger and weaker sides of the body. It is important to place greater emphasis on the affected side without neglecting the nonaffected side. If there is nerve innervation on the weakened side, a resistance-training program should result in measurable improvement in strength. Individuals with hemiplegia may require active-assistive resistance exercise on the affected side and standard exercises on the nonaffected side.
3. Spasticity results in an exaggerated contractile response to stretch [38]. It is often seen in persons who have damage to their central nervous system, such as individuals with cerebral palsy, stroke, MS, and SCI. It might be helpful for the rehabilitation specialist to identify the amount of spasticity as mild, moderate, or severe and to plan a program based on a greater or lesser need in various muscle groups. Flexibility training should be combined with resistance training to mitigate the effects of spasticity.
4. Several types of physical disabilities reduce joint flexibility. When a joint is immobile for long periods of time, a contracture can develop [38]. Contractures occur when a body part (eg, an arm or a leg) is placed in a fixed position over an extended period of time (weeks or months). This situation often cannot be avoided due to the neurologic involvement, whereas at other times it can be prevented by constantly stretching the

muscle group. Contractures may be permanent or temporary depending on the severity of spasticity and the length of time that the joint has been placed in a fixed or static position. Flexibility training might be helpful to some individuals with contractures, but it is important to first consult with a rehabilitation specialist to determine the extent of the contracture and whether or not it should be targeted in a physical activity plan. Contractures in older adults with physical disabilities can be a greater problem than in younger individuals because of the higher risk of sustaining a fracture when a flexibility program is initiated due to the lower bone mineral density in later adulthood.

5. At certain times in the person's life, it may be necessary to temporarily stop the exercise program because of an exacerbation. Exacerbations can occur frequently or infrequently depending on the individual pathology. After an exacerbation, it is often necessary to start out at a lower training volume because of the complications that may result from the exacerbation. Upon resuming activity, the instructor should contact the client's physician to determine the appropriate training volume and progression. Although the person may be unable to reestablish the same level of strength or aerobic capacity as before the exacerbation, it is important that the instructor reassure the client that strength, flexibility, and cardiorespiratory endurance can be improved from the new entry point. Strength and aerobic function should be reassessed to establish a new baseline. Clients who have exacerbations should understand that the goal is to maintain the highest possible level of strength, flexibility, and aerobic function.

6. Damage to sensory nerves occurs with many types of physical disabilities. This results in the inability to detect pressure against the skin, which, if left untreated, could result in a pressure ulcer. Because many people with physical disabilities use braces or wheelchairs, they have a high risk of incurring a pressure ulcer. It is important for the therapist or trainer to frequently check all parts of the body for skin irritations that may result from a new exercise or use of a new piece of exercise equipment.

7. Muscle groups may be functional, partially functional (paresis), or nonfunctional (paralysis) depending on type and length (number of years) of the disability. There may also be some joint dysfunction that needs to be considered in the exercise prescription. For example, individuals with cerebral palsy often have hip dislocations due to the strong pull of the adductor muscles. If a person has a history of hip displacement, the instructor needs to check with the client's physician to determine if modifications need to be made to the training program.

8. It is important to keep detailed records on each client. Because there are often several associated conditions that accommodate a physical disability (eg, spasticity, hypertension, joint pain, exacerbations, and pressure ulcers), maintaining records and noting new health issues

during the training program lowers the risk of injury associated with the exercise program.

9. Two primary secondary conditions reported in people with physical disabilities are fatigue and chronic pain [9]. These conditions can often result in reduced physical activity participation resulting from a fear or perception that exercise would increase fatigue and pain. It is important that the physical activity regimen does not worsen these symptoms and that the program include physical activity regimens that may reduce fatigue or chronic pain.

10. Certain types of physical disabilities (eg, stroke and traumatic brain injury [TBI]) are often accommodated by cognitive impairments. Individuals with TBI often have cognitive, behavioral, or emotional changes [39]. These conditions could lead to mood swings, memory deficits, depression, frustration, and anxiety. Individuals with TBI and other cognitive disorders (eg, mental retardation) may require adaptations to compensate for the loss in judgment, memory, and motor planning. Understanding the magnitude of cognitive impairments must be done on an individual basis because there is great variability between individuals who sustain a similar type of head injury and among individuals with various physical/cognitive impairments depending on what part of the brain is affected.

Cognitive impairments are also observed in aging individuals with Parkinson disease and Alzheimer disease. Although Alzheimer disease results in more severe cognitive impairments at a much faster decline than Parkinson disease, both conditions can lead to a progressive, irreversible declines in memory, performance of routine tasks, time and space orientation, language and communication skills, abstract thinking, and judgment. An exercise training program for individuals with cognitive impairments faces three major challenges: (i) problems arising from the declining physical and mental health of the participant, (ii) behavioral changes that may cause the client to become agitated or lose interest with the exercise program or the exercise setting, and (iii) caregivers' willingness to continue bringing the person to the exercise program as the condition increases in severity. The cornerstone of an exercise program for persons with limited cognitive function is consistency and patience. Simple exercise routines, such as walking and performing light calisthenics, are easier than performing more complex routines. Reinforcement stratagies should be used to increase compliance to the program.

11. Individuals with limb loss must make sure that the prescribed exercise is not causing skin irritation or skin breakdown [40]. Stump socks should be changed daily and should fit properly over the residual limb to avoid skin irritation. Because a high percentage of individuals with limb loss have cardiovascular disease (eg, peripheral vascular disease or diabetes),

it is important that the participant is approved by his/her physician before initiating the exercise program.

Boxes 1 and 2 provide general exercise guidelines for endurance (cardiorespiratory) and resistance (strength) training for persons aging with a physical disability.

Areas for future research

There is a need to conduct various types of research related to physical activity and persons with physical disabilities. The literature demonstrating the enormous benefits that can accrue from a physically active lifestyle has usually excluded individuals with disabilities.

Need for prospective longitudinal studies on effective physical activity interventions for aging adults with disabilities

There is a need for prospective longitudinal studies that examine the long-term impact of exercise aimed at enhancing health and overall function in persons aging with a physical disability. Although a few small, non-randomized exercise studies with disabled subjects have been supportive of the clinical benefits of exercise in improving mobility, functional capacity, and balance in various cohorts with physical disabilities [31–35], these studies are generally not long enough to determine the viability of sustaining these health benefits over a longer period of time.

Establishing appropriate doses of exercise for various cohorts with disabilities

The lack of randomized controlled trials has resulted in limited data for establishing standard exercise guidelines for persons with physical disabilities. Previous studies involving persons with disabilities indicate that there is substantial variability in responses to increased physical activity at a prescribed level of duration or intensity [36,41]. Because of the heterogeneity of physical disability in terms of involvement (impairment), health, and function, it is important to identify optimal doses of exercise from evidenced-based outcomes that delineate the safety of the activity and the specific health outcomes achieved by various exercise regimens for this population. Randomized controlled exercise trials with adequate power are needed to establish the appropriate dose(s) required to achieve maximum cardiovascular, musculoskeletal, and functional health benefits in persons with disabilities. This information is important for rehabilitation and other health care providers to have available to establish the appropriate training regimen that will have the greatest benefit to the individual at the lowest risk level.

Establish a better understanding of responders versus nonresponders

There is a need to identify responders versus nonresponders to various doses of physical activity. Nonresponders—individuals who receive little or no benefit (ie, little or no change in functional aerobic capacity) from physical activity—may become discouraged with their progress and stop exercising. This situation might be remedied by increasing the dose of exercise in nonresponders. For some individuals with disabilities, a higher threshold of training (volume or intensity) may be necessary to achieve similar health outcomes as in early responders. Given the implications of exercise nonresponse, it is important to identify factors that differentiate between high responders and low or nonresponders among persons with disabilities and to determine if alternative exercise treatment strategies in nonresponders can achieve desirable gains in functional capacity.

Establishing public health recommendations appropriate to persons with disabilities

Although major public health organizations recommend 30 minutes of moderate physical activity most days of the week [17,18], these recommendations have been established from longitudinal data sets on nondisabled populations. It is unclear how this recommended dose of exercise would affect the health of individuals with physical disabilities. Another problem with public health guidelines is that the common recommendation is to walk more often. It is unclear if this is the most ideal mode or dose of physical activity for people with joint pain or balance impairments (eg, those with severe arthritis, cerebral palsy, MS, and others forms of disability that result in limited ability to walk for sustained periods of time).

Age-related versus disability-related loss in function

It is important to determine how common age-related declines in function affect the overall health status of people with disabilities. Several studies have reported low levels of strength and cardiorespiratory endurance among individuals with physical disabilities [25,41]. How this lower functional level interacts with the natural aging process is unclear. The synergistic effects of aging-related decline in combination with the progression of secondary conditions (eg, pain, fatigue, or generalized weakness) associated with the disability could lead to a substantial loss in function at a much earlier stage of life. The onset of aging-related loss in function compounds the decline in function associated with the person's disability. It is unclear how much of an impact physical activity can have in offsetting the loss in functional mobility.

Box 1. General guidelines for endurance training in aging persons with physical disabilities

- Use Rating of Perceived Exertion (RPE) along with heart rate to gauge the intensity of the exercise.
- Be aware that beta-blockers blunt heart rate response to aerobic exercise.
- The most accurate method for establishing target heart rate during aerobic activity is from a graded exercise test.

Aerobic guidelines for persons with paralysis
- In persons with paraplegia, arm exercise elicits heart rates 10 to 20 beats/min^{-1} lower than for leg exercise.
- Avoid autonomic dysreflexia by monitoring blood pressure before, during, and after exercise.
- Make sure bladder and bowel have been voided before exercise.
- When an individual is severely deconditioned, exercise should be in 5- to 10-minute increments with interspersed rest intervals.
- Monitor fatigue and pain carefully and make sure the training is safe and beneficial.

Sample aerobic exercise machines for wheelchair users and persons with lower extremity impairments
- Nu-Step recumbent stepper (arms only)
- Schwinn Air-Dyne (arms only)
- Upper arm cycle ergometer
- Wheelchair ergometer
  or
- Wheelchair exercise videos

Thermoregulatory guidelines
- External temperature must be carefully monitored to avoid hyper- or hypothermia.
- Control body temperature with fans, water, etc., especially in warm gyms.
- Appropriate clothing should be worn according to temperature.

Common overuse injuries in wheelchair users
- Blisters, abrasions, and lacerations
- Carpal tunnel syndrome
- Rotator cuff strain/shoulder impingement

Reducing injury in wheelchair users
- Use workout gloves with adequate padding.
- Push rims should be padded.
- Push rims should be positioned to provide the most comfortable and efficient push angle.
- Legs may need to be securely strapped.
- Avoid overuse injuries by varying the exercise routine (eg, cross-training, using different types of exercise equipment that focus on different joints and muscle groups).
- Vary exercise routines on alternate days.

More information on specific guidelines for various disabilities is available at www.ncpad.org.

Prevalence of overuse injury

There is a need to examine the prevalence of overuse injuries among persons with physical disabilities. Individuals who use manual wheelchairs are at risk for repetitive motion (overuse) injuries [42,43]. Several studies have noted that people who use manual wheelchairs have a higher incidence of shoulder pain compared with the general population [44,45]. Over time, independently propelling a manual wheelchair can result in repetitive motion injuries at the shoulder, elbow, or wrist. If cardiovascular exercise uses similar movements and muscle groups as wheelchair propulsion (eg, an arm or wheelchair ergometer), the possibility of a repetitive motion injury may increase [46].

Several studies have reported that arm ergometry and wheelchair ergometry often precipitate upper extremity injuries that compromise a wheelchair user's ability to perform various ADLs [47,48]. These concerns have challenged investigators to find alternative exercises for improving cardiovascular fitness [46,48]. There is a lack of commercial cardiovascular exercise equipment that is accessible to people with lower extremity impairments.

Need for valid and reliable instruments for measuring physical activity in persons with disabilities

Although many physical activity instruments have been validated on specific subgroups of the general population (eg, children or adults), these instruments often do not capture low levels of reported physical activity and contain questions that have little or no relationship to the lifestyles of many people with disabilities (eg, "During the past month, did you participate in any physical activities such as jogging, calisthenics, or golf?"). One function of a survey instrument is to capture baseline measures so changes in

Box 2. Guidelines for resistance exercise training in aging persons with physical disabilities

General resistance training guidelines—understanding the disability
- Identify the associated and secondary conditions that underlie each disability.
- Determine if the condition is progressive or nonprogressive.
- Determine which muscle groups are functional.
- Determine if there is noticeable weakness on one side of the body (hemiplegia).
- Consult with the client's physician to determine the client's bone integrity (eg, any indications for osteoporosis with a moderate to high risk for fractures).

Training volume
- Varies in persons with similar and different disabilities.
- Depends on the amount of muscle mass that is functional.
- Progressive disorders (eg, postpolio syndrome, MS, ALS) must start at low levels and be carefully monitored.
- The greater the level of impairment, the lower the training volume (higher rest interval, fewer reps, fewer sets).

Training progression
- Varies according to health status.
- Active-assistive exercise may be necessary in certain individuals or for certain muscle groups.

Asymmetrical weakness (hemiplegia)
- Common in stroke and cerebral palsy.
- Determine if there is nerve innervation on the hemiplegic side.
- Develop a separate training regimen for the weaker side.
- Adaptive devises (eg, gloves or mitts to attach the hand to a weight or a weight machine) may be required.

Spasticity
- A spastic muscle can be strengthened and should not cause higher levels of spasticity.
- Strengthen the opposing muscle group.
- Spastic muscle groups that are incapable of being strengthened should be stretched.
- Consult with a therapist to determine how to safely stretch spastic muscles or contractures.

More information on specific exercise guidelines for various disabilities is available at www.ncpad.org.

behavior or performance can be tracked over time. Instruments that start at higher levels of physical activity than are generally observed in aging disabled populations (eg, sport, high level recreational activities) miss lower levels of physical activity (eg, housework, moving around, standing). The failure to capture low levels of activity results in floor effects and sample data that are not normally distributed [49].

Objective measures (eg, pedometers, accelerometers, and ambulatory monitors) represent an alternative approach to measuring physical activity. These measurement tools have shown promise in their ability to predict energy expenditure and cardiovascular fitness compared with self-report instruments [50,51]. The use of objective methods of physical activity measurement, however, has its limitations. Among individuals with mobility impairments, particularly those who use wheelchairs and similar assistive devices, accelerometers, pedometers, and ambulatory monitoring devices, fail to accurately capture the types of physical movement these individuals perform because these instruments were designed to capture lower extremity movement.

Understanding barriers to physical activity

There are many barriers to physical activity experienced by people with physical disabilities. One of the most significant barriers faced by many individuals aging with a physical disability is the lack of information about programs that are available in their community [52]. Historically, most health care providers have not actively promoted such wellness programming for people with disabilities and do not maintain information about specific physical activity programs for their clientele or patients [53]. More research on the types of barriers experienced by people aging with a physical disability would be useful for developing appropriate physical activity regimens that have a greater likelihood of compliance [54].

A one-stop resource on physical activity and disability: The National Center on Physical Activity and Disability

The National Center on Physical Activity and Disability (NCPAD) (www.ncpad.org) is a national information center funded by the CDC. NCPAD has developed several initiatives to assist professionals with locating information on physical activity and disability. Through the Center's toll-free hotline (800-900-8086), anyone nationwide can obtain information about how to develop exercise programs for people with various types of disabilities (eg, limb loss, MS, or SCI) or where to find an accessible fitness facility in their community. NCPAD has online directories of adaptive equipment vendors, conferences, organizations, and programs and facilities that provide opportunities for accessible physical activity.

Summary

The relationship between physical functioning and physical activity is a reciprocal one; physical functioning provides the individual with the capability to engage in physical activities, and physical activity helps to maintain and in some cases improve physical functioning. This reciprocal relationship, coupled with the high prevalence of physical inactivity among persons aging with a disability, has profound implications for rehabilitation practice, especially in evaluating intermediate and long-term outcomes of clinical practice. For rehabilitation to play a role in the long-term maintenance and enhancement of physical functioning among persons with disabilities, increasing participation in various types of physical activity in the community must be part of the recovery and maintenance continuum [12,22]. There is also a critical need to identify specific doses of physical activity for specific disabilities and secondary conditions. HMOs and other health insurers will require evidence-based outcomes before establishing reimbursement procedures for physical activity programs for persons aging with a physical disability.

References

[1] Rejeski WJ, Brawley LR, Haskell WL. The prevention challenge: an overview of the supplement. Am J Prev Med 2003;25:107–9.
[2] Manton KG, Vaupel JW. Survival after the age of 80 in the United States, Sweden, France, England, and Japan. N Engl J Med 1995;333:1232–5.
[3] Campbell ML, Sheets D, Strong PS. Secondary health conditions among middle-aged individuals with chronic physical disabilities: Implications for unmet needs for services. Assistive Tech 1999;11:105–22.
[4] Hicks AL, Martin KA, Ditor DS, Latimer AE, Craven C, Bugaresti J, et al. Long-term exercise training in persons with spinal cord injury: effects on strength, arm ergometry performance and psychological well-being. Spinal Cord 2003;41:34–43.
[5] Petrella RJ. Exercise for older patients with chronic disease. Phys Sports Med 1999;27:1–14.
[6] Turk MA, Scandale J, Rosenbaum PF, Weber RJ. The health of women with cerebral palsy. Phys Med Rehab Clin North Am 2001;12:153–68.
[7] Roller S. Health promotion for people with chronic neuromuscular disabilities. In: Krotoski DM, Nosek MA, Turk MA, editors. Women with disabilities: achieving and maintaining health and well-being. Baltimore: Paul H. Brookes; 1996. p. 431–40.
[8] Kemp B, Mosqueda L. Aging-related conditions. In: Fuhrer MJ, editor. Assessing medical rehabilitation practices. Baltimore: Paul H. Brookes; 1997. p. 393–411.
[9] Wilber N, Mitra M, Walker DK, Allen DA, Meyers AR, Tupper P. Disability as a public health issue: findings and reflections from the Massachusetts survey of secondary conditions. Millbank Q 2002;80:393–421.
[10] Rejeski WJ, Focht BC. Aging and physical disability: on integrating group and individual counseling with the promotion of physical activity. Exerc Sport Sci Rev 2002;30:166–70.
[11] Turk MA. The impact of disability on fitness in women: musculoskeletal issues. In: Krotoski DM, Nosek MA, Turk MA, editors. Women with disabilities: achieving and maintaining health and well-being. Baltimore: Paul H. Brookes; 1996. p. 391–406.
[12] Rimmer JH. Health promotion for persons with disabilities: the emerging paradigm shift from disability prevention to prevention of secondary conditions. Phys Ther 1999;79: 495–502.

[13] Smith RD. Promoting the health of people with physical disabilitie: a discussion of the financing and organization of public health services in Australia. Health Promot Int 2000; 15:79–86.

[14] Haskell WL. Physical activity and disease prevention: past, present and future. A personal perspective. Exerc Sport Sci Rev 2003;31:109–10.

[15] Shephard RJ. How much physical activity is needed for good health? Int J Sports Med 1999; 20:23–7.

[16] Healthy people 2010: conference edition, vol. II. Washington, DC: US Department of Health and Human Services; 2000.

[17] Pate RR, Pratt M, Blair SN, Haskell WL, Macera CA, Bouchard C, et al. Physical activity and public health: a recommendation from the Centers for Disease Control and Prevention and the American College of Sports. JAMA 1995;273:402–7.

[18] Physical activity and health: a report of the Surgeon General. Atlanta (GA): US Department of Health and Human Services, Centers for Disease Control and Prevention, National Center for Chronic Disease Prevention and Health Promotion; 1996.

[19] Heath GW, Fentem PH. Physical activity among persons with disabilities: a public health perspective. Exerc Sport Sci Rev 1997;25:195–234.

[20] Rimmer JH, Rubin SS, Braddock D, Hedman G. Physical activity patterns of African-American women with physical disabilities. Med Sci Sports Exerc 1999;31:613–8.

[21] Morey CM, Zhu CW. Improved fitness narrows the symptom-reporting gap between older men and women. J Womens Health 2003;12:381–90.

[22] Rimmer JH. Health promotion for individuals with disabilities: the need for a transitional model in service delivery. Dis Manage Health Outcomes 2002;10:337–43.

[23] Rimmer JH, Braddock D. Health promotion for people with physical, cognitive and sensory disabilities: an emerging national priority. Am J Health Prom 2002;16:220–4.

[24] Freedman VA, Martin LG. Understanding trends in functional limitations among older Americans. Am J Public Health 1999;88:1457–62.

[25] Lexell J. Muscle structure and function in chronic neurological disorders: the potential of exercise to improve activities of daily living. Exerc Sport Sci Rev 2000;28:80–4.

[26] Morey MC, Pieper CF, Cornoni-Huntley J. Physical fitness and functional limitations in community-dwelling older adults. Med Sci Sports Exerc 1998;30:715–23.

[27] Huang Y, Macera CA, Blair SN, Brill PA, Kohl HW, Kronenfeld JJ. Physical fitness, physical activity, and functional limitation in adults aged 40 and older. Med Sci Sports Exerc 1998;30:1430–5.

[28] Binder EF, Burge SJ, Spina R. Peak aerobic power is an is an important component of physical performance in older women. J Gerontol Med Sci 1999;54A:M353–6.

[29] Lawrence RH, Jette AM. Disentangling the disablement process. J Gerontol Soc Sci 1996; 51B:5173–82.

[30] Stessman J, Hammerman-Rozenberg R, Maaravi Y, Cohen A. Effect of exercise on ease in performing activities of daily living and instrumental activities of daily living from age 70 to 77: the Jerusalem longitudinal study. J Am Geriatr Soc 2002;50:1934–8.

[31] Rimmer JH, Riley B, Creviston C, Nicola T. Exercise training in a predominantly African-American group of stroke survivors with multiple comorbidities. Med Sci Sports Exerc 2001; 32:1990–6.

[32] Aitkens SG, McCrory MA, Kilmer DD, Bernauer EM. Moderate resistance exercise program: its effect in slowly progressive neuromuscular disease. Arch Phys Med Rehabil 1993;74:711–5.

[33] Brown M, Sinacore DR, Ehsani AA, Binder EF, Holloszy JO, Kohrt WM. Low-intensity exercise as a modifier of physical frailty in older adults. Arch Phys Med Rehabil 2000;81:960–5.

[34] Petajan JH, Gappmaier E, White AT, Spencer MK, Mino L, Hicks RW. Impact of aerobic training on fitness and quality of life in multiple sclerosis. Ann Neurol 1996;39:432–41.

[35] Eng JJ, Chu KS, Maria Kim C, Dawson AS, Carswell A, Hepburn KE. A community-based group exercise program for persons with chronic stroke. Med Sci Sports Exerc 2003;35: 1271–8.

[36] Macko RF, Smith GV, Dobrovolny CL, Sorkin JD, Goldberg AP, Silver KH. Treadmill training improves fitness reserve in chronic stroke patients. Arch Phys Med Rehabil 2001; 82:879–84.

[37] Kilmer DD. Response to resistive strengthening exercise training in humans with neuromuscular disease. Am J Phys Med Rehabil 2002;81:S121–6.

[38] Krivickas LS. Training flexibility. In: Frontera WR, editor. Exercise in rehabilitation medicine. Champaign (IL): Human Kinetics; 1999. p. 83–102.

[39] Palmer KP, Harbst K, Harbst T. Brain injury. In: Myers JN, Herbert WG, Humphrey R, editors. ACSM's resources for clinical exercise physiology: musculoskeletal, neuromuscular, neoplastic, immunologic, and hematologic conditions. Baltimore: Lippincott Williams & Wilkins; 2002. p. 98–108.

[40] Pitetti KH, Manske RC. Amputation. In: Myers JN, Herbert WG, Humphrey R, editors. ACSM's resources for clinical exercise physiology: musculoskeletal, neuromuscular, neoplastic, immunologic, and hematologic conditions. Baltimore: Lippincott Williams & Wilkins; 2002. p. 170–6.

[41] Rimmer JH. Physical fitness levels of persons with cerebral palsy. Dev Med Child Neurol 2001;43:208–12.

[42] Olenik LM, Laskin JJ, Burnham R, Wheeler GD, Steadward RD. Efficacy of rowing, backward wheeling and isolated scapular retractor exercise as remedial strength activities for wheelchair users: application of electromyography. Paraplegia 1995;33:148–52.

[43] Rodgers MM, Keyser RE, Rasch EK, Gorman PH, Russell PJ. Influence of training on biomechanics of wheelchair propulsion. J Reh Res Develop 2001;38:505–11.

[44] Burnham RS. Shoulder pain in wheelchair athletes: the role of muscle imbalance. Am J Sports Med 1993;21:238–42.

[45] Fullerton HD, Borckardt JJ, Alfano AP. Shoulder pain: a comparison of wheelchair athletes and nonathletic wheelchair users. Med Sci Sports Exerc 2003;35:1958–61.

[46] Jacobs PL, Nash MS, Rusinowski JW. Circuit training provides cardiorespiratory and strength benefits in persons with paraplegia. Med Sci Sports Exerc 2001;33:711–7.

[47] Burnham RS, Steadward RD. Upper extremity peripheral nerve entrapments among wheel-chair athletes: prevalence, location, and risk factors. Arch Phys Med Rehabil 1994;75:519–24.

[48] Curtis KA, Drysdale GA, Lanza RD. Shoulder pain in wheelchair users with tetraplegia and paraplegia. Arch Phys Med Rehabil 1999;80:453–7.

[49] Rimmer JH, Riley BB, Rubin SS. A new measure for assessing the physical activity behaviors of persons with disabilities and chronic health conditions: The Physical Activity and Disability Survey. Am J Health Promot 2001;16:34–45.

[50] McDermott MM, Liu K, O'Brien E. Measuring physical activity in peripheral arterial disease: a comparison of two physical activity questionnaires with an accelerometer. Angiology 2000;51:91–100.

[51] Poston CW, Suminski RR, Jackson AS. Non-equivalence of self-report and Caltrac measures of energy expenditure. Med Sci Sports Exerc 1998;30:12.

[52] Rimmer JH, Riley B, Wang E, Rauworth A, Jurkowski J. Physical activity participation among persons with disabilities: barriers and facilitators. Am J Prev Med 2004;26:419–25.

[53] Lawlor DA, Hanratty B. The effect of physical activity advice given in routine primary care consultations: a systematic review. J Public Health Med 2001;23:219–26.

[54] Taylor WC, Baranowski T, Young DR. Physical activity interventions in low-income, ethnic minority, and populations with disability. Am J Prev Med 1998;15:334–43.

Phys Med Rehabil Clin N Am
16 (2005) 57–90

ELSEVIER
SAUNDERS

PHYSICAL MEDICINE
AND REHABILITATION
CLINICS OF
NORTH AMERICA

Practical considerations in the assessment and treatment of pain in adults with physical disabilities

Adrian Cristian, MD[a,b,*], Jodi Thomas, MD[a,b],
Michelle Nisenbaum, MD[a], LilyAnn Jeu, PharmD[b]

[a]Department of Rehabilitation Medicine, Mount Sinai School of Medicine,
One Gustave L. Levy Place, New York, NY 10029, USA
[b]Bronx Veterans Affairs Medical Center, 130 West Kingsbridge Road, Bronx,
NY 10468, USA

In recent years, there has been a growing interest in pain experienced by adults with various disabilities [1]. Various surveys have reported on the prevalence of pain, types of pain, and the impact of painful conditions on the activities of daily living (ADL) of adults living with physical disabilities.

Pain is common in physically disabled persons. It is often varied in nature and can be present in multiple sites. There have been few randomized trials to assess the effectiveness of the treatments commonly used. This article provides an overview of this common symptom in physically disabled adults and practical considerations in its assessment and treatment.

Epidemiology of pain in adults with disabilities

In this section the prevalence and type of pain present are described for some common types of physical disabilities, such as amputation, Parkinson disease (PD), stroke, and traumatic brain injury (TBI). The prevalence of pain in cerebral palsy, multiple sclerosis (MS), polio, and spinal cord injury is discussed in greater detail elsewhere in this issue.

* Corresponding author. Bronx Veterans Affairs Medical Center, Room 3d-16 526/117 Bronx VAMC, 130 West Kingsbridge Road, Bronx NY 10468.
E-mail address: adrian.cristian@med.va.gov (A. Cristian).

1047-9651/05/$ - see front matter © 2004 Elsevier Inc. All rights reserved.
doi:10.1016/j.pmr.2004.06.008
pmr.theclinics.com

Amputation

Among amputees, there is a high prevalence of phantom limb pain (51% to 80%) and residual limb pain (22% to 74%). Severe phantom pain can be disabling, interfering with ADL, level of function, ambulation, and employment, and is associated with a poorer quality of life (QOL) and depression [2–7]. It is troublesome long after the surgery is performed [8]. In spite of its high prevalence, amputees receive varied and often inadequate information from their health care providers [9].

Multiple areas of pain are common for lower-limb amputees. Back pain is common (52% to 71%) [10–12], as is pain in the hips, buttocks, knee, opposite foot, neck, and shoulders. In one study, 33% of the participants had pain in three or more locations [11]. Osteoarthritis has also been described in amputees [12], as has the role of total knee arthroplasty in its treatment [14].

Parkinson disease

Patients with PD complain of sensory symptoms such as burning, coldness, numbness, cramplike, and aching. Symptoms are intermittent and poorly localized [15,16]. Migraine headaches have been reported to be more prevalent in this disease [17].

Traumatic brain injury

More than 50% of people living with the sequelae of a TBI complain of pain [18]. Twenty-four percent of TBI survivors have pain daily 6 months after discharge [19]. Headache is the most common symptom, with 47% of patients (mild TBI) and 34% of patients (moderate-severe TBI) reporting it [19]. Musculoskeletal pain involving the neck, shoulders, low back, and limbs has been described [19,20]. Pain that interferes with ADL has been reported by 95% of patients with mild TBI and 22% of patients with moderate-severe TBI [20].

An overlap in symptoms has been described between chronic pain patients and mild TBI [21–23]. These symptoms include poor concentration and memory, inadequate sleep, fatigue, myofascial pain syndromes, dizziness, anxiety, and depression. Both groups often seek care from multiple medical providers, have had extensive medical work-ups, and have legal problems [21]. Anderson reported that 11% of patients referred to a chronic pain program had evidence of brain injury [22].

Stroke

Several types of pain have been described in stroke survivors, the most common being central post-stroke pain, nociceptive pain, and headaches [24]. Post-stroke pain can be chronic, with some studies describing it 1 to 2 years after stroke onset [24,25]. Central pain is located in the area of total or partial thermo-sensory deficits after the stroke. It is believed to be caused by a lesion of the spinal-thalamic-cortical pathway [26–28]. It has been proposed that symptoms are caused by spontaneous discharges of injured thalamic or cortical neurons [26]. Two percent to eight percent of stroke survivors (especially younger ones) are believed to be affected by it [24,25,29,30]. Affected patients have described the pain as a "stabbing," "aching," "dull," "burning," "troublesome," "annoying," "lacerating," or "pinching" sensation [24,31]. It is continuous and is worsened by cold, touch, or physical or emotional stress [24,31,32]. Nociceptive pain has been described as "cramping," "troublesome," "annoying," and "tiring" [24]. Shoulder pain is a significant source of pain for many stroke survivors, especially when it is associated with lost motion [24].

Guillain Barré syndrome

Pain was reported to be common in people living with Guillain Barré syndrome, with a prevalence rate of 89%. Forty-seven percent of the patients with pain described it as "distressing," "horrible," and "excruciating." The pain was described as deep, aching, dysesthetic, and affecting the back and legs [33].

Facioscapulohumeral muscular dystrophy

Muscle pain was described in four case reports of patients with facioscapulohumeral muscular dystrophy with no objective evidence for their pain. The pain was daily and was associated with disturbed sleep [34].

The aging process and its challenges in the management of pain

People aging with disabilities face the challenges of normal aging and challenges caused by aging with a disability. It is relevant to review the normal aging changes that can affect the diagnosis and management of pain in the elderly persons with physical disabilities. The most pertinent organs in the management of pain are the kidneys, liver, brain, and intestines. Kidney function decreases at a rate of 1% per year over the age of 50. A reduction in aldosterone and renin release leads to an increased risk of hyperkalemia. The liver decreases in size, has a reduction in blood flow and metabolism, and has a reduction in mono-oxygenase and cytochrome enzymes [35]. There is reduced protein binding. Gastrointestinal (GI) peristalsis is also reduced, thereby predisposing to constipation [36].

Other changes include an overall increase in body fat, which increases the volume of distribution of lipophilic medications [36], thereby affecting the elimination of these medications. Because elderly patients typically take many medications, there is the possibility of significant drug interactions [36]. Atrophy of cortical and subcortical brain tissue and neuronal loss accompanied by a reduction in cerebral blood flow can lead to altered pain response and perception of pain. The age-related decrease in baroreceptor response can lead to increased risk of orthostatic hypotension [36].

Pain in the elderly population

Pain is a common complaint among elderly persons living in the community and in nursing homes [37]. Pain is commonly associated with conditions that affect the musculoskeletal system (eg, osteoarthritis, vertebral compression fractures), the nervous system (eg, neuropathies), and the cardiovascular system (eg, angina, peripheral vascular disease) [36]. Eighteen percent of elderly Americans take medication for pain on a regular basis and seek help from physicians to address pain [37].

Pain is prevalent in nursing homes, with rates reported to be between 45% and 80% [38,39]. The most common sources of pain are attributed to conditions of the nervous and musculoskeletal systems (eg, low back, shoulder, foot, hip, and neck pain; previous fractures; neuropathies) and claudication [38]. In this population, the presence of pain has been associated with impaired leisure activity, impaired ADL, difficulties with ambulation, depression, and anxiety.

There are significant challenges in the treatment and diagnosis of pain in nursing homes. The patients are typically frail and have multiple medical problems, polypharmacy, and cognitive impairments. The facilities may have limited diagnostic equipment and pain medications on formulary in the pharmacy. Staff may have limited knowledge about the diagnosis and treatment of pain [38]. Some authors feel that pain is undertreated in the nursing home setting [40].

The assessment of pain in people with physical disabilities

Barriers to the assessment of pain in adult with disabilities

In evaluating pain in adults with disabilities, the practitioner faces several barriers, especially in the older adult with a disability. Cognitive or communicative impairments can make the collection of pertinent information difficult (eg, cerebral palsy) [1]. The older adult may harbor fears of possible serious terminal diagnoses uncovered, discomfort associated with diagnostic tests, side effects of prescribed medications, addiction, and the high cost of treatments and therefore may not be forthcoming with information [36].

Elderly individuals may de-emphasize pain due to the over-riding significance of other life stressors, such as loss of a spouse, finances, and independence. They may choose not to report pain so as not to be identified as complainers or burdens to others [39]. Health care providers may feel reluctant to address this issue due to inadequate training in the diagnosis and management of pain in this population.

History

Pain is a subjective experience with no objective markers. It is influenced by social, personal, and cultural factors. The patient's previous experiences and fears and the presence of depression can affect their perception of pain [36].

A detailed history is important in the evaluation of pain in adults with disabilities. There are four general areas that should be addressed: (1) characteristics of the pain and its impact on the functionality of the disabled person, (2) a pertinent review of systems, (3) a review of previous diagnostic tests, and (4) previously tried interventions for the management of the pain and their effectiveness.

Pain characteristics and the impact of pain on functionality

Characteristics of pain to be recorded include location, type of pain (eg, burning, electrical, dull, achy), intensity, radiation, frequency, duration, pattern (eg, constant, intermittent), and aggravating and alleviating factors [36,37].

The disabled or elderly person may not readily volunteer information about pain but may be prompted by questions about "discomfort," "aching," "heaviness," "soreness," or "tightness" [37,41], especially with activities such as transfers, dressing, or pushing a wheelchair.

There are several ways to assess severity of pain. The McGill Pain Questionnaire, the visual analog scale (VAS), numerical pain rating scales, verbal descriptor scales (ie, that use terms such as "mild," "moderate," and "severe"), face scales, pain thermometers, and pain interviews are commonly used.

Regardless of the instrument used, it is important that a patient's cognitive, visual, or manual dexterity limitations (eg, difficulty holding a pen) be taken into consideration (eg, for visual impairment, the scale could be written in large print). The cognitively impaired individual may have difficulty with severity scales that require abstract thinking (eg, the McGill pain questionnaire, VAS, and verbal descriptor scales). The pain thermometer may be more appropriate for this type of patient [41]. Observation of behavior (eg, crying, moaning, agitation, groaning, and withdrawing), facial expressions, and surrogate reporting can be used for the individual with severe cognitive deficits [36,37,41].

Pain diaries can be helpful to identify the intensity, pattern, and aggravating or alleviating factors that contribute to the pain over a period of time. They can be used to record the effectiveness of the prescribed interventions. Aggravating and alleviating factors should be recorded, especially those that affect ADL (eg, shoulder pain in a wheelchair user that makes it difficult to dress, perform transfers, or push the wheelchair). Questions should address changes in daily routines that contribute to the pain. For example, a move to a new neighborhood that requires walking for long distances for food shopping can aggravate underlying chronic back pain in a polio survivor. Problems with a power wheelchair may necessitate the use of a manual wheelchair for long distances, thereby leading to pain in the arms.

It is important to ask the patient if their pain is worse throughout the day or around the time when the effect of the pain medication wears off.

Previous diagnostic tests

All pertinent diagnostic tests should be recorded, preferably in chronologic order. Radiologic tests are commonly used in the evaluation of pain; therefore, the clinician should attempt to obtain reports of such tests when they are available (eg, CT scans, MRIs, x-rays, discograms, myelograms). Electrodiagnostic tests (eg, EMG/NCS, SSEPs), pertinent lab tests (eg, CBC, ESR, rheumatologic tests), and history of nerve blocks can be beneficial.

In the patient with a history of an injury or disease process affecting the central nervous system (eg, stroke, TBI, MS), it is important to determine the extent of the injury. Radiologic tests of the head and spinal cord (eg, CT scan, MRI, MRA reports) and neuropsychologic evaluations can provide useful information about the extent of the injury.

Previous treatments

Given the multitude of treatments available for the treatment of pain, it is important for the clinician to perform a thorough review of all the treatments tried by the patient for their pain. A review of medications should include information about the dosage, route, and duration of time that the patient tried the medication. Appropriate questions should probe for effectiveness of the medication and side effects that affected functionality (eg, Did the medication worsen constipation in a patient with a neurogenic bowel? Did the medication cause drowsiness that affected wheelchair propulsion?) or QOL. The effectiveness of an intervention may not be seen by a reduction in the intensity of pain but may be demonstrated through an increase in functionality (eg, wheelchair propulsion, ambulation distance), improvement in QOL (eg, better sleep), or a decrease in the frequency or duration of the pain itself.

Nonpharmacologic interventions should receive the same scrutiny for effectiveness and side effects as pharmacologic interventions. The clinician should ask the patient about physical therapy, massage, acupuncture, homeopathy, chiropractic, nutritional supplements, magnet therapy, transcutaneous electrical nerve stimulation (TENS) units, and orthotics. Reasons for the discontinuation of such therapies can provide valuable information. Was it due to lack of transportation, lack of finances, interference with functionality, or poor fit (eg, an ill-fitting brace)?

Social history

It is important to assess the individual's social support network [41]. Does the patient live alone or with a family or friends? Is someone available to bring them for therapy? How accessible is the transportation where they live? Do they have financial resources to cover travel or medication expenses?

Physical examination

Because most pain complaints in disabled patients are musculoskeletal or neurologic in nature, a thorough examination of these systems is important. Key aspects of the physical examination include inspection (eg, for joint or limb deformities, scoliosis, kyphosis, swelling, pressure ulcers, an ill-fitting orthotic, or obesity), palpation (tender areas or trigger points), range-of-motion—passive and active (joint laxity, limitation of movement, pain with motion, contractures), strength, and sensory testing.

Sensory testing typically includes light touch, pinprick, and proprioception. The clinician should check for sensory loss, hyperpathia, or allodynia. Pertinent "special" tests should be performed (eg, shoulder impingement signs) as necessary. Gait analysis can yield important information about painful structures with motion.

Wheelchair users are at risk for painful overuse syndromes of the upper extremities and pain in the low back, hips, and lower extremities if not properly seated. It is therefore beneficial for the clinician to evaluate the patient's wheelchair. Special attention should be given to the seat cushion and the patient's seated position in the wheelchair. An inappropriate cushion can lead to pain in the lower back, hips, and upper posterior thighs. A sling back chair may contribute to back pain. An inappropriately sized wheelchair can make it difficult for a smaller individual to propel it, thereby contributing to arm pain.

Amputees should have their residual limbs checked for tender areas or evidence of an ill-fitting prosthesis (eg, erythema or skin breaks in pressure-sensitive areas). The prosthesis should be checked for signs of excessive wear and broken parts. The peripheral vascular system should be assessed for evidence of vascular compromise (eg, faint distal pulses, dependent rubor).

Given the possibility of cognitive deficits, it is advisable to include a mini-mental status examination as part of the physical examination of a neurologically impaired individual presenting with pain when cognitive limitations are suspected. An instrument to assess for depression can be of benefit.

Need for diagnostic tests

Once the history and physical examination are completed, the necessity of ordering diagnostic tests or procedures is often considered. Diagnostic tests or procedures (eg, nerve blocks) can be useful in localizing the source of the pain. However, they can place additional burdens and potential risks on the physically disabled person. The clinician should carefully consider the potential benefit of the procedure against the potential risks and burdens to the patient. The question of how the results of the test will influence management options should be discussed with the patient.

The patient may have limited access to transportation, and the trip to the test may be burdensome to the patient and family. Financial factors, such as the cost of the transportation or out-of-pocket costs for the test, can be considerable for someone with limited financial resources. When a patient has to undergo more than one diagnostic test or procedure, scheduling the procedures on the same day can reduce the transportation burden. The clinician should attempt to implement interventions to address the pain while awaiting the results of the diagnostic tests.

Lab tests can provide useful information about the function of the kidneys and liver. Baseline values should be obtained for review before inception of a medication that could adversely affect these organs.

The management of pain in physical disability

An accurate diagnosis is essential to the proper treatment of a patient's pain [36,37]. This can be challenging in the adult with a physical disability. There may be more than one diagnosis. For example, an ill-fitting prosthesis may be the direct cause of residual limb pain but may indirectly aggravate a hip with advanced osteoarthritis and lumbar spinal stenosis in an elderly amputee.

General principles

Adults with disabilities face considerable barriers in the treatment of their pain, many of which are beyond their control. Limited transportation can make it difficult to attend outpatient physical therapy and physician visits. Limited finances can place constraints on the use of certain medications or treatments. Lack of access to appropriate specialists can further limit their choices. Individuals with cognitive impairment face additional challenges, such as the undertreatment of their pain by health care providers.

Given these limitations, it is important for the clinician to discuss with the patient and his/her family their preferences for the various treatment options being considered. For example, it has been reported that elderly patients do not like interventions such as medications (fear of side effects), physical therapy, or exercise (fear of falls or injury). They do like home remedies, massage, topical agents, physical modalities (heat and cold), music, humor, and prayer [42]. Other factors to discuss with the patient include their fears about the various treatment options being considered (eg, addiction to narcotics, side effects of medications).

Davis defined the goal of pain management as "pain reduction associated with improved function reflected in ADL, sleep and socialization, and not necessarily complete absence of pain or the use of minimal analgesic medication" [36]. To accomplish this goal he emphasized three principal elements of pain management: (1) a comprehensive assessment of the pain with a clear understanding of its etiology, (2) use of pharmacologic and nonpharmacologic therapy, and (3) age- and function-adjusted pharmacology [36].

Pharmacologic management of pain

There have been few well-designed studies on the use of medications for the treatment of pain in this population. Therefore, the primary considerations for the use of medications lies in choosing agents with the least potential for adverse effects while maximizing their analgesic potential. This section provides guidelines and considerations regarding the use of commonly prescribed pain medications in adults with disabilities.

Key points to consider when prescribing medications for pain management in elderly patients and in patients with disabilities include the following: (1) Choose medications that minimize the risk of side effects, drug–drug interactions, and drug–disease interactions. (2) Treat as many pain symptoms with one medication as possible. (3) Choose only one drug per class. Combining small doses of different drug classes can be effective and can minimize side effects [37]. (4) Reduced doses based on a reduction in the function of key organs responsible for the metabolism of medications. (5) Start medications at the lowest doses and gradually increase the dose as tolerated. In anticipation of age-related increased sensitivity to the effects and duration of effects of various medications, use a low dose and increase the interval frequency. (6) Use an as-needed schedule as opposed to a standing order whenever possible. (7) Educate patients and caregivers about the mechanism of action, common (and also potentially serious) side effects, desired outcome, and time until onset of action or duration of effects of analgesics. Patients and caregivers should be counseled about precautions to take with analgesics, such as the avoidance of alcohol use with medications that may cause sedation or hepatotoxicity.

For mild to moderate nociceptive pain, non-opioid analgesics such as acetaminophen and nonsteroidal anti-inflammatory drugs (NSAIDs) continue to be first-line agents. Doses of these agents are limited by ceiling analgesic effect or the propensity for side effects that may be prominent in elderly patients. For more severe pain, opioids may be used in combination with nonopioids or as monotherapy. Neuropathic pain may be treated with adjunctive pain medications, including antidepressants, antiepileptic agents, skeletal muscle relaxants, and anesthetics. Precautions for the use of commonly used agents in each class are described below. Drug–drug interactions and precautions for special populations and adverse effects of medications are summarized in Tables 1 and 2, respectively.

Table 1
Adverse effects and precautions for the use of pain medications in physically disabled patients

Population at risk	Medications	Adverse effects and precautions

Physical disabilities
  MS
  TBI
	Opioids	Sedation, dizziness, falls risk, impaired mental function, delirium, confusion

Cerebral palsy Cerebrovascular accident	Tricyclic antidepressants, trazodone	Sedation, dizziness, lightheadedness, seizure risk, confusion
PD Polio	Antiepileptics	Sedation, drowsiness, dizziness, fatigue, falls risk, ataxia, seizure risk, confusion
Elderly with gait abnormalities	NSAIDs	Dizziness, confusion, delirium
	Skeletal muscle relaxants	Sedation, ataxia, drowsiness, dizziness, falls risk
	Lidocaine/mexiletene	Seizure risk, nervousness, tremors, irritability
	Tramadol	Increased risk of seizures
Hepatic dysfunction Cirrhosis/liver disease Chronic alcohol use	Opioids	Reduced metabolism to active metabolites or reduced ability to inactivate active drug to inactive metabolites
	Acetaminophen	Risk of hepatotoxicity. Reduce dose or avoid acetaminophen in these patients
	Tramadol	Reduced elimination. Reduce initial dose of tramadol in these patients
	Tricyclic antidepressants	Reduced metabolism to active metabolites and reduced efficacy of some agents
	Phenytoin, carbamazepine	Potential hepatotoxicity
Renal dysfunction Reduced renal function	NSAIDs	Acute renal failure or worsening chronic renal dysfunction
	Opioids, gabapentin, tramadol	Reduced elimination of active drug or metabolites
Cardiovascular disease Hypertension Chronic heart failure Arrhythmia	Opioids	Hypotension
	NSAIDs	Elevation of blood pressure, worsening of heart failure symptoms
	Tricyclic antidepressants	Orthostatic hypotension, tachycardia, cardiac conduction defects
	Lidocaine/mexiletene, carbamazepine	Cardiac conduction abnormalities

Table 1 (continued)

Population at risk	Medications	Adverse effects and precautions
Decreased pulmonary reserve COPD Cor pulmonale Sleep apnea	Opioids	Respiratory depression
GI disorders Peptic ulcer disease Neurogenic bowel	NSAIDs Opioids Tricyclic antidepressants, trazodone	Dyspepsia, ulceration of gastric mucosa Constipation, nausea/vomiting Constipation, anorexia, dry mouth
Genitourinary disorders Benign prostatic hypertrophy Erectile dysfunction	Opioids Tricyclic antidepressants, trazodone	Urinary retention Urinary retention, priapism
Substance abuse history Chronic alcohol use Heroin or cocaine use	Opioids, tramadol, skeletal muscle relaxants	Addiction potential

Abbreviations: MS, multiple sclerosis; TBI, traumatic brain injury; PD, Parkinson disease; NSAID, nonsteroidal anti-inflammatory drug; COPD, chronic obstructive pulmonary disease; GI, gastrointestinal.

Nonsteroidal anti-inflammatory drugs

Commonly used in the treatment of musculoskeletal pain and inflammatory disorders, NSAIDs are associated with numerous potentially serious adverse effects when used for long-term treatment in elderly patients with disabilities. NSAIDs exert analgesic, antipyretic, and anti-inflammatory properties through the inhibition of prostaglandin synthesis via inhibition of cyclooxygenase-1 and -2 (COX-1 and COX-2) isoenzymes. Some evidence suggests that at low doses NSAIDs have primarily an analgesic effect, whereas at higher doses there is a more pronounced anti-inflammatory effect [36,37,43]. Thus, it is important to know the intended role of the NSAID in the treatment plan. NSAIDs may be better for inflammatory arthritis than for mechanical osteoarthritic conditions. In addition, the analgesic effects start within several hours of administration, whereas the anti-inflammatory benefits may take several days to weeks to take effect [36,37,44].

Dyspepsia or GI intolerance associated with NSAID use is a common side effect that can be minimized by instructing patients to take these medications on a full stomach [45]. The risk of mucosal lesions and ulceration may result from the inhibition of production of prostaglandins in the gastric mucosa. Although less likely with ibuprofen, meloxicam, or etodolac due to a relatively higher selectively for the COX-2 isoenzyme, the risk of GI bleeding may be reduced by the addition of a proton pump

Table 2
Drug–drug interactions for pain medications in physically disabled patients

Population at risk	Medication combinations	Adverse interactions

Physical disabilities
MS
TBI
Cerebral palsy
Cerebrovascular accident
PD
	Tricyclic antidepressants
	+ Baclofen,
	  diphenhydramine,
	  or opioids
	+ Phenytoin
	Opioids
		Increased sedation, dizziness,
		  confusion, and ataxia;
		  increased anticholinergic
		  effects; impaired motor
		  function or skills
		Increased risk of ataxia,
		  tremors, and nystagmus

Polio
Elderly with gait
  abnormalities
	+ Sedatives or
	  antiepileptic drugs
		Increased sedation, dizziness,
		  and confusion; additional
		  impairment in motor
		  function or skills

Hepatic dysfunction
Cirrhosis/liver disease
 	
Chronic alcohol use
	Acetaminophen
	+ Phenytoin or
	  carbamazepine
		Increased potential for
		  hepatotoxicity

Renal dysfunction
Reduced renal function
	NSAIDs
	+ Angiotensin-converting
	  enzyme inhibitors
		Acute or worsening renal
		  failure, hyperkalemia, or
		  elevated blood pressure

Cardiovascular disease
Hypertension
Chronic heart failure
Arrhythmia
	NSAIDs
	+ Antihypertensive
	  agents
	+ Warfarin, aspirin,
	  or clopidogrel
	Tricyclic antidepressants
	+ Warfarin
	
	+ Antiarrhythmic agents
	
	Carbamazepine
	+ Warfarin
		Reduced antihypertensive
		  effects
		Increased bleeding risk
		
		Increased bioavailability of
		  warfarin and bleeding risk
		Increased risk of cardiac
		  conduction abnormalities
		
		Decreased bioavailability of
		  warfarin and anticoagulation

Neurologic impairment
Seizure history
	Tricyclic antidepressants
	+ Phenytoin
	
	+ Valproic acid
	
	Carbamazepine
	+ Tricyclic
	  antidepressants
		Risk of ataxia, tremors,
		  nystagmus
		Increased serum
		  concentrations of
		  amitriptyline and
		  nortriptyline
		
		Decreased efficacy of tricyclic
		  antidepressants; increased
		  seizure risk

Table 2 (*continued*)

Population at risk	Medication combinations	Adverse interactions
Decreased pulmonary reserve	NSAIDs	
COPD	+ Prednisone	Increased risk dyspepsia and gastric ulceration
Cor pulmonale	Carbamazepine	
Sleep apnea	+ Prednisone	Decreased effectiveness of prednisone
GI or genitourinary disorders	NSAIDs	
Peptic ulcer disease	+ Warfarin, aspirin, or clopidogrel	Increased risk of gastric ulcers
Neurogenic bowel	Opioids	
Urinary retention	+ Tricyclic antidepressants	Increased risk of constipation and urinary retention
Mood disorders	Tramadol or tricyclic antidepressants	
Major depressive disorder	+ Selective serotonin inhibitors,	Risk of serotonin syndrome
Bipolar disorder	or monoamine oxidase inhibitors	
	Carbamazepine	
	+ Selective serotonin inhibitors	Increased risk of ataxia, nystagmus, headache, or seizures

Abbreviations: MS, multiple sclerosis; TBI, traumatic brain injury; PD, Parkinson disease; NSAID, nonsteroidal anti-inflammatory drug; COPD, chronic obstructive pulmonary disease; GI, gastrointestinal.

inhibitor or prostaglandin analog for patients at risk. These include patients with peptic ulcer disease or patients concurrently taking other medications (eg, systemic corticosteroids, oral potassium) that may be erosive to the gastric mucosa [45,46].

Because NSAIDs affect platelet function, they must also be used cautiously in patients with bleeding disorders and in patients taking other medications with bleeding risk. Among patients with physical disabilities, these may include patients taking clopidogrel for secondary stroke prevention or patients taking warfarin or aspirin for antithrombotic therapy or cardiovascular protection. In addition, because most NSAIDs are primarily eliminated renally, patients with renal disease may require reduced doses. Hepatic dysfunction should also be considered for agents that require this route of elimination [47].

NSAIDs should be used with caution in patients with renal dysfunction, hypertension, and heart failure. NSAID-induced inhibition of renal prostaglandin production may reduce renal blood flow and glomerular filtration.Thus, antihypertensive effects of diuretics, beta-blockers, and angiotensin-converting enzyme inhibitors may be diminished, and blood pressure elevation or peripheral edema may result. Furthermore, the risk of acute renal failure and hyperkalemia among patients receiving potassium-sparing agents or potassium supplements with NSAIDs is a potential concern and should be monitored. Clinicians may consider using shorter-acting agents (given BID) (eg, ibuprofen) instead of longer-acting preparations in anticipation of potential effects on renal function [48].

Cyclooxygenase-2 inhibitors

Although COX-2 inhibitors have become popular medications for the treatment of osteoarthritis and rheumatoid arthritis, there has been little written about their efficacy in people with physical disabilities. Piovesan et al [49] reported on three cases of idiopathic stabbing headache post stroke that was successfully treated with celecoxib. Although COX-2 inhibitors are associated with a lower incidence of significant GI side effects (eg, upper GI ulcers) when compared with nonselective NSAIDs [50–54], the risk is not eliminated [55,56]. In addition, the risks of cardiovascular and renal side effects of COX-2 inhibitors, such as elevated blood pressure, peripheral edema, and renal failure, are considerable [45,57]. Due to concerns about increased risk of heart disease and stroke, rofecoxib has been recently pulled off the market. This has led to greater scrutiny of COX-2 inhibitors in general. Because COX-2 inhibitors do not inhibit platelet aggregation, patients taking low-dose aspirin for cardioprotective effects should be instructed to continue aspirin with the COX-2 inhibitor.

Acetaminophen

Unlike NSAIDs, acetaminophen has analgesic and antipyretic effects but lacks anti-inflammatory properties. Also unlike NSAIDs, acetaminophen does not have effects on gastric mucosa and has no renal effects. Because acetaminophen is primarily metabolized by conjugation in the liver, rather than via cytochrome P450 (CYP 450) enzymes, acetaminophen has relatively few drug–drug interactions. However, patients with liver dysfunction or a history of alcohol abuse should use acetaminophen with caution. The maximum recommended daily dosage for patients without hepatic dysfunction is 4000 mg per day divided in four to six doses [47].

Opioids

Opioids exhibit a wide therapeutic index [58], with analgesic effects mediated primarily by binding to μ receptors [59,60]. Some evidence suggests that opioids may have anti-inflammatory properties, although they have limited efficacy for neuropathic pain [61]. Goals of chronic opioid therapy include dosage titration for analgesia or improvement in functioning, initiation with short-acting preparations on an as-needed basis and change to long-acting preparations for baseline pain management with supplemental doses for breakthrough pain [36], and minimization of adverse effects [59–61]. Although it is beyond the scope of this article to provide a full review of the role of opioids in the management of pain, key aspects of their usefulness and limitations when prescribed to adults with disabilities are explored.

Potential side effects associated with opioid use include sedation, dizziness, delirium, confusion, respiratory depression, hypotension, nausea/vomiting, constipation, urinary retention, pruritus, and physical or psychologic dependence [47]. Although patients may develop tolerance to many side effects (eg, sedation and nausea), most patients do not develop tolerance to constipation and should be placed on a prophylactic bowel regimen that includes a stimulant laxative. Opioid-related side effects present a special concern to elderly adults with disabilities. For example, patients with neurogenic bowel may need to avoid opioids or use them with caution due to the potential for constipation. Because opioids have direct effects on brainstem respiratory and cough centers and because their use may lead to respiratory depression, caution should also be used when prescribing opioids to patients with underlying chronic obstructive pulmonary disease, cor pulmonale, sleep apnea, or substantially decreased pulmonary reserve (eg, severe kyphoscoliosis) [60]. Due to potential respiratory depression and hypotension, fentanyl, in particular, should not be used immediately post-operatively or via the transdermal route for opioid-naive patients. Pentazocine, meperidine, and propoxyphene are associated with significant neurologic (eg, seizures) and cardiac toxicity [36]. Dizziness and sedation may impair balance or gait in patients with limited ambulation due to physical disabilities.

Hepatic or renal failure can affect the metabolism and elimination of opioids, thereby increasing their duration and the incidence of side effects [36,60]. Because a number of agents require hepatic metabolism to produce active metabolites or undergo hepatic elimination, opioids must be used with caution in patients with hepatic dysfunction. For prodrugs that require metabolism to an active metabolite (eg, codeine, oxycodone), patients unable to convert the parent drug may not receive adequate analgesia and may be at risk for adverse effects. For active compounds, lack of hepatic elimination may result in the accumulation of the parent compound and the risk for adverse effects. Although patients with liver failure should avoid using codeine, pentazocine, or pethidine (a.k.a. meperidine), morphine and fentanyl have been reported to be safer to use in these patients [36]. Because many opioids or their active metabolites require renal excretion, it is prudent to reduce doses or interval frequency for opioids such as codeine, fentanyl, oxycodone, meperidine, propoxyphene, and morphine [36,47].

Tramadol

Tramadol is a centrally acting agent that binds to μ receptors and blocks the reuptake of serotonin and norepinephrine [48]. Showing weak opioid effects, tramadol is less likely to cause constipation, confusion, and respiratory depression and has less abuse potential than opioids. It has been reported to be useful in the treatment of moderate-to-severe osteoarthritic pain [48] and diabetic peripheral polyneuropathy [62,63]. The maximum daily dosage is 400 mg in divided doses every 6 to 8 hours [48,63]. For patients with renal or hepatic dysfunction or age >75 years, starting dose should be 50 mg every 12 to 24 hours [36]. Tramadol should be avoided in patients with a history of seizures [64,65] or who may be taking selective serotonin reuptake inhibitors, monoamine oxidase inhibitors, or serotonergic agents due to risk for serotonin syndrome [66,67].

Tricyclic antidepressants and trazodone

Tricyclic antidepressants (TCAs) and trazodone are commonly used in the treatment of neuropathic pain. TCAs inhibit the reuptake of serotonin and norepinephrine into presynaptic terminals [36,62,63], whereas trazodone affects serotonin accumulation. These agents have been found to produce an analgesic effect at doses much lower than those required for the treatment of depression [36,62]. However, antagonist effects at other receptors (histaminergic, cholinergic and alpha-adrenergic, dopaminergic) may result in adverse side effects [63], including impaired motor and mental function; worsening constipation and urinary retention; potential tachycardia, orthostatic hypotension, and cardiac conduction defects; and seizure risk in susceptible patients [47,68]. Among patients with physical disabilities, those with neurologic impairments are at increased risk of falls and should receive these agents with caution [47,69]. Secondary amines such as desipramine and nortriptyline have a lower incidence of side effects [36], although amitriptyline is hepatically metabolized to nortriptyline and desipramine to imipramine. Trazodone also requires hepatic metabolism to an active metabolite [47].

Antiepileptics

Ahmad et al [63] provide a review of the use of antiepileptics for treatment of neuropathic pain. However, the role of antiepileptic agents in the treatment of pain conditions in adults with disabilities remains unclear. These agents are believed to work by blocking sodium channels, stabilizing neuronal membranes, and decreasing neuronal excitability [63]. Carbamazepine, gabapentin, valproic acid, lamotrigine, valproic acid, and phenytoin have been used [47]. In addition to having the potential for cognitive (eg, sedation, confusion) and motor (eg, ataxia, dizziness) side effects, antiepileptic agents have the potential for pharmacodynamic drug interactions between other agents with similar side effects (eg, sedation with opioids and antiepileptics) or pharmacokinetic interactions because some are inducers, inhibitors, or substrates of the hepatic CYP 450 system. Doses of antiepileptics may need to be reduced among patients with reduced hepatic or renal function (eg, gabapentin) to reduce the risk of accumulation and side effects. Although doses should be increased gradually to reduce the risk of side effects, all agents should be tried with dose escalation for several weeks before declaring treatment failure with particular agents. Idiosyncratic side effects should be taken into consideration when choosing antiepileptic agents among patients with comorbid conditions (eg, severe rash and Stevens-Johnson syndrome with lamotrigine, nephrolithiasis with topiramate) [68].

Local anesthetics

Anesthetic effects of lidocaine have been explored using intravenous, oral (eg, mexiletine), and transdermal (eg, Lidoderm patches) routes of administration. The proposed mechanism of action is the reduction of spontaneous neuronal discharges in damaged nerves. Although the systemic use of lidocaine has been associated with an increased risk of seizures, dizziness, irritability, tremors, and nervousness [36], Lidoderm patches may be safer and more tolerable in elderly patients with peripheral neuropathies. Lidocaine (5%) patches are available for treatment of allodynia and postherpetic neuralgia [47].

Capsaicin

Capsaicin is believed to work by depleting substance P. Substance P facilitates the transmission of pain information from the peripheral nervous system to the central nervous system. Topical capsaicin has been useful for treating neuralgia, neuropathy, and arthritis [47]. However, it is messy, requires several applications per day, requires several weeks before noticeable improvements occur, and may cause localized burning sensations. Therefore, capsaicin may be cumbersome to use among patients with limited hand dexterity or who live alone [36,62].

Skeletal muscle relaxants

Baclofen is a GABA-B analog commonly used in the treatment of spasticity. It has been reported to have a role in the management of painful neuropathic conditions such as trigeminal neuralgia. Intrathecal baclofen has also been reported to be of benefit for the treatment of pain [70]. Ataxia, dizziness, confusion, and drowsiness may result in a risk for falls and impaired cognitive function. Abrupt discontinuation may result in seizures and hallucinations. Carisoprodol and its active metabolite meprobamate are no longer routinely recommended skeletal muscle relaxants because of the potential for dependence. Cyclobenzaprine is structurally similar to tricyclic antidepressants and may have similar side effects to other analgesics, including drowsiness, ataxia, confusion, and anticholinergic effects [47].

Noninvasive/nonpharmacologic approaches to pain management

Cognitive/behavior modification

Coping skills, relaxation training, assertiveness training, effective communication, and problem-solving skills have been described as helpful for adults living with chronic pain [71]. There is limited research on this topic in adults with physical disabilities.

Physical therapy

Physical therapy (PT) is an important component of pain management. The combination of exercises to regain mobility, strength, and function, with modalities such as heat, cold, and electrical stimulation, can be effective. Minimal reported side effects are an inherent advantage of the use of PT for elderly and physically disabled patients. These populations are often familiar with the treatment approaches and the potential benefits of the various interventions. Some drawbacks include the often short-lived benefits and transportation difficulties for patients. There have been few studies to assess the effectiveness of modalities for the treatment of painful conditions in adults with disabilities.

Heat therapy

Heat therapy is believed to relieve pain by inducing analgesia and sedation and by increasing local blood flow. These effects help to clear the region of toxins and metabolites [44], decrease muscle spindle sensitivity, and relax muscles that are in spasm. Examples of heat therapy include hot packs, paraffin (conduction), hydrotherapy, fluidotherapy (convection), and ultrasound (conversion). Hydrotherapy can be useful for painful contractures or pain over large body surfaces [44]. Heat is indicated for pain associated with osteoarthritis, muscle spasm, and joint contractures. It is contraindicated in the acute phase of an inflammatory condition, insensate skin, malignancy, pregnant uterus, regions of poor arterial circulation, or direct application over a pacemaker [72].

Cold therapy

Cold therapy has been reported to increase endorphin production and decrease local blood flow, to decrease muscle spindle firing rate, and to have a numbing effect on sensory nerve fibers [44,72]. Examples of cold therapy include cold packs (conduction) and fluoromethane spray (conversion). It can be useful in acute inflammatory conditions, osteoarthritic pain, and muscle spasm. Contraindications include Raynaud disease/phenomenon, cold insensitivity, ischemia, and cryoglobulinemia [72].

The use of TENS is based on the gate control theory of pain. The electrical stimulation of large nerve fibers blocks the gate opened by the input from painful smaller nerve fibers, thereby reducing the pain. Low-frequency TENS has been associated with the production of endorphins and enkephalins. The indications for TENS includes pain associated with osteoarthritis, rheumatoid arthritis, diabetic neuropathy, myofascial pain, phantom limb pain, adhesive capsulitis, and post herpetic neuralgia. Its role in the management of central pain and psychogenic pain has been disputed [73]. Contraindications include application of the TENS electrodes near the carotid sinus or epiglottis or using it in patients with arrhythmias, pacemakers, or pregnant women [72].

Exercise

Exercise is an integral part of pain management. Range-of-motion exercises can help to regain lost motion in the spine and limbs due to painful conditions. Strengthening exercises can help to regain strength lost due to the secondary deconditioning effects of chronic pain. Endurance training exercises can help to improve the stamina necessary for everyday activities. Passive therapy (eg, modalities, passive range of motion, and massage) is beneficial for acutely painful conditions. Active therapy (active range of motion, progressive resistive exercises, and endurance training) are integral parts of chronic pain programs. It is believed that exercise and modalities should be used together for the effective management of pain.

Orthotics

Orthotics are commonly used in the care of adults with various disabilities. By immobilizing, supporting, or restricting the motion of a body part, pain can be decreased. However, there are several disadvantages that may limit patient compliance. They are often difficult to put on or take off. They can irritate the skin or damage clothing and, depending on the body region immobilized, can increase energy consumption or decrease respiratory function. Their use may also be limited by their often uncosmetic appearance.

Complimentary approaches

Krauss et al [74] surveyed adults with disabilities regarding their use of alternative therapies. Fifty-seven percent of adults with disabilities were found to use alternative therapies. The most common reasons were pain management, anxiety, insomnia, headache, and depression. Of patients with SCI responding to a survey, 40.3% reported using at least one complementary medicine technique to manage chronic pain. The most common reason cited was dissatisfaction with standard interventions. Acupuncture, massage, chiropractic care, and herbs were the most frequently used interventions. Acupuncture was the least preferred, and massage was most preferred [75].

There is a paucity of well-designed controlled studies to evaluate the benefit of complimentary approaches for the treatment of pain in adults with disabilities. A discussion of the commonly available therapies is beyond the scope of this article; the reader is referred elsewhere [76]. Because acupuncture and massage are commonly used complimentary interventions, they are briefly discussed them here.

Acupuncture. Acupuncture is a discipline of oriental medicine that is based on the premise that a patient's illness is the result of an internal homeostatic imbalance that can be corrected by the placement and manipulation of needles in appropriately selected acupuncture points. There have been few well-designed studies to assess its efficacy in adults with disabilities. Nayak [75,77] reported on 25 patients with SCI who received 15 acupuncture treatments after a baseline 7.5-week period without acupuncture. Forty-six percent of the participants had an improvement in pain intensity scores. Acupuncture has been associated with an acute elevation of blood pressure; therefore; it is advisable to monitor for autonomic dysreflexia during treatments [78]. Dyson-Hudson [79] compared the effectiveness of acupuncture and Trager therapy for chronic shoulder pain in wheelchair users in a randomized study. Although both treatments were considered effective at 1 month postintervention, the group that received the Trager therapy seemed to have more sustained results [79].

Massage. Massage has been defined as "the systematic, mechanical stimulation of the soft tissues of the body by means of rhythmically applied pressure and stretching for therapeutic purposes" [80]. It has been used for thousands of years and has recently seen a resurgence in interest due to the interest of clinicians and patients in alternative medicine. There are several techniques commonly used, including the Swedish technique, which uses different strokes (effleurage, pétrissage, tapotement, vibration, and friction) applied to muscles. Massage has been reported to work by increasing local blood flow, serve as a counterirritant to painful stimuli, and induce relaxation in muscles. Indications include various musculoskeletal complaints (eg, low back pain), juvenile rheumatoid arthritis, tendinitis, tension headaches, and post-op pain. Contraindications include skin infections (cellulitis, abscess), open wounds, cancer, and varicose veins. Adverse effects include localized bruising and swelling. Massage has not been studied for the pain relief in adults with disabilities, although it is commonly used by them [74]. Massage therapy may be of substantial benefit for the management of pain in disabled adults given its limited number of adverse effects and wide acceptance among patients as a therapeutic modality. Caution should be used when massaging over insensate skin because the patient may not be able to feel excessive pressure, and tissue injury may occur. Proper positioning of the patient during the massage is essential. Contracted joints should also be massaged with caution.

Interventional options

Invasive modalities

There are two main advantages of invasive modalities in the treatment of pain. First, they can be helpful in localizing the source of the pain (eg, local nerve block). Second, they can reduce or eliminate the need for systemic medications and their potential side effects and therefore can be useful in the treatment of pain in fragile populations [81]. Little information has been published on the role of many interventional techniques in the management of pain in elderly and physically disabled patients. This section reviews some of the known risks and benefits of some of these procedures.

Intra-articular injections

Intra-articular steroids, morphine, and hyaluronan have been used and studied in patients with painful knee osteoarthritis [82–92]. Nonarthroscopic joint lavage and intra-articular steroids were noted to decrease pain but not improve function. A series of four intra-articular steroid injections improved range of motion and decreased pain when compared with placebo [83]. The benefit was less evident after 2 years, even with continued injections every 3 months [83]. Intra-articular morphine for knee osteoarthritis has been reported to lead to significant pain relief that lasted for at least 1 week [84].

Hyaluronic acid is a long polysaccharide chain that represents one of the main components of synovial fluid. It contributes to the viscosity and elasticity of synovial fluid. The molecular weight and concentration of hyaluronic acid is decreased in osteoarthritic joints. There have been several studies done to evaluate intra-articular joint injections with hyaluronic acid. Studies of hylan GF-20, also known as Synvisc, have shown favorable results. Placebo-controlled trials have demonstrated the superior efficacy of hylan GF-20 to placebo. A dosage schedule of three injections at weekly intervals was shown to be significantly better than injections twice a week, 2 weeks apart [92]. Evanich et al [85] discovered that intra-articular hylan GF-20 was most effective in the older patient population with mild radiographic disease. A series of 750-kD hyaluronan injections, known as Hyalgan, has shown to be effective in the treatment of knee osteoarthritis with symptomatic benefit lasting for about 6 months [86–89]. Intra-articular hyaluronan may pose less risk than NSAIDs with respect to the GI system [87]. However, lack of efficacy of 750-kD hyaluronan has been shown in the treatment of knee osteoarthritis [90]. The medical literature is not in agreement on the efficacy of intra-articular hyaluronic acid for knee osteoarthritis. Ultrasound guided intra-articular injections of hyaluronic acid in osteoarthritic hips have been studied with positive results [91].

Many studies of intra-articular injections of hyaluronic acid have reported adverse effects, the most common being local and transient pain or swelling [85–87,90,93]. Others adverse effects that have been reported include acute arthritis, inflammatory flares of synovitis, acute chondrocalcinosis, pseudogout, and gout [94–98]. These were acute and resolved. Patients and physicians must be aware of these complications before intra-articular injections are used. There have been no reported long-term adverse effects.

Injections for painful shoulder

Injections for painful shoulder in adults with disabilities are commonly used by physicians [99]; however, there have been few studies on their effectiveness in adults with disabilities. Yelnick et al [100] reported on three stroke patients who had a reduction of shoulder pain after injection of the subscapularis muscle with botulinum toxin a. A multicenter randomized trial that compared three triamcinolone acetonide injections versus normal saline (placebo) in 37 patients with post-stroke hemiplegic pain failed to show a statistically significant advantage for the triamcinolone group. A trend toward significance was noted [101]. A similar benefit was reported in another small study [102].

Although few studies have assessed the role of shoulder corticosteroid injections in the elderly population in general, there is some evidence attesting to their benefit [103,104]. The proper placement of the needle has been associated with a better outcome [105].

Botulinum toxin injections

Botulinum toxin injections have been used in the treatment of chronic myofascial pain syndromes. A description of their role is beyond the scope of this article. The reader is referred elsewhere for information [13,106–108].

Epidural steroid injection

Low back pain with or without radicular pain is a frequent complaint among the elderly patients and adults with physical disabilities. Common causes include herniated nucleus pulposus disease, osteoarthritis of the spine, spinal stenosis, and spondylolisthesis. Epidural steroid injections (ESIs) have been used in the management of spinal pain.

The use of lumbar epidural steroid injections for the management of pain from lumbar spinal stenosis or herniated disks is controversial and not completely supported by the medical literature. Their role in the care of adults with physical disabilities is unknown. Differing diagnoses, injection types, injection techniques, and varying lengths of follow-up times make it difficult to draw conclusions about their efficacy. Some studies have revealed positive outcomes [109,110], especially for temporary relief [111,112], whereas other studies have not proven long-term efficacy [111,113].

ESIs are generally known to be safe, but complications have been reported for fluoroscopically guided and nonfluoroscopically guided injections. The most common complications reported are transient headache (3.1%) and discomfort at the injection site (2.4%), both of which resolve within 24 hours. Less common complications are increases in leg pain, facial flushing, rashes, transient subjective leg weakness, dizziness, a transient increase in blood glucose, and an increase in blood pressure requiring medication. The overall incidence of minor complications per injection has been reported to be 9.6% [114]. More significant complications from nonfluoroscopically guided ESIs include spinal epidural abscess, iatrogenic Cushing syndrome, suppression of the pituitary-adrenal axis, steroid myopathy, chemical meningitis, acute retinal necrosis, and retinal hemorrhage [115–121].

Dural puncture is the most common technical complication in ESIs, with a 5% incidence [122]. Other reported technical complications include the injection of a local anesthetic into the subdural space causing hypotension, sensory loss in the lower trunk and legs that resolved, and a post-epidural headache from injection of air into the subdural space [123,124].

Few studies have examined the role of intrathecal opioids in the management of refractory pain in physically disabled patients. Nevertheless, there are several advantages to their use when other measures have been exhausted: (1) A lower dose of medication is needed, (2) there are fewer systemic side effects, and (3) medications are administered closer to their potential site of action.

Complications associated with the use of intrathecal narcotics, in addition to those described for opioids in general, include puncture headache, migration of the catheter from the intrathecal space, obstruction of the catheter, and cerebrospinal fluid (CSF) tracking along the catheter with seroma formation.

Spinal cord stimulation has been used to help alleviate chronic intractable pain. It is usually used as a last resort. Its role in the treatment of pain in adults with disabilities is unknown. Few studies on spinal cord stimulation incorporate the older disabled population. Some studies do not list the ages of the participants [125–129]. When age has been reported, it seems that spinal cord stimulation has been studied mostly in patients younger than 65 years of age. It is therefore difficult to draw conclusions on the safety and efficacy of spinal cord stimulation in elderly and physically disabled persons.

Spinal cord stimulation has been shown to be effective for a variety of pain syndromes. Successes have been shown in phantom limb pain [130,131], peripheral nerve pain [130], chronic sciatica [131], residual limb pain [126,131], pain from peripheral vascular disease [129,131], pain from diabetic amyotrophy [126], and failed back surgery syndrome [125,128,132,133]. Some studies have shown phantom limb pain and failed back surgery syndrome to respond poorly [125,127].

Complications from spinal cord stimulation may be technical or biologic. Most complications seem to be technical. Those reported include electrode dislocation and breakage, faulty receivers or transmitters, broken or displaced electrodes, connector failure, lead migration or breakage, generator failure, and battery depletion [128,132,134–138]. Biologic complications include wound infections [125,127,128,130,132,136–138] (which could be dangerous in a geriatric disabled population), CSF leaks [130], transient or prolonged leg weakness [127,130], pulmonary embolus [127,137], and discomfort at the implantation site [125,137].

Spinal cord stimulation should be used with caution and in a select group when implanted in the older population until more studies in this age group are available.

Efficacy of treatments in various populations with disabilities

Although pain is common in adults with physical disabilities and there are many reported interventions, there is a paucity of well-designed studies to evaluate their efficacy. Much of the literature is limited by study design or by the small number of patients. This section provides a brief review of the efficacy of treatments for various disabilities.

Amputees

Phantom pain and residual limb pain are common sources of pain for amputees. Although there have been numerous treatments described for phantom pain, few have been reported to be effective [139–141]. In one study, 68 treatments were identified, and 50 were in current use [141]. Among the most effective treatments reported were nerve blocks, relaxation training, acupuncture, biofeedback, stump conditioning, ultrasound, prosthetic revision, and multidisciplinary pain centers. Among the least effective were most surgical procedures and TENS [140]. Case reports have reported good response from the use of chlorpromazine [142] and electroconvulsive therapy [143]. There have been few controlled placebo studies on interventions for the treatment of phantom pain. One study reported some potential benefit from morphine [144], whereas another reported no benefit from amitriptyline [145]. The role of pre-operative epidural blockade was studied for the prevention of postoperative phantom and residual limb pain in several studies, with mixed results reported [146–149]. Residual limb pain has also been treated with capsaicin [150].

Parkinson disease

A case report described the successful use of Tramadol for pain in PD [151]. Severe osteoarthritic joint pain has been successfully treated with total hip arthroplasty in a multi-center study [152]. Acupuncture was reported to provide pain relief, improve sleep, and decrease anxiety in a small pilot study [153]. In some patients, adjustment of doses of antiparkinsonian agents may relieve pain [154].

Traumatic brain injury

Two small controlled studies for the treatment of post-traumatic headaches found no significant long-lasting benefit from amitriptyline [155] or manual therapy [156]. Symptoms of post-traumatic stress disorder (PTSD) were noted in adults with TBI, implying that coping mechanisms to reduce PTSD might help with the pain [19].

Stroke

Central pain

Patients often describe inadequate pain relief for this stroke or no treatment at all [24]. Several potentially useful treatments that have been described for central pain include the use of amitriptyline, carbamazepine

[29,164], lamotrigine [157], IV lidocaine [158], mexiletine [159], ketamine [165], acupuncture [160], motor cortex stimulation [161], and TENS [162]. Naloxone was no better than placebo in a double-blind study [163].

Nociceptive pain

Shoulder pain is a common source of pain for stroke survivors. In one study, less than 50% of participants got relief from a subacromial injection [166].

Cerebral palsy

Exercise and heat have been reported to help relieve pain [167] in patients with cerebral palsy. Cognitive strategies are more commonly used than physical strategies [1]. The use of prayer has also been described as a helpful coping strategy [168].

Polio

There have been few well-designed studies for the treatment of pain in polio survivors. One randomized study found benefit from a home exercise program with lifestyle modifications for overuse syndromes in patients with shoulder pain [169]. Total knee arthroplasty, dynamic water exercises, and appropriate orthotics have been described as beneficial for the management of pain in this population [170–172].

Spinal cord injury

The management of musculoskeletal pain is covered elsewhere in this issue. This section addresses the evidence for efficacy of various treatments for neuropathic pain in SCI. Although pain is a major complaint in adults with SCI, patients have reported dissatisfaction with their pain management [173]. Large-scale controlled trials are needed to evaluate pharmacologic and nonpharmacologic treatments. Clinical trials assessing the efficacy of medications are limited by small study samples. Most available evidence includes case reports and uncontrolled trials.

Several anticonvulsant medications have been studied for efficacy in treating SCI neuropathic pain. Gabapentin has a low side-effect profile and does not require frequent monitoring of serum levels. Studies that have examined the effects of gabapentin in SCI neuropathic pain have reported a benefit [174,175]. Other anti-epileptic medications that have been investigated with some potential benefit include valproate [176] and lamotrigine [177]. Medications found not to be beneficial include tricyclic antidepressants [178] and mexiletine [179]. The combination of amitriptyline and carbamazepine was reported to be helpful in a case report [180].

There is minimal evidence to support use of opioids in the treatment of neuropathic SCI pain. Nevertheless, in a patient survey, opioids were reported as the "most helpful" medications [181]. Siddall et al [182] found that the intrathecal combination of morphine and clonidine produced significantly greater relief of neuropathic SCI pain than saline placebo [182]. Pain in MS and polio is covered elsewhere in this issue.

Future areas of research

There is a need for well-designed, randomized studies with adequate patient samples to assess the efficacy of various treatment interventions for the management of pain in adults with physical disabilities. Interventional procedures, pharmacologic agents, and complimentary approaches could benefit from such studies.

Summary

Adults aging with physical disabilities experience a variety of pain disorders that affect their functionality and QOL. It is important that clinicians caring for this population be knowledgeable about this common symptom and be able to perform a thorough history and physical examination. In addition, it is imperative to have a good working knowledge of the strengths and limitations of the treatments available.

Acknowledgments

The authors thank Eliane Zuller-Cristian and Alexis Renta, MD, for their insightful comments and critique.

References

[1] Ehde DM, Jensen MP, Engel JM, Turner JA, Hoffman AJ, Cardenas DD. Chronic pain secondary to disability. Clin J Pain 2003;19:3–17.
[2] Van der Schans CP, Geertzen JH, Schoppen T, Dijkstra PU. Phantom pain and health related quality of life in lower limb amputees. J Pain Symptom Manage 2002;24:429–36.
[3] Kooijman CM, Dijkstra PU, Geertzen JHB. Phantom pain and phantom sensations in upper limb amputees: an epidemiological study. Pain 2000;87:33–41.
[4] Whyte AS, Carroll LJ. A preliminary examination of the relationship between employment, pain and disability in an amputee population. Disabil Rehabil 2002;24:462–70.
[5] Lindesay JE. Multiple pain complaints in amputees. J Royal Soc Med 1985;78:452–5.
[6] Hill A, Niven CA, Knussen C. The role of coping in adjustment to phantom limb pain. Pain 1995;62:79–86.
[7] Jensen MP, Ehde DM, Hoffman AJ, Patterson DR, Czerniecki JM, Robinson LR. Cognitions, coping and family environment predict adjustment. Pain 2002;95:133–42.
[8] Jensen TS, Krebs B, Nielsen J, Rasmussen P. Immediate and longterm phantom limb pain in amputees: incidence, clinical characteristics and relationships to pre-amputation limb pain. Pain 1985;21:267–78.

[9] Mortimer CM, Steedman WM, McMillan IR, Martin DJ, Ravey J. Patient information on phantom limb pain: a focus group study of patient experiences, perceptions and opinions. Health Educ Res 2002;17:291–304.

[10] Smith D, Ehde DM, Legno MW. Phantom limb, residual limb and back pain after lower extremity amputations. Clin Orthop 1999;361:29–38.

[11] Ehde DM, Smith DG, Czerniecki JM, Campbell KM, Malchow DM, Robinson LR. Back pain as a secondary disability in persons with lower limb amputations. Arch Phys Med Rehabil 2001;82:731–4.

[12] Burke MJ, Roman V, Wright W. Bone and joint changes in lower limb amputees. Ann Rheum Dis 1978;37:252–4.

[13] Raj PP. Botulinum toxin therapy in pain management. Anesthesiol Clin North Am 2003; 21:715–31.

[14] Crawford JR, Coleman N. Total knee replacement in a below knee amputation. J Arthroplasty 2003;18:662–5.

[15] Kolle WC. Sensory symptoms in Parkinson's disease. Neurology 1984;34:957–9.

[16] Snider SR. Primary sensory symptoms in Parkinsonism. Neurology 1976;26:423–9.

[17] Lorentz IT. A survey of headache in Parkinson's disease. Cephalgia 1989;9:83–6.

[18] Lahz S, Bryant RA. Incidence of chronic pain following traumatic brain injury. Arch Phys Med Rehabil 1996;77:889–91.

[19] Bryant RA, Marosszesky JE, Crooks J, Baguley IJ, Gurka JA. Interaction of post-traumatic stress disorder and chronic pain following traumatic brain injury. J Head Trauma Rehab 1999;14:588–94.

[20] Uomoto J, Esselman P. Traumatic brain injury and chronic pain: differential types and rates by head injury severity. Arch Phys Med Rehabil 1993;74:61–4.

[21] Andary MT, Crewe N, Ganzel S, Haines-Pepi C, Kulkarni MR, Stanton DF. Traumatic brain injury and chronic pain syndrome: a case comparison study. Clin J Pain 1997;13: 244–50.

[22] Anderson J, Kaplan M. Brain injury obscured by chronic pain: a preliminary report. Arch Phys Med Rehabil 1990;71:703–8.

[23] Smith-Seemiller L, Fow NR, Kant R, Franzen MD. Presence of post-concussion syndrome symptoms in patients with chronic pain vs. mild traumatic brain injury. Brain Injury 2003; 17:199–206.

[24] Wider M, Samuelsson L, Karlsson-Tivenius S. Long-term pain conditions after a stroke. J Rehabil Med 2002;34:165–70.

[25] Andersen G, Vestergaard K, Ingeman NM, Jensen TS. Incidence of central post-stroke pain. Pain 1995;61:187–93.

[26] Vestergaard K, Nielsen J, Andersen G, Ingeman-Nilesen M, Arendt-Nielsen L, Jensen TS. Sensory abnormalities in consecutive unselected patients with central post-stroke pain. Pain 1995;61:177–86.

[27] Boivie J, Leijon G, Johansson I. Central post stroke pain: a study of the mechanisms through analyses of the sensory abnormalities. Pain 1989;37:173–85.

[28] Holmgren H, Leijon G, Boivie J, Johansson I, Ilievska L. Central post stroke pain: somatosensory evoked potential in relation to location of the lesion and sensory signs. Pain 1990;40:43–52.

[29] Bowster D. The management of central post-stroke pain. Postgrad Med J 1995;71:598–604.

[30] Kumral E, Kocaer T, Ertubey N, Kumral K. Thalamic hemorrhage: a prospective study of one hundred patients. Stroke 1995;26:964–70.

[31] Leijon G, Boivie J, Johansson I. Central post stroke pain: neurological symptoms and pain characteristics. Pain 1989;36:13–25.

[32] Bowsher D. Central pain: clinical and physiological characteristics. J Neurol Neurosurg Psychiatry 1996;61:62–9.

[33] Moulin DE, Hagen N, Feasby TE, Amireh R, Hahn A. Pain in Gullian Barre Syndrome. Neurology 1997;48:328–31.

[34] Bushby KM, Pollitt C, Johnson MA, Rogers MT, Chinnery PF. Muscle pain as a prominent feature of fascioscapulohumeral muscular dystrophy (FSHD): four illustrative case reports. Neuromuscul Disord 1998;8:574–9.
[35] Tumer N, Scarpace PJ, Lowenthal DT. Geriatric pharmacology: basic and clinical considerations. Annu Rev Pharmacol Toxicol 1992;32:271–302.
[36] Davis MP, Srivastava M. Demographics, assessment and management of pain in the elderly. Drugs Aging 2003;20:23–57.
[37] Clinical practice guidelines: the management of chronic pain in older persons. JAGS 1998; 46:635–51.
[38] Stein WM. Pain in the nursing home. Clin Geriatr Med 2001;17:575–93.
[39] Helme RD, Gibson SJ. The epidemiology of pain in elderly people. Clin Geriatr Med 2001; 17:417–31.
[40] Weiner DK, Hanlon JT. Pain in nursing home residents: management strategies. Drugs Aging 2001;18:13–29.
[41] Herr KA, Garand L. Assessment and measurement of pain in older adults. Clin Geriatr Med 2001;17:457–77.
[42] Lansbury G. Chronic pain management: a qualitative study of elderly people's preferred coping strategies and barriers to management. Disabil Rehabil 2000;22:2–14.
[43] Sager DS, Bennett RM. Individualizing the risk/benefit ratio of NSAID's in older adults. Geriatrics 1992;47:24–31.
[44] Gloth MJ, Matesi AM. Physical therapy and exercise in pain management. Clin Geriatr Med 2001;17:525–35.
[45] Micklewright R, Laine S, Linley W, McQuade C, Thompson F, Maskrey N. NSAIDs, gastroprotection and cyclo-oxygenase-II-selective inhibitors. Aliment Pharmacol Ther 2003;17:321–32.
[46] Graham DY, Agrawal NM, Campbell DR, Haber MM, Collis C, Lukasik NL, et al. Ulcer prevention in long-term users of non-steroidal anti-inflammatory drugs: results of a double-blind, randomized, multicenter, active- and placebo-controlled study of misoprostol vs. lansoprazole. Arch Intern Med 2002;162:169–75.
[47] Barkin RL, Barkin D. Pharmacologic management of acute and chronic pain: focus on drug interactions and patient-specific pharmacotherapeutic selection. South Med J 2001;94: 756–812.
[48] McCarberg BH, Herr KA. Osteoarthritis: how to manage pain and improve pain function. Geriatrics 2001;56:14–24.
[49] Piovesan EJ, Zukerman E, Kowacs PA, Werneck LC. COX-2 inhibitor for the treatment of idiopathic stabbing headache secondary to cerebrovascular diseases. Cephalgia 2002;22: 197–200.
[50] Bombardier C, Laine L, Recin A, Shapiro D, Burgos-Vargas R, Davis B, et al. Comparison of upper gastrointestinal toxicity of rofecoxib and naproxen in patients with rheumatoid arthritis. N Engl J Med 2000;343:1520–8.
[51] Silverstein FE, Faich G, Goldstein JL, Simon LS, Pincus T, Whelton A, et al. Gastrointestinal toxicity with celcoxib vs. nonsteroidal anti-inflammatory drugs for osteoarthritis and rheumatoid arthritis: the CLASS study-a randomized controlled trial. JAMA 2000;284:1247–55.
[52] Goldstein JL, Eisen G, Bensen W. SUCCESS in osteoarthritis (OA) trial: celecoxib significantly reduces the risk of upper gastrointestinal (UGI) hospitalizations compared to diclofenac and naproxen in 13,274 randomized patients with OA. Presented at the European League Against Rheumatism. Prague, Czech Republic, June 13–16, 2001.
[53] Geba GP, Lisse JR, Polis AB. Gastrointestinal tolerability in primary care patients treated with naproxen or rofecoxib for osteoarthritis (OA): the ADVANTAGE trial. Presented at the European League Against Rheumatism. Prague, Czech Republic, June 13–16, 2001.
[54] Scheiman JM. Outcome studies of the gastrointestinal safety of cyclooxygenase-2 inhibitors. Cleve Clin J Med 2002;69(Suppl 1):SI40–6.

[55] Stollberger C, Finsterer J. Side effects of conventional non-steroidal anti-inflammatory drugs and celecoxib: more similarities than differences. South Med J 2004;97:209.

[56] Crawford AS, White JG. Celecoxib-induced upper gastrointestinal hemorrhage and ulceration. South Med J 2002;95:1444–6.

[57] Chan FK, Hung LC, Suen BY, Wu JC, Lee KC, Leung VK, et al. Celecoxib versus diclofenac and omeprazole in reducing the risk of recurrent ulcer bleeding in patients with arthritis. N Engl J Med 2002;347:2104–10.

[58] Fine P. Opioid analgesic drugs in older people. Clin Geriatr Med 2001;17:479–85.

[59] Holdcroft A, Power I. Management of pain. BMJ 2003;326:635–9.

[60] Portenoy RK. Chronic opioid therapy in nonmalignant pain. J Pain Symptom Manage 1990;5:S46–62.

[61] Przewlocki R, Przewlocka B. Opioids in chronic pain. Eur J Pharmacol 2001;429:79–91.

[62] Lipman AG. Analgesic drugs for neuropathic and sympathetically maintained pain. Clin Geriatr Med 1996;12:501–15.

[63] Ahmad M, Goucke CG. Management strategies for the treatment of neuropathic pain in the elderly. Drugs Aging 2002;19:929–45.

[64] Jick H, Derby LE, Vasilakis C, Fife D. The risk of seizures associated with tramadol. Pharmacotherapy 1998;18:607–77.

[65] Gardner JS, Blough D, Drinkard CR, Shatin D, Anderson G, Graham D, et al. Tramadol and seizures: a surveillance study in a managed care population. Pharmacotherapy 2000;20: 1423–31.

[66] Lange-Asschenfeldt C, Weigmann H, Hienmke C, Mann K. Serotonin syndrome as a result of fluoxetine in a patient with tramadol abuse: plasma level-correlated symptomatology. J Clin Psychopharmacol 2002;22:440–1.

[67] Ripple MG, Pestaner JP, Levine BS, Smialek JE. Lethal combination of tramadol and multiple drugs affecting serotonin. Am J Forensic Med Pathol 2000;21:370–4.

[68] Dworkin RH, Backonja M, Rowbotham MC, Allen RR, Argoff CR, Bennett GJ, et al. Advance in neuropathic pain: diagnosis, mechanisms, and treatment recommendations. Arch Neurol 2003;60:1524–34.

[69] Dallocchio C, Buffa C, Mazzarello P, Chiroli S. Gabapentin vs. amitriptyline in painful diabetic neuropathy: an open-label pilot study. J Pain Symptom Manage 2000; 20:280–5.

[70] Warms CA, Turner JA, Marshall HM, Cardenas DD. Treatments for chronic pain associated with spinal cord injuries: many are tried, few are helpful. Clin J Pain 2002;18: 154–63.

[71] Kerns RD, Otis JD, Marcus KS. Cognitive-behavioral therapy for chronic pain in the elderly. Clin Geriatr Med 2001;17:503–23.

[72] Nguyen DMT. The role of physical medicine and rehabilitation in pain management. Clin Geriatr Med 2001;17:517–29.

[73] Thorsteinsson G. Chronic pain: use of TENS in the elderly. Geriatrics 1987;42:75–82.

[74] Krauss HH, Godfrey C, Kirk J, Eisenberg DM. Alternative health care: its use by individuals with physical disabilities. Arch Phys Med Rehabil 1998;79:1440–7.

[75] Nayak S, Matheis RJ, Agostinelli S, Shifleft SC. The use of complementary and alternative therapies for chronic pain following spinal cord injury: a pilot survey. J Spinal Cord Med 2001;24:54–62.

[76] Wainapel SF, Fast A, editors. Alternative medicine and rehabilitation: a guide for practitioners. New York: Demos Medical Publishing; 2003.

[77] Nayak S, Shiflett SC, Schenberger NE, Agostinelli SA, Kirshblum S, Averill A, et al. Is acupuncture effective in the treatment of chronic pain following spinal cord injury? Arch Phys Med Rehabil 2001;82:1578–86.

[78] Averill A, Cotter AC, Nayak S, Matheis RJ, Shiflett SC. Blood pressure response to acupuncture in a population at risk for autonomic dysreflexia. Arch Phys Med Rehabil 2000;81:1494–7.

[79] Dyson-Hudson T, Shiflett SC, Kirschblum S, Bowen JE, et al. Acupuncture and Trager in the treatment of shoulder pain in spinal cord injury. Arch Phys Med Rehabil 2001;82: 1038–46.

[80] Tan JC. Massage as a form of complementary and alternative healing modality for physical manipulation. In: Wainapel SF, Fast A, editors. Alternative medicine and rehabilitation: a guide for practitioners. New York: Demos Medical Publishing; 2003. p. 77–97.

[81] Prager JP. Invasive modalities for the diagnosis and treatment of pain in the elderly. Clin Geriatr Med 1996;12:549–61.

[82] Ravaud P, Moulinier L, Giraudeau B, Ayral X, Guerin C, Noel E, et al. Effects of joint lavage and steroid injection in patients with osteoarthritis of the knee: results of a multi center, randomized, controlled trial. Arthritis Rheum 1999;42:475–82.

[83] Raynauld JP, Buckland-Wright C, Ward R, Choquette D, Haraoui B, Martel-Pelletier J, et al. Safety and efficacy of long-term intraarticular steroid injections in osteoarthritis of the knee: a randomized, double-blind, placebo-controlled trial. Arthritis Rheum 2003;48: 370–7.

[84] Likar R, Schafer M, Paulak F, Sittl R, Pipam W, Schalk H, et al. Intraarticular morphine analgesia in chronic pain patients with osteoarthritis. Anesth Analg 1997;84: 1313–7.

[85] Evanich JD, Evanich CJ, Wright MB, Rydlewicz JA. Efficacy of intraarticular hyaluronic acid injections in knee osteoarthritis. Clin Orthop 2001;390:173–81.

[86] Huskisson EC, Donnelly S. Hyaluronic acid in the treatment of osteoarthritis of the knee. Rheumatology (Oxford) 1999;38:602–7.

[87] Altman RD, Moskowitz R. Intraarticular sodium hyaluronate (Hyalgan) in the treatment of patients with osteoarthritis of the knee: a randomized clinical trial. Hyalagan Study Group. J Rheumatol 1998;25:2203–12.

[88] Miltner O, Schneider U, Siebert CH, Niedhart C, Niethard FU. Efficacy of intraarticular hyaluronic acid in patients with osteoarthritis: a prospective clinical trial. Osteoarthritis Cartilage 2002;10:680–6.

[89] Lohmander LS, Dalen N, Englund G, Hamalainen M, Jensen EM, Karlsson K, et al. Intra-articular hyaluronan injections in the treatment of osteoarthritis of the knee: a randomized, double blind, placebo controlled multicentre trial. Hyaluronan Multicentre Trial Group. Ann Rheum Dis 1996;55:424–31.

[90] Henderson EB, Smith EC, Pegley F, Blake DR. Intra-articular injections of 750 kD hyaluronan in the treatment of osteoarthritis: a randomized single centre double-blind placebo-controlled trial of 91 patients demonstrating lack of efficacy. Ann Rheum Dis 1994; 53:529–34.

[91] Migliore A, Martin LS, Alimonti A, Valente C, Tormenta S. Efficacy and safety of viscosupplementation by ultrasound-guided intra-articular injection in osteoarthritis of the hip. Osteoarthritis Cartilage 2003;11:305–6.

[92] Yacyshyn EA, Matteson EL. Gout after intraarticular injection of hylan GF-20 (Synvisc). J Rheumatol 1999;26:2717.

[93] Adams ME. An analysis of clinical studies of the use of crosslinked hyaluronan, hylan, in the treatment of osteoarthritis. J Rheumatol (Suppl) 1993;39:16–8.

[94] Maillefert JF, Hirschhorn P, Pascaud F, Piroth C, Tavernier C. Acute attack of chondrocalcinosis after an intraarticular injection of hyaluronan. Rev Rhum Eng Ed 1997;64:593–4.

[95] Puttick MP, Wade JP, Chalmers A, Connell DG, Rangno KK. Acute local reactions after intraarticular hylan for osteoarthritis of the knee. J Rheumatol 1995;22:1311–4.

[96] Luzar MJ, Altawil B. Pseudogout following intraarticular injection of sodium hyaluronate. Arthritis Rheum 1998;41:939–40.

[97] Pullman-Mooar S, Mooar P, Sieck M, Clauburne G, Schumacher HR. Are there distinctive inflammatory flares of synovitis after hyalan FG intra-articular injections [abstract]? Arthritis Rheum 1999;42(Suppl):S55.

[98] Bernardeau C, Bucki B, Liote F. Acute arthritis after intra-articular hyaluronate injection: onset of effusions without crystal. Ann Rheum Dis 2001;60:518–20.

[99] Snels IA, Beckerman H, Lankhorst GJ, Bouter LM. Treatment of hemiplegic shoulder pain in the Netherlands: results of a national survey. Clin Rehabil 2000;14:20–7.

[100] Yelnick AP, Colle FM, Bonan IV. Treatment of pain and limited movement of the shoulder in hemiplegic patients with botulinum toxin a in the subscapular muscle. Eur Neurol 2003; 50:91–3.

[101] Snels IA, Beckerman H, Twisk JW, Dekker JH, DeKoning P, Koppe PA. Effect of triamcinolone acetonide injections on hemiplegic shoulder pain: a randomized clinical trial. Stroke 2000;31:2396–401.

[102] Dekker JH, Wagenaar RC, Lankhorst GJ, deJong BA. The painful hemiplegic shoulder: effects of intra-articular triamcinolone acetonide. Am J Phys Med Rehabil 1997;76:43–8.

[103] Blair B, Rokito A, Cuomo F, Jarolem K, Zuckerman J. Efficacy of injections of corticosteroids for subacromial impingement syndrome. J Bone Joint Surg Am 1996;78A: 1685–9.

[104] Hay EM, Thomas E, Paterson SM, Dziedzic K, Croft PR. A pragmatic randomised controlled trial of local corticosteroid injection and physiotherapy for the treatment of new episodes of unilateral shoulder pain in primary care. Ann Rheum Dis 2003;62:394–9.

[105] Eustace JA, Brophy DP, Gibney RP, Bresnihan B, FitzGerald O. Comparison of the accuracy of steroid placement with clinical outcome in patients with shoulder symptoms. Ann Rheum Dis 1997;56:59–63.

[106] Lan AM. Botulinum toxin type A in chronic pain disorders. Arch Phys Med Rehabil 2003; 84(Suppl):569–73.

[107] DeAndres J, Cerda-Olmedo G, Valia JC, Monsalve V, Lopez-Alarcon MA. The use of botulinum toxin in the treatment of chronic myofascial pain. Clin J Pain 2003;19: 269–75.

[108] Royal MA. Botulinum toxins in pain management. Phys Med Rehabil Clin North Am 2003;14:805–20.

[109] Papagelopoulos PJ, Petrou HG, Triantafyllidis PG, Vlamis JA, Psomas-Pasalis M, Korres DS, et al. Treatment of lumbosacral radicular pain with epidural steroid injections. Orthopedics 2001;24:145–9.

[110] Botwin KP, Gruber RD, Bouchlas CG, Torres-Ramos FM, Sanelli JT, Freeman ED, et al. Fluoroscopically guided lumbar transforaminal epidural steroid injections in degenerative lumbar stenosis: an outcome study. Am J Phys Med Rehabil 2002;81:898–905.

[111] Rosen CD, Kahanovitz N, Bernstein R, Viola K. A retrospective analysis of the efficacy of epidural steroid injections. Clin Orthop 1998;228:270–2.

[112] Cuckler JM, Bernini PA, Wiesel SW, Booth RE, Rothman RH, Pickens GT. The use of epidural steroid in the treatment of radicular pain. J Bone Joint Surg Am 1985;67:63–6.

[113] Fukusaki M, Kobayashi I, Hara T, Sumikawa K. Symptoms of spinal stenosis do not improve after epidural steroid injection. Clin J Pain 1998;14:148–51.

[114] Botwin KP, Gruber RD, Bouchlas CG, Torres-Ramos FM, Freeman TL, Slaten WK. Complications of fluoroscopically guided transforaminal lumbar epidural injections. Arch Phys Med Rehabil 2000;81:1045–50.

[115] Kushner FH, Olson JC. Retinal hemorrhage as a consequence of epidural steroid injection. Arch Ophthalmol 1995;113:310–3.

[116] Browning DJ. Acute retinal necrosis following epidural steroid injections. Am J Ophthalmol 2003;136:192–4.

[117] Gutknecht DR. Chemical meningitis following epidural injections of corticosteroids. Am J Med 1987;82:570.

[118] Boonen S, Van Distel G, Westhovens R, Dequeker J. Steroid myopathy induced by epidural triamcinolone injection. Br J Rheumatol 1995;34:385–6.

[119] Kay J, Findling JW, Raff H. Epidural triamcinolone suppresses the pituitary-adrenal axis in human subjects. Anesth Analg 1994;79:501–5.

[120] Tuel SM, Meythaler JM, Cross LL. Cushing's syndrome from epidural methylpredniso-lone. Pain 1990;40:81–4.

[121] Chan ST, Leung S. Spinal epidural abscess following steroid injection for sciatica. Spine 1989;14:106–8.

[122] National Health and Medical Research Council. Epidural use of steroids in the management of back pain. Canberra, Australia: National Health and Medical Research Council; 1994.

[123] Lehmann LJ, Pallares VS. Subdural injection of a local anesthetic with steroids: complication of epidural anesthesia. South Med J 1995;88:467–9.

[124] Katz JA, Lukin R, Bridenbaugh PO, Gunzenhauser L. Subdural intracranial air: an unusual cause of headache after epidural steroid injection. Anesthesiology 1991;74:615–8.

[125] Wester K. Dorsal column stimulation in pain treatment. Acta Neurol Scand 1987;75:151–5.

[126] Richardson RR, Siqueira EB, Cerullo LJ. Spinal epidural neurostimulation for treatment of acute and chronic intractable pain: initial and long term results. Neurosurgery 1979;5: 344–8.

[127] Devulder J, Vermeulen H, DeColvenaer L, Rolly G, Calliauw L, Caemaert J. Spinal cord stimulation in chronic pain: evaluation of results, complications, and technical consid-erations in sixty-nine patients. Clin J Pain 1991;7:21–8.

[128] Burton CV. Session on spinal cord stimulation: safety and clinical efficacy. Neurosurgery 1977;1:214–5.

[129] Augustinsson LE. Epidural spinal electrical stimulation in peripheral vascular disease. Pace 1987;10:205–6.

[130] Nielson KD, Adams JE, Hosobuchi Y. Experience with dorsal column stimulation for relief of chronic intractable pain: 1968–1973. Surg Neurol 1975;4:148–52.

[131] Vogel HP, Heppner B, Humbs N, Schramm J, Wagner C. Long-term effects of spinal cord stimulation in chronic pain syndromes. J Neurol 1986;233:16–8.

[132] North RB, Ewend MG, Lawton MT, Kidd DH, Piantadosi S. Failed back surgery syndrome: 5-year follow-up after spinal cord stimulator implantation. Neurosurgery 1991; 28:692–9.

[133] Turner JA, Loeser JD, Bell KG. Spinal cord stimulation for chronic low back pain: a systematic literature synthesis. Neurosurgery 1995;37:1088–95.

[134] Urban BJ, Nashold BS. Percutaneous epidural stimulation of the spinal cord for relief of pain. J Neurosurg 1978;48:323–8.

[135] De La Porte C, Van de Kelft E. Spinal cord stimulation in failed back surgery syndrome. Pain 1993;52:55–61.

[136] Koeze TH, Williams AC de C, Reiman S. Spinal cord stimulation and the relief of chronic pain. J Neurol Neurosurg Psychiatry 1987;50:1424–9.

[137] Mittal B, Thomas DGT, Walton P, Calder I. Dorsal column stimulation (DCS) in chronic pain: report of 31 cases. Ann Roy Coll Surg Eng 1987;69:104–9.

[138] Simpson BA. Spinal cord stimulation in 60 cases of intractable pain. J Neurol Neurosurg Psychiatry 1991;54:196–9.

[139] Sherman RA, Sherman CJ, Parker L. Chronic phantom and stump pain among veterans: results of a survey. Pain 1984;18:83–95.

[140] Sherman RA, Sherman CJ, Gall NG. A survey of current phantom limb pain treatment in the United States. Pain 1980;8:85–99.

[141] Sherman RA, Sherman CJ. A comparison of phantom sensations among amputees whose amputation were of civilian and military origins. Pain 1985;21:91–7.

[142] Logan TP. Persistent phantom limb pain: dramatic response to chlorpromazine. South Med J 1983;76:1585.

[143] Rasmussen KG, Rummans TA. Electroconvulsive therapy for phantom limb pain. Pain 2000;85:297–9.

[144] Huse E, Larbig W, Flor H, Birbaumer N. The effect of opioids on phantom limb pain and cortical reorganization. Pain 2001;90:47–55.

[145] Robinson LR, Czerniecki JM, Ehde DM, Edwards WT. Trial of amitriptyline for relief of pain in amputees: results of a randomized control trial. Arch Phys Med Rehabil 2004;85: 1–6.

[146] Lambert AW, Dashfield AK, Cosgrove C, Wilkins DC, Walker AJ, Ashley S. Randomized prospective study comparing pre-operative epidural intra-operative perineural analgesia for the prevention of post-operative stump and phantom limb pain following major amputation. Reg Anesth Pain Med 2001;26:316–21.

[147] Bach S, Noreng MF, Tjellden Nu. Phantom limb pain in amputees during the first twelve months following limb amputation after pre-operative lumbar epidural blockade. Pain 1988;33:297–301.

[148] Nikolajsen L, Ilkjaer S, Christensen JH, Kroner K, Jensen TS. Randomized trial of epidural bupivacaine and morphine in the prevention of stump and phantom pain in lower limb amputation. Lancet 1997;350:1353–7.

[149] Nikolajsen L, Ilkjaer S, Jensen TS. Effect of pre-operative extradural bupivacaine and morphine on stump sensations in lower limb amputees. Br J Anaesth 1998;81:348–54.

[150] Cannon DT, Wu Y. Topical capsaicin as an adjunct analgesic for the treatment of traumatic amputee neurogenic residual limb pain. Arch Phys Med Rehabil 1998;79:591–3.

[151] Stein WM, Read S. Chronic pain in the setting of Parkinson's disease and depression. J Pain Sympt Manage 1997;14:255–8.

[152] Weber M, Cabarela ME, Sim FH, Frassica FJ, Harmsen WS. Total hip replacement in patients with Parkinson's Disease. Int Orthop 2002;26:66–8.

[153] Shulman LM, Wen X, Weiner WJ. Acupuncture therapy for the symptoms of Parkinson's Disease. Mov Disord 2002;17:799–802.

[154] Sage JI. Pain in Parkinson's disease. Curr Treat Options Neurol 2004;6:191–200.

[155] Saran A. Antidepressants not effective in headache associated with minor closed head injury. Int J Psychiatry Med 1988;18:75–83.

[156] Jensen O, Nielsen FF, Vosmar L. An open study comparing manual therapy with the use of cold packs in the treatment of post-traumatic headache. Cephalgia 1990;10:241–5.

[157] Vestergaard K, Andersen G, Gottrug H. Lamotrigine for central post-stroke pain. Neurology 2001;56:184–90.

[158] Attal N, Gaude V, Brasseur GL, Dupuy M, Guirimand F, Parker F, et al. IV lidocaine in central pain. Neurology 2000;54:564–74.

[159] Awerbuch GI, Sandy KR. Mexiletine for thalamic pain syndrome. Int J Neurosci 1990;55: 129–33.

[160] Yen HL, Chan W. An east-west approach to the management of central post stroke pain. Cerebrovasc Dis 2003;16:27–30.

[161] Nandi D, Smith H, Owen S, Joint C, Stein J, Aziz T. Peri-ventricular grey stimulation vs. motor cortex stimulation for post-stroke neuropathic pain. J Clin Neurosci 2002;9:557–61.

[162] Leijon G, Boivie J. Central post-stroke pain: the effect of high and low frequency TENS. Pain 1989;38:187–91.

[163] Bainton T, Fox M, Bowster D, Welb C. A double blind trial of naloxone in central post stroke pain. Pain 1992;48:159–62.

[164] Leijon G, Bovie J, Johansson I. Central post-stroke pain: a controlled trial of amitriptyline and carbamazepine. Pain 1989;36:27–36.

[165] Vick PG, Lamer TJ. Treatment of central post-stroke pain with oral ketamine. Pain 2001; 92:311–3.

[166] Joynt RI. The source of shoulder pain in hemiplegia. Arch Phys Med Rehabil 1992;73: 409–13.

[167] Schwartz L, Engel J, Jensen M. Pain in persons with cerebral palsy. Arch Phys Med Rehabil 1999;80:1243–6.

[168] Engel J, Schwartz L, Jensen M, Johnson D. Pain in cerebral palsy-the relation of coping strategies to adjustment. Pain 2000;88:225–30.

[169] Kelin MG, Whyte J, Esquenazi A, Keenan MA. A comparison of the effects of exercise and lifestyle modification on the resolution of overuse syndromes of the shoulder in polio survivors: a preliminary study. Arch Phys Med Rehabil 2002;83: 708–13.

[170] Giori NJ, Lewallen DG. Total knee replacement in limbs affected by poliomyelitis. J Bone Joint Surg Am 2002;84-A:1157–61.

[171] Willen C, Sunnerhagen KS, Grimbi G. Dynamic water exercise in individuals with late poliomyelitis. Arch Phys Med Rehabil 2001;82:66–72.

[172] Waring WP, Maynard F, Grady W, Grady R, Boyles C. Influence of appropriate lower extremity orthotic management on ambulation, pain and fatigue in a post-polio population. Arch Phys Med Rehabil 1989;70:371–5.

[173] Murphy D, Reid DB. Pain treatment satisfaction in spinal cord injury. Spinal Cord 2001; 39:44–6.

[174] Tai Q, Kirshblum S, Chen B, Millis S, Johnston M, DeLisa JA. Gabapentin in the treatment of neuropathic pain after spinal cord injury: a prospective, randomized, double-blind, crossover trial. J Spinal Cord Med 2002;25:100–5.

[175] Ahn SH, Park HW, Lee BS, Moon HW, Jang SH, Sakong J, et al. Gabapentin effect on neuropathic pain compared among patients with spinal cord injury and different durations of symptoms. Spine 2003;28:341–6.

[176] Drewes AM, Andreasen A, Poulsen LH. Valproate for treatment of chronic central pain after spinal cord injury: a double blind crossover study. Paraplegia 1994;32:565–9.

[177] Finnerup NB, Sindrup SH, Bach FW, Johannsen IL, Jensen TS. Lamotrigine in spinal cord injury pain: a randomized controlled trial. Pain 2002;96:375–83.

[178] Cardenas DD, Warms CA, Turner JA, Marshall H, Brooke MM, Loeser JD. Efficacy of amitriptyline for relief of pain in spinal cord injury: results of a randomized controlled trial. Pain 2002;96:365–73.

[179] Chiou-Tan FY, Vennix MJ, Dinh T, Robinson LR. Effect of mexiletine on spinal cord injury dysesthetic pain. Am J Phys Med Rehabil 1996;75:84–7.

[180] Sandford PR, Lindblom LB, Haddox JD. Amitriptyline and carbamazepine in the treatment of dysesthetic pain in spinal cord injury. Arch Phys Med Rehabil 1992;73:300–1.

[181] Warms CA, Turner JA, Marshall HM, Cardenas DD. Treatments for chronic pain associated with spinal cord injuries: many are tried, few are helpful. Clin J Pain 2002;18: 154–63.

[182] Sidall PJ, Molloy AR, Walker S, Mather LE, Rutkowski SB, Cousins MJ. The efficacy of intrathecal morphine and clonidine in the treatment of pain after spinal cord injury. Anesth Analg 2000;91:1493–8.

ELSEVIER
SAUNDERS

Phys Med Rehabil Clin N Am
16 (2005) 91–108

PHYSICAL MEDICINE
AND REHABILITATION
CLINICS OF
NORTH AMERICA

Fatigue in the elderly population

Ashok Poluri, MD[a], John Mores, MS[a],
Dane B. Cook, PhD[a,b],
Thomas W. Findley, MD, PhD[a,c,d,*],
Adrian Cristian, MD[e,f]

[a]War-Related Illness and Injury Study Center, Department of Veteran Affairs,
385 Tremont Avenue, East Orange, NJ 07018, USA
[b]Department of Radiology, University of Medicine and Dentistry of New Jersey-New Jersey
Medical School, 185 South Orange Avenue, Newark, NJ 07101, USA
[c]Center for Healthcare Knowledge Management, School of Health Related Professions,
University of Medicine and Dentistry of New Jersey, 65 Bergen Street, University Heights,
Newark, NJ 07107-3001, USA
[d]Center for Healthcare Knowledge Management, Department of Veteran Affairs,
385 Tremont Avenue, East Orange, NJ 07018, USA
[e]Department of Rehabilitation Medicine, Bronx Veterans Affairs Medical Center,
130 West Kingsbridge Road, Bronx, NY 10468, USA
[f]Department of Rehabilitation Medicine, Mount Sinai School of Medicine, One Gustave
L. Levy Place, New York, New York 10029, USA

The number of persons 65 years of age and older continues to rise in the United States. The number of persons over 65 years of age is expected to increase from approximately 35 million in 2000 to an estimated 71 million by 2030 [1], and the number of persons over 80 years, the fastest growing segment, is expected to increase from 9.3 million in 2000 to 19.5 million by 2030 [1,2]. The amount of national medical care resources consumed by the elderly population is disproportionate to their numbers among the population. In 1995, 12.8% of the total population represented individuals aged 65 years and above in the United States, but these individuals accounted for nearly one third of total personal health care dollars ($310 billion) [3]. This interaction of demographic, health, and income trends will result in a tripling of the number of elderly persons requiring nursing home care by the year 2030, compared with a 200% increase in the elderly

* Corresponding author. War-Related Illness and Injury Study Center, Department of Veterans Affairs, New Jersey Health Care System Mail Box #129, 385 Tremont Ave, East Orange, NJ 07018.
E-mail address: tfindley@njneuromed.org (T.W. Findley).

1047-9651/05/$ - see front matter © 2004 Elsevier Inc. All rights reserved.
doi:10.1016/j.pmr.2004.06.006   pmr.theclinics.com

population during this period [4]. Aging is associated with a decline in the reserve capacity of organ systems, apparent only during periods of maximal exertion or stress; blunting of thermoregulatory systems; a decline in baroreceptor sensitivity; a decreased ability to adapt to different environments; and a decreased capacity to respond to stress [5]. This additional burden requires physicians to become proficient in the diagnosis, evaluation, and management of concerns unique to this population group.

Definition of fatigue

Fatigue has been defined as a subjective state of overwhelming, sustained exhaustion and a decreased capacity for physical and mental work that is not relieved by rest [6]. It has two components: physical and mental. Physical or muscle fatigue can be defined as impairment in the ability to exert force or power regardless of whether the task itself can still be performed successfully. Mental fatigue can be defined as fatigue arising as a consequence of mental effort. The psychophysical construct of fatigue has received scant scientific attention.

Epidemiology of fatigue

Approximately 20% of men and 30% of women in the United States population complain of frequent tiredness [7]. There are no clear gender differences: Some studies find fatigue more common in women [8], whereas others find it more common in men [9]. The prevalence of clinically significant fatigue depends on the threshold chosen for severity and persistence [10]. In the general population, persons older than 65 years suffer significantly more from fatigue than their younger counterparts [11]. Fatigue, specifically in the elderly population, has been associated with many chronic diseases. Almost 75% of elderly persons (age 65 and over) have at least one chronic illness, and about 50% have at least two chronic illnesses [12]. Chronic conditions, along with acute conditions such as spinal cord injury (SCI), traumatic brain injury (TBI), hip fractures, and stroke can lead to severe and immediate disabilities and to progressive disability that slowly erodes the ability of elderly people to care for themselves [13]. Fatigue is one of the most common symptoms associated with these disabilities. These include people with cancer during radiotherapy or chemotherapy or after surgery [14–21], congestive heart failure [22], anemia [23], thyroid disorders, infections (endocarditis, hepatitis, pneumonias), chronic obstructive pulmonary disease, multiple sclerosis (MS) [24], dialysis [25], lupus [26], and osteoarthritis [27]. Fatigue is described elsewhere in this issue for adults with post-polio syndrome and cerebral palsy It has also been associated with pain [21,28], depression [29,30], physical dysfunction [21,28], sleep disturbance [31], psychologic problems, and other quality of life issues [32,33]. Many medications, including antihistamines [34], sedatives, and beta-blockers [35,36], contribute significantly to side effects of fatigue. This has a great impact on the already compromised population and leads to a vicious cycle of fatigue and disability. Gender differences seem to exist in patients with SCI, with women reporting more fatigue than men associated with anemia [37]. Women also report more fatigue among TBI patients along with a worse outcome [38]. Table 1 lists the prevalence of fatigue in various medical conditions.

Pathophysiology and mechanism

Because fatigue is a symptom of an underlying pathophysiologic process rather than an independent entity, it is difficult to isolate a single cause for it. Many substances and disease processes correlate with the presence of fatigue.

Table 1
Prevalence of fatigue

Condition	Fatigue reported	Instruments used	Sample size	Age (yr) (mean ± SD)	Data from reference
Elderly in a residential care facility	98%	Modified Piper Fatigue scale	199	87.8 ± 4.9	[99]
Post-stroke: 2-yr follow-up	39.2%	Riks-Stroke questionnaire	3667	71.8	[100]
Malignancy		Fatigue Severity scale	227	66.0 (range 30–89)	[101]
Breast	15%				
Prostate	16%				
Lung	50%				
Advanced cancer (inpatient palliative care)	78%				
Age-matched elderly control subjects[a]	6%		98	68.0 (range 41–85)	
Parkinson disease	44.2%	NHP, 7-point fatigue scale	233	73.6 ± 8.4	[19]
Depressive disorders in a French primary care study	4.5%	Fatigue as a presenting complaint	900	Range 55–64	[102]
MS	14% to 55%	Fatigue Impact scale	85	44.8 ± 10	[103]
SLE	58.6%	Fatigue Severity scale	29	35.6 ± 8.9	[24]
Rheumatoid arthritis	100%	MAF, POMS	51	43.6 ± 8.9	[21]

Abbreviations: NHP, Nottingham Health Profile; MS, multiple sclerosis; SLE, systemic lupus erythematosus; MAF, Multidimensional Assessment of Fatigue; POMS, Profile of Mood States.

[a] UK adult population with 49% being overweight or obese and 50% having at least one medical problem (eg, arthritis, chronic airflow limitation, or hypertension).

Mechanisms common to all age groups

Insufficient oxygen transport to muscles mainly caused by anemia, insufficient pumping of blood to the muscles caused especially by anti-neoplastic and cardiotoxic drugs [39,40], and severe muscle mass atrophy from the catabolic effects of sedentary habits and long-term bed rest [41] can contribute to fatigue in all age groups.

Mechanisms in specific disorders

It was initially thought that the fatigue in MS was the result of a reduction of central nervous system conduction velocity and conduction block. Clinical and electrophysiologic evidence of demyelination is likely the reason for the development of frequency-dependent conduction block and subsequent fatigue. However, transcranial magnetic stimulation used to examine the primary motor pathways of a limb undergoing fatigue has shown little evidence to suggest that the fatigue is the result of increased central motor dysfunction due to frequency-dependent conduction block [42]. Inflammatory mediators such as interleukin (IL)-1, tumor necrosis factor (TNF)-α, and IL-6 may play an important role in fatigue, and it has been correlated with active inflammation in rheumatoid arthritis [43]. Recent studies by Tartaglia et al [44] using MRI to examine the relationship between axonal injury and fatigue in patients with MS have failed to show any association between fatigue and levels of clinical disability and disease burden. In accordance with the disease process of MS, diffuse neuronal injury seems to be one of the many likely causes of fatigue.

Diffuse axonal injury is the distinguishing feature of TBI. It is primarily responsible for the initial loss of consciousness [45]. Incomplete recovery of the disrupted axons, gray matter contusion, brain edema leading to depressed metabolic activity of intact neurons, and depressed neural activity due to anticonvulsant medication may contribute to fatigue in this specific group of patients.

Mechanisms probably different in the elderly population

Several factors, including pain, sleep deprivation, and the stress of illness or surgery, could contribute to the fatigue experienced by elderly persons. Pain may contribute to fatigue by increasing heart rate, blood pressure, respiratory rate, muscle tone, and oxygen consumption. Sleep deprivation results in limited non-rapid eye movement phase of sleep, decline in protein synthesis, and a slower rate of healing [46].

Elderly persons suffer more from disabilities than their younger counterparts, and the energy required for rehabilitation contributes to fatigue. Patients with lower extremity injury, surgery, or weakness must learn to ambulate with the support of walkers. For those with restricted weight bearing, the arms must support the body weight. Mechanical work performed by the unaffected limb is increased, and the energy cost of walking may approach maximal oxygen consumption [47].

Age-related alterations in the structure of skeletal muscle, such as losses in muscle mass, motor unit and fiber number, and motor unit remodeling, have been well described in the literature [48–51]. The functional consequences of these age-related alterations include substantial loss of strength and slowed contractile characteristics, and it has been proposed that with advanced age (>70 years), type I fibers contribute proportionally more to force generation than in younger adults [50]. Aging has also been shown to result in decreased cortical [52] and muscle membrane excitability [53], uncoupling of excitation-contraction mechanisms [53], and altered metabolic capacity [54]. However, specific effects of these changes on fatigue in the elderly population have not been well studied, with the exception of maximal oxygen uptake (Vo_2max), which declines progressively with age. It is also unclear whether some of these changes are due to aging or to prolonged decreased physical activity.

Central and peripheral causes of fatigue

Basic mechanisms of fatigue can be divided into two categories: (1) peripheral fatigue produced by changes at or distal to the neuromuscular junction, and (2) central fatigue defined as a progressive reduction in voluntary activation of muscle during exercise by factors proximal to the neuromuscular junction [55].

Recent studies comparing peripheral and central fatigue in young (approximately 25 years of age) and elderly (70–85 years of age) subjects showed that peripheral fatigue may develop more slowly in elderly than in young subjects, whereas central fatigue may be more prominent in elderly subjects. Peripheral fatigue has multiple mechanisms: force loss through the accumulation of metabolites, substrate depletion, and accumulation of electrolytes and their effects on excitation-contraction coupling [56]. With aging, there is evidence of muscle fiber atrophy, with a reduction of type II fiber area of approximately 20% between 20 and 70 years of age. Results from normalized voluntary fatigue protocols using intermittent maximal isometric or isokinetic contractions in a variety of muscles suggest no discernible difference in the amount or rate of fatigue between young and elderly subjects [57,58]. The manifestation of central fatigue seems to be task dependent and may be mediated by intrinsic motoneuronal, spinal (including the intrinsic behavior of the motoneuron, recurrent inhibition, and reflex inputs reaching alpha and gamma motoneurons and their presynaptic modulation), and supraspinal factors, which include the descending corticospinal tracts to the motoneurons [55,59,60]. Voluntary activation has been assessed using the twitch interpolation (peripheral stimulation) technique on a variety of muscles, including the quadriceps [60,61], tibialis anterior [62–64], and elbow flexors [65–68], but the results are inconclusive as to whether elderly subjects are able to activate their muscles to the same extent as younger adults. Studies in young adults suggest that sustained maximum voluntary contraction protocols induce an increased excitation and increased inhibition in the motor cortex using transcranial magnetic stimulation suggest that central fatigue may develop from inadequate neural drive upstream of the motor cortex [69].

There are other factors that may be involved, but specific evidence is limited for which age. As the intensity of exercise increases, the rate of energy consumption exceeds the aerobic capacity, and muscle cells become highly dependent on anaerobic metabolism. Anaerobic breakdown of glycogen results in the accumulation of inorganic acids, mainly lactic acid, which dissociates into lactate and hydrogen ions. Lactate ions have little effect on muscle contraction [70], whereas the increase in hydrogen ions has been considered an important cause of muscle fatigue. If lactic acid has an effect on fatigue, it might be via inducing central fatigue by reflex inhibition of spinal motoneurons or by inhibition of voluntary supraspinal motor activity due to perceived discomfort from exercising muscles.

There have been a few studies examining the role of cytokines in the etiology of fatigue. In patients with chronic disease, red blood cells have a shorter survival than those of healthy people. This may be due to the increased concentrations of IL-1 and TNF-α in the circulation [71,72]. Increased concentrations of cytokines are associated with fatigue; they are observed in fatigue related to cancer and cancer treatment and in fatigue syndrome unrelated to cancer. For example, when IL-6 is administered to healthy subjects, it induces fatigue and poor mental concentration [73]. TNF-α has been noted to be elevated in postdialysis fatigue [74]. Tumor growth factor-beta has been shown to be associated with fatigue in patients with chronic fatigue [75]. Decreased natural killer cell activity has also been noted in a family with chronic fatigue syndrome [76].

Some studies have suggested that serotonin might be involved in the pathogenesis of fatigue and depression [77–79]. Subjects suffering from chronic fatigue had an increased amount of tryptophan in the circulation after physical exercise. Fatigue does not seem to be associated with an increased sensitivity of the hypothalamo-hypophyseal axis to 5-hydroxytryptamine [77], and attempts to control fatigue with serotonin re-uptake inhibitors have not achieved desired results.

Tools for studying fatigue

Fatigue has been studied with various tools proposed in different clinical settings. None of these instruments has been validated sufficiently in the elderly population. Recommendations must be based on principles rather than direct evidence. Several factors should be considered when measuring fatigue in elderly patients. Fatigue should be measured as a state rather than as a trait because it tends to fluctuate over time. It may also be closely associated with pain, sleep, depression, medications, and other comorbid diseases. A scale that captures most of these aspects is needed.

Portenoy and Itri [80] have suggested the use of three questions to assess fatigue severity and impact over time in a practice setting where time is of major concern. These have been used exclusively in patients with cancer, although they can be applied to the elderly population for screening purposes.

1. Are you experiencing any fatigue?
2. If so, how severe has it been, on average, during the past week? (If fatigue is present, a 0–10 rating scale can be used [eg, 0–3 is mild fatigue, 4–6 moderate, and 7–10 severe].)
3. How does fatigue interfere with your ability to function?

These questions are easy to administer and can give the health care provider a baseline status for future follow-up of the elderly patient. The main drawback of this scale is that it provides a uni-dimensional assessment of fatigue.

Some of the other widely used scales that may be easily used for identifying undiagnosed fatigue especially in elderly patients are listed in Box 1.

Fatigue Severity scale

The Fatigue Severity scale [24] provides a unitary measure of global fatigue severity. This scale has been used to assess fatigue in a number of medical conditions (SLE, MS, Parkinson disease, brain injury, chronic hepatitis, sleep disorders, and amyotrophic lateral sclerosis) and has been validated in patients with advanced cancer. The internal consistency of this scale was found to be 0.94 in 95 patients with advanced cancer and 0.88 in 98 control subjects [81].

Brief Fatigue Inventory

The Brief Fatigue Inventory [82] is comprised of nine items measured on a 10-point scale. It assesses the severity of fatigue and its effects on the

---

Box 1. Scales for identifying fatigue

- Fatigue Severity scale (9 items)
- Brief Fatigue Inventory (9 items)
- Fatigue Questionnaire (11 items)
- Fatigue Symptom Inventory (13 items)
- Multidimensional Fatigue Inventory (20 items)
- Modified Piper Fatigue scale (22 items)
- Fatigue Assessment Instrument (29 items)

patient's ability in activities of daily living. This scale has been used in assessing fatigue in cancer patients and has a high internal consistency (Cronbach's alpha = 0.96). Its main drawback is its uni-dimensional measure of fatigue.

Fatigue Questionnaire

The Fatigue Questionnaire [83] is an 11-item questionnaire with a yes/no response or four-point Likert scale measuring physical and mental fatigue. It has good clinical validity supported by a study of fatigue in the general population [84]. Elderly patients (older than 60 years) comprised around 22% of the subject population. It seems to be a useful tool for assessing fatigue in a variety of medical disorders, such as HIV, cancer, MS, and disorders in Gulf war veterans. It has an internal consistency rate of 0.88 to 0.90.

Fatigue Symptom Inventory

The Fatigue Symptom Inventory [85] is a 13-item self-report. It measures the intensity and duration of fatigue and its impact on quality of life. The psychometric properties of the scale assessed in women with breast cancer had good internal consistency, with alpha coefficients above 0.90.

Multidimensional Fatigue Inventory

The Multidimensional Fatigue Inventory [86] covers five areas: general fatigue, physical fatigue, reduced activity, reduced motivation, and mental fatigue. It consists of 20 items. It has shown good reliability in assessing fatigue in the general population (Cronbach's alpha = 0.65–0.80).

Modified Piper Fatigue scale

The Modified Piper Fatigue scale [87] covers four subjective dimensions (cognitive, sensory, behavioral, and affective) and includes three open-ended questions with respect to cause, other symptoms, and relief measures. The scale contains 22 items scored on a scale of 0 to 10. Test-retest reliability assessed by Cronbach's alpha was at least 0.89. The length could be a major drawback for this comprehensive and multi-dimensional scale.

Fatigue Assessment Instrument

The Fatigue Assessment Instrument [88] is an expanded version of the one-dimensional Fatigue Severity scale, with items added to assess additional aspects of fatigue. It has been validated in a sample of outpatients at neurology and rheumatology clinics with a variety of diagnoses. It has four subscales: fatigue severity, situation specificity, consequences of fatigue, and responsiveness to rest/sleep, with extra dimensions providing information on situational aspects of fatigue. It has been used for assessing fatigue in Lyme disease, chronic fatigue syndrome, SLE, and MS and has an internal consistency of 0.29 to 0.69.

Diagnostic work-up and differential diagnosis of fatigue

The nature of fatigue is vital to the diagnosis, and it is therefore important to elucidate patient's complaints. A comprehensive history facilitates in isolating the causes of fatigue and excludes possible causes. The history should cover

- Systemic inquiry for diseases associated with fatigue
- Symptoms of depression, anxiety, and sleep disorder
- Patient's understanding of their illness and how they cope with it
- Current social stressors
- Medications and their interactions

A detailed physical and mental examination must be performed in each case to identify medical and psychiatric diagnoses associated with fatigue. A standard set of routine investigations to identify the most common cause of fatigue should be ordered (Box 2), followed by special investigations (eg, sleep studies for recognizing obstructive sleep apnea and narcolepsy, imaging studies to rule out neurologic or cardiac causes of fatigue). It is important to inquire fully about the patient's understanding of their illness. Patients may be worried that the fatigue is a symptom of a severe undiagnosed disease or that activity will cause a worsening of their condition.

Cancer-related fatigue has been studied extensively, and a detailed guide to approach and management can be obtained from the NCCN 2002 cancer-related fatigue guidelines [89].

Treatment options

As an initial approach to fatigue, efforts should be made to correct potential treatable etiologies: treating anemia if present; identifying medication interactions, any sleep disorder, metabolic abnormalities, or

---

Box 2. Screening tests for fatigue

- Complete blood count with differential erythrocyte sedimentation rate/C reactive protein
- Liver function tests
- Complete metabolic profile
- Thyroid function tests
- Urine analysis for protein and glucose
- Pulmonary function tests

psychiatric disorders; and devising an appropriately tailored exercise prescription. Many of these interventions are relatively simple and are routinely used in the primary care setting with minimal risk to the elderly patient. Pharmacologic therapies for fatigue, associated with medical illnesses or not, have not been rigorously evaluated in controlled trials. However, there is evidence to support the use of a few drug classes. Psychostimulants, such as methylphenidate, pemoline, and dextroamphetamine, have been well studied for the treatment of opioid-related somnolence and cognitive impairment [90] and depression in elderly and medically ill patients [90–92].

Role of exercise in elderly patients

The US Preventive Services Task Force, which rigorously reviewed the evidence that exercise promotes health and prevents illness, concluded that clinicians should counsel patients to engage in a program of regular physical activity that is tailored to their health status and personal lifestyles [93]. With the elderly population, the framework for recommending exercise is potentially broader. A key issue is whether some types of exercise can be recommended to prevent age-related decline in health status and loss of independence. In this context, the ability of exercise to affect specific aspects of health status, such as mobility and risk of fall, assumes great importance.

Muscle strength declines by 15% per decade after age 50 and 30% per decade after age 70; however, resistance training can result in 15% to 100%, or more, strength gains in older adults. It is beneficial to prescribe a range of exercise intensities that patients can match to their energy or functional level on any given day. In spite of the increased likelihood of chronic pre-existing conditions, elderly individuals can obtain benefits from regular endurance training that are similar to those observed in younger adults [94]; for example, Vo_2max can increase significantly in sedentary older individuals when they engage in regular endurance activity. A sustained exercise program leads to physiologic adaptations that likely contribute to reduce fatigue. These include increases in cardiac output and distribution to muscle, oxygen transport and use, oxidative enzyme activity and capacity, and lean body mass; decreases in heart rate, fat mass, and lactate production; and improved blood lipid profiles [95]. The initial exercise prescription should be tailored to this population to prevent adverse consequences from a poorly performed exercise program.

Before initiating an exercise program, the elderly patient should undergo a history and physical examination directed at identifying cardiac risk factors and physical limitations. The American College of Sports Medicine (ACSM) recommends exercise stress testing for all sedentary or minimally active older adults who plan to begin exercising at a vigorous intensity. Elderly persons can safely begin a moderate aerobic and resistance-training program without stress testing if they begin slowly and gradually increase their level of activity. They should be counseled to discontinue exercise and seek medical advice if they experience major warning signs or symptoms (eg, chest pain, palpitations, or light-headedness) [96].

The exercise prescription

The three essential components of an exercise program for any age group consist of cardiorespiratory endurance, muscular strength and endurance, and flexibility. The exercise prescription includes the appropriate modes, intensity, duration, frequency, and progression of physical activity [97]. Specific exercise recommendations for a given person depend on existing comorbidities and on a baseline level of physical activity [96].

Cardiorespiratory endurance

The elderly patient should be encouraged whenever possible to meet the ACSM, the Centers for Disease Control and Prevention, and the President's Council on Physical Fitness and Sports recommendations put forth in 1995 to accumulate at least 30 minutes of moderate intensity exercise on most and preferably all days of the week. Evidence has shown that regular participation in moderate-intensity physical activity is associated with health benefits even when aerobic fitness (eg, Vo_2max) remains unchanged. This can be accomplished with activities such as brisk walking, biking, gardening, yard work, housework, climbing stairs, and active recreational pursuits. Exercise duration need not be continuous to produce benefits; thus, those who have difficulty sustaining exercise for 30 minutes or who prefer shorter bouts of exercise can be advised to exercise for 10-minute periods or less at different times throughout the day [97]. Sedentary adults should begin at a low level and gradually progress to a goal of moderate activity [96]. To avoid injury and to ensure safety, older adults should initially increase exercise duration rather than intensity. For those achieving this level, additional benefits may be obtained with longer-duration, moderate-intensity exercise following the traditional ACSM intensity guidelines and precautions established for cardiorespiratory fitness [97].

Intensity can be defined as using a percentage of maximum heart rate, heart rate reserve, and Vo_2 ranges. A rating of perceived exertion (RPE) scale can be used, such as the original Borg scale, and one can identify activities that require the appropriate intensity of effort based on the average energy expenditure required to do the activity [98]. The ACSM recommends an intensity of exercise corresponding to between 55% and 65% to 90% of maximum heart rate, or between 40% and 50% to 85% of heart rate reserve. The average RPE range associated with physiologic adaptation to exercises is 12 to 16 ("somewhat hard" to "hard") on the category Borg scale [97]. Adults can exercise at the maximal intensity at which they are able to comfortably carry on a conversation (the "talk test"). This may require some trial and error [96]. The frequency recommended is three to five workouts per week. The duration of exercise recommended is 20 to 60 minutes of continuous or intermittent aerobic activity (minimum of

10-minute bouts) accumulated throughout the day [97]. Moderate intensity can be defined as 60% to 79% of maximal heart rate, 50% to 74% of heart rate reserve, or an RPE rating of 12 to 13 on the Borg scale [98].

Warm-up and cool-down periods

The format for an exercise session should include warm-up and cool-down periods, especially for persons exercising at a moderate intensity. Warm-up facilitates the transition from rest to exercise, augments blood flow, and increases the metabolic rate from the resting level to the aerobic requirements for endurance training. A warm-up may reduce the susceptibility to musculoskeletal injury by increasing connective tissue extensibility, improving joint range of motion and function, and enhancing muscular performance. A warm-up session should begin with 5 to 10 minutes of low-intensity, calisthenic-type exercises and 5 to 10 minutes of progressive aerobic activity sufficient to approach the lower limit of the prescribed heart rate for endurance training. For example, persons who use brisk walking during the endurance phase might conclude the warm-up period with slow walking. Similarly, brisk walking serves as an ideal warm-up for persons who jog slowly during the endurance phase [97]. Flexibility exercises can be included in the warm-up period but should always be preceded by some type of warm-up activity (calisthenics or aerobic activity) to increase circulation and internal body temperature. The cool-down period provides a gradual recovery from the endurance/games phase and includes exercise of diminishing intensities—for example, slower walking or jogging, calisthenics and flexibility exercises and in some cases, or alternate activities (eg, yoga, tai chi, or relaxation training). The cool-down permits appropriate circulatory adjustments and return of the heart rate and blood pressure to near resting values; enhances venous return, thereby reducing the potential for postexercise hypotension and dizziness; facilitates the dissipation of body heat; promotes more rapid removal of lactic acid than stationary recovery; and combats the potential, deleterious effects of the postexercise rise in plasma catecholamines [97].

Strength training

Elderly patients should be encouraged to supplement aerobic exercise and an active lifestyle with strength-developing exercises. Muscular fitness may allow performance of activities of daily living with less effort and extend functional independence by living the latter years in a self-sufficient, dignified manner. Individualization of the strength training prescription is essential and should be based on the health or fitness status of the participant [97]. Sedentary or irregularly active older adults should start slowly and then gradually advance the intensity of their training regimen. Participants can start with resistive bands/tubing, light weights (eg, 1- or 2-lb hand weights or a can of food), or simple exercise (eg, repeatedly rising from a chair) [96]. This allows for adaptations of the connective tissue elements, allows time to improve their exercise techniques, and reduces possible postexercise pain and soreness. The first several strength training sessions should be closely supervised by trained personnel. Participants should maintain their normal breathing pattern, and all exercises should be performed in a manner in which the speed is controlled. General guidelines for intensity, frequency, and duration of a strength training program are as follows [97]:

- Frequency—Strength training should be performed at least twice a week, with at least 48 hours of rest between sessions.
- Intensity—Perform at least one set of 10 to 15 repetitions before reaching fatigue or an intensity that elicits a RPE on the Borg scale of 12 to 13 (somewhat hard), and, as a training effect occurs, achieve an overload initially by increasing the number of repetitions and then by increasing the resistance (initially you can start with as few as five repetitions and increase to 15). All of the major muscle groups should be included in the exercise selection.
- Duration—Adherence to the guidelines set forth here should permit individuals to complete a total body strength training program within 20 to 30 minutes.

Flexibility

An adequate range of motion in all body joints is important to maintaining an acceptable level of musculoskeletal function, balance, and agility in older adults. A well-rounded program of stretching should include exercises for every major joint in the body. Guidelines pertaining to stretching by older adults are as follows (always precede stretching exercises with a warm-up activity to increase circulation and internal body temperature) [97]:

- Frequency—Stretching exercises should be performed a minimum of 2 to 3 days a week and should be included as an integral part of the warm-up and cool down exercises.
- Intensity—Exercises should incorporate slow movement (eg, static stretches that are sustained for 10–30 seconds), no bouncing, and at least four repetitions per muscle group. The degree of stretch achieved should not cause pain, but rather mild discomfort.
- Duration—The stretching phase of an exercise session should last long enough to stretch all the major muscle groups.

Regulatory barriers need to be revised to maximize convenience, benefit, and compliance and to minimize cost and disability.

Future research questions

Intervention studies specific to the elderly population that measure the multidimensionality of fatigue are required. Future research needs to focus on ways to manage symptoms, such as alterations in nutrition, oxygenation, and pain; modulation of environmental factors to reduce disruption of sleep-wake cycle; and patient self-education to reduce anxiety. Exercise seems to be the most efficacious treatment, and randomized controlled trials need to be conducted to validate its role in combating fatigue.

Summary

Fatigue in the elderly population is a complex phenomenon. Although a number of factors contributing to the fatigue have been identified, its basic mechanism remains elusive. Additional research on prevalence, identification, diagnosis, severity of fatigue, and associated factors and the role of exercise as an effective treatment modality could lead to a better understanding of the causal factors.

Reference

[1] US Census Bureau. International database. Table 094. Midyear population, by age and sex. U.S. Census Bureau, Population Division, Population Projections Branch. 2004.

[2] Williams ME, Hadler NM. Sounding board: the illness as the focus of geriatric medicine. N Engl J Med 1983;308:1357–60.

[3] Anonymous. Special focus. Healthy aging: preventing the diseases of aging. Chron Dis Notes Rep 1999;12. 1999. p. 1–4.

[4] Polednak AP. Projected numbers of cancers diagnosed in the US elderly population, 1990 through 2030. Am J Public Health 1994;84:1313–6.

[5] Clark GS, Siebens HC. Rehabilitation of the geriatric patient. In: DeLisa JA, Gans BM, editors. Rehabilitation medicine: principles and practice. Philadelphia: Lippincott; 1993. p. 642–65.

[6] Cella D, Peterman A, Passik S, Jacobsen P, Breitbart W. Progress toward guidelines for the management of fatigue. Oncology (Huntingt) 1998;12:369–77.

[7] Hjermstad MJ, Fayers PM, Bjordal K, Kaasa S. Health-related quality of life in the general Norwegian population assessed by the European Organization for Research and Treatment of Cancer Core Quality-of-Life Questionnaire: the QLQ = C30 (+ 3). J Clin Oncol 1998; 16:1188–96.

[8] Chen MK. The epidemiology of self-perceived fatigue among adults. Prev Med 1986;15: 74–81.

[9] David A, Pelosi A, McDonald E, Stephens D, Ledger D, Rathbone R, et al. Tired, weak, or in need of rest: fatigue among general practice attenders. BMJ 1990;301:1199–202.

[10] Cathebras PJ, Robbins JM, Kirmayer LJ, Hayton BC. Fatigue in primary care: prevalence, psychiatric comorbidity, illness behavior, and outcome. J Gen Intern Med 1992;7:276–86.

[11] Cella D, Lai JS, Chang CH, Peterman A, Slavin M. Fatigue in cancer patients compared with fatigue in the general United States population. Cancer 2002;94:528–38.

[12] Calkins E. New ways to care for older people: building systems based on evidence. New York: Springer; 1999.

[13] Fried LP, Guralnik JM. Disability in older adults: evidence regarding significance, etiology, and risk. J Am Geriatr Soc 1997;45:92–100.

[14] Irvine D, Vincent L, Graydon JE, Bubela N, Thompson L. The prevalence and correlates of fatigue in patients receiving treatment with chemotherapy and radiotherapy: a comparison with the fatigue experienced by healthy individuals. Cancer Nurs 1994;17:367–78.

[15] Portenoy RK, Thaler HT, Kornblith AB, Lepore JM, Friedlander-Klar H, Coyle N, et al. Symptom prevalence, characteristics and distress in a cancer population. Qual Life Res 1994;3:183–9.

[16] King KB, Nail LM, Kreamer K, Strohl RA, Johnson JE. Patients' descriptions of the experience of receiving radiation therapy. Oncol Nurs Forum 1985;12:55–61.
[17] Nail LM, Jones LS, Greene D, Schipper DL, Jensen R. Use and perceived efficacy of self-care activities in patients receiving chemotherapy. Oncol Nurs Forum 1991;18: 883–7.
[18] Friedman J, Friedman H. Fatigue in Parkinson's disease. Neurology 1993;43:2016–8.
[19] Karlsen K, Larsen JP, Tandberg E, Jorgensen K. Fatigue in patients with Parkinson's disease. Mov Disord 1999;14:237–41.
[20] Krupp LB, Pollina DA. Mechanisms and management of fatigue in progressive neurological disorders. Curr Opin Neurol 1996;9:456–60.
[21] Belza BL. Comparison of self-reported fatigue in rheumatoid arthritis and controls. J Rheumatol 1995;22:639–43.
[22] Friedman MM, King KB. Correlates of fatigue in older women with heart failure. Heart Lung 1995;24:512–8.
[23] Yellen SB, Cella DF, Webster K, Blendowski C, Kaplan E. Measuring fatigue and other anemia-related symptoms with the Functional Assessment of Cancer Therapy (FACT) measurement system. J Pain Symptom Manage 1997;13:63–74.
[24] Krupp LB, LaRocca NG, Muir-Nash J, Steinberg AD. The fatigue severity scale: application to patients with multiple sclerosis and systemic lupus erythematosus. Arch Neurol 1989;46:1121–3.
[25] Srivastava RH. Fatigue in end-stage renal disease patients. Key aspects of comfort: management of pain, fatigue, and nausea. New York: Springer; 1989.
[26] Krupp LB, LaRocca NG, Muir J, Steinberg AD. A study of fatigue in systemic lupus erythematosus. J Rheumatol 1990;17:1450–2.
[27] Wolfe F, Hawley DJ, Wilson K. The prevalence and meaning of fatigue in rheumatic disease. J Rheumatol 1996;23:1407–17.
[28] Belza BL, Henke CJ, Yelin EH, Epstein WV, Gilliss CL. Correlates of fatigue in older adults with rheumatoid arthritis. Nurs Res 1993;42:93–9.
[29] Piper BF. The development of an instrument to measure the subjective dimension of fatigue. In: Funk SG, Tornquist EM, Champagne MT, et al, editors. Key aspects of comfort: management of pain, fatigue, and nausea. New York: Springer; 1989. p. 199–208.
[30] Piper BF, Lindsey AM, Dodd MJ. Fatigue mechanisms in cancer patients: developing nursing theory. Oncol Nurs Forum 1987;14:17–23.
[31] Krupp LB, Jandorf L, Coyle PK, Mendelson WB. Sleep disturbance in chronic fatigue syndrome. J Psychosom Res 1993;37:325–31.
[32] Camarillo MA. The oncology patient's experience of fatigue. In: Whedon M, editor. Quality of life: a nursing challenge. Philadelphia: Meniscus; 1991. p. 39–44.
[33] Ferrell BR, Grant M, Funk B, Ly J. Bone tired: the experience of fatigue and its impact on quality of life. Oncol Nurs Forum 1996;23:1539–47.
[34] Kay GG, Berman B, Mockoviak SH, Morris CE, Reeves D, Starbuck V, et al. Initial and steady-state effects of diphenhydramine and loratadine on sedation, cognition, mood, and psychomotor performance. Arch Intern Med 1997;157:2350–6.
[35] Head A, Kendall MJ, Ferner R, Eagles C. Acute effects of beta blockade and exercise on mood and anxiety. Br J Sports Med 1996;30:238–42.
[36] Gullestad L, Dolva LO, Aase O, Kjekshus J. Interaction of naloxone and timolol on maximal exercise capacity and the subjective perception of fatigue. Int J Sports Med 1989; 10:259–63.
[37] Shackelford M, Farley T, Vines CL. A comparison of women and men with spinal cord injury. Spinal Cord 1998;36:337–9.
[38] Edna TH, Cappelen J. Late post-concussional symptoms in traumatic head injury: an analysis of frequency and risk factors. Acta Neurochir (Wien) 1987;86:12–7.
[39] Dimeo FC. Effects of exercise on cancer-related fatigue. Cancer 2001;92(Suppl):1689–93.
[40] Keefe DL. Trastuzumab-associated cardiotoxicity. Cancer 2002;95:1592–600.

[41] Germain P, Guell A, Marini JF. Muscle strength during bedrest with and without muscle exercise as a countermeasure. Eur J Appl Physiol Occup Physiol 1995;71:342–8.

[42] Sheehan GL, Murray NM, Rothwell JC, Miller DH, Thompson AJ. An electro-physiological study of the mechanism of fatigue in multiple sclerosis. Brain 1997;120: 299–315.

[43] Elliott MJ, Maini RN, Feldmann M, Kalden JR, Antoni C, Smolen JS, et al. Randomised double-blind comparison of chimeric monoclonal antibody to tumour necrosis factor alpha (cA2) versus placebo in rheumatoid arthritis. Lancet 1994;344:1105–10.

[44] Tartaglia MC, Narayanan S, Francis SJ, Santos AC, De Stefano N, Lapierre Y, et al. The relationship between diffuse axonal damage and fatigue in multiple sclerosis. Arch Neurol 2004;61:201–7.

[45] Denny-Brown D, Russell WR. Experimental cerebral concussion. Brain 1941;64:93–164.

[46] McDowell JA, Mion LC, Lydon TJ, Inouye SK. A nonpharmacologic sleep protocol for hospitalized older patients. J Am Geriatr Soc 1998;46:700–5.

[47] Gussoni M, Margonato V, Ventura R, Veicsteinas A. Energy cost of walking with hip joint impairment. Phys Ther 1990;70:295–301.

[48] Doherty TJ, Vandervoort AA, Brown WF. Effects of ageing on the motor unit: a brief review. Can J Appl Physiol 1993;18:331–58.

[49] Luff AR. Age-associated changes in the innervation of muscle fibers and changes in the mechanical properties of motor units. Ann N Y Acad Sci 1998;854:92–101.

[50] Roos MR, Rice CL, Vandervoort AA. Age-related changes in motor unit function. Muscle Nerve 1997;20:679–90.

[51] Vandervoort AA. Aging of the human neuromuscular system. Muscle Nerve 2002;25s: 17–25.

[52] Eisen A, Siejka S, Schulzer M, Calne D. Age-dependent decline in motor evoked potential (MEP) amplitude: with a comment on changes in Parkinson's disease. Electroencephalogr Clin Neurophysiol 1991;81:209–15.

[53] Hicks AL, Cupido CM, Martin J, Dent J. Muscle excitation in elderly adults: the effects of training. Muscle Nerve 1992;15:87–93.

[54] Pastoris O, Boschi F, Verri M, Baiardi P, Felzani G, Vecchiet J, et al. The effects of aging on enzyme activities and metabolite concentrations in skeletal muscle from sedentary male and female subjects. Exp Gerontol 2000;35:95–104.

[55] Gandevia SC. Spinal and supraspinal factors in human muscle fatigue. Physiol Rev 2001; 81:1725–89.

[56] Fitts RH. Cellular mechanisms of muscle fatigue. Physiol Rev 1994;74:49–94.

[57] Green HJ. Mechanisms of muscle fatigue in intense exercise. J Sports Sci 1997;15:247–56.

[58] McLester JR Jr. Muscle contraction and fatigue: the role of adenosine 5'-diphosphate and inorganic phosphate. Sports Med 1997;23:287–305.

[59] Gandevia SC. Neural control in human muscle fatigue: changes in muscle afferents, motoneurones and motor cortical drive. Acta Physiol Scand 1998;162:275–83.

[60] Roos MR, Rice CL, Connelly DM, Vandervoort AA. Quadriceps muscle strength, contractile properties, and motor unit firing rates in young and old men. Muscle Nerve 1999;22:1094–103.

[61] Stackhouse SK, Stevens JE, Lee SC, Pearce KM, Snyder-Mackler L, Binder-Macleod SA. Maximum voluntary activation in nonfatigued and fatigued muscle of young and elderly individuals. Phys Ther 2001;81:1102–9.

[62] Connelly DM, Rice CL, Roos MR, Vandervoort AA. Motor unit firing rates and contractile properties in tibialis anterior of young and old men. J Appl Physiol 1999;87:843–52.

[63] Kent-Braun JA, Ng AV. Specific strength and voluntary muscle activation in young and elderly women and men. J Appl Physiol 1999;87:22–9.

[64] Vandervoort AA, McComas AJ. Contractile changes in opposing muscles of the human ankle joint with aging. J Appl Physiol 1986;61:361–7.

[65] Allman BL, Rice CL. Incomplete recovery of voluntary isometric force after fatigue is not affected by old age. Muscle Nerve 2001;24:1156–67.

[66] De Serres SJ, Enoka RM. Older adults can maximally activate the biceps brachii muscle by voluntary command. J Appl Physiol 1998;84:284–91.

[67] Klein CS, Rice CL, Marsh GD. Normalized force, activation, and coactivation in the arm muscles of young and old men. J Appl Physiol 2001;91:1341–9.

[68] Yue GH, Ranganathan VK, Siemionow V, Liu JZ, Sahgal V. Older adults exhibit a reduced ability to fully activate their biceps brachii muscle. J Gerontol Med Sci 1999; 54A:M249–53.

[69] Taylor JL, Gandevia SC. Transcranial magnetic stimulation and human muscle fatigue. Muscle Nerve 2001;24:18–29.

[70] Posterino GS, Dutka TL, Lamb GD. L(+)-lactate does not affect twitch and tetanic responses in mechanically skinned mammalian muscle fibres. Pflugers Arch 2001;442: 197–203.

[71] Zucker S. Anemia in cancer. Cancer Invest 1985;3:249–60.

[72] Salvarani C, Casali B, Salvo D, Brunati C, Macchioni PL, Massai G, et al. The role of interleukin 1, erythropoietin and red cell bound immunoglobulins in the anaemia of rheumatoid arthritis. Clin Exp Rheumatol 1991;9:241–6.

[73] Spath-Schwalbe E, Hansen K, Schmidt F, Schrezenmeier H, Marshall L, Burger K, et al. Acute effects of recombinant human interleukin-6 on endocrine and central nervous sleep functions in healthy men. J Clin Endocrinol Metab 1998;83:1573–9.

[74] Dreisbach AW, Hendrickson T, Beezhold D, Riesenberg LA, Sklar AH. Elevated levels of tumor necrosis factor alpha in postdialysis fatigue. Int J Artif Organs 1998;21:83–6.

[75] Bennett AL, Chao CC, Hu S, Buchwald D, Fagioli LR, Schur PH, et al. Elevation of bioactive transforming growth factor-beta in serum from patients with chronic fatigue syndrome. J Clin Immunol 1997;17:160–6.

[76] Levine PH, Whiteside TL, Friberg D, Bryant J, Colclough G, Herberman RB. Dysfunction of natural killer activity in a family with chronic fatigue syndrome. Clin Immunol Immunopathol 1998;88:96–104.

[77] Sharpe M, Hawton K, Clements A, Cowen PJ. Increased brain serotonin function in men with chronic fatigue syndrome. BMJ 1997;315:164–5.

[78] Bakheit AM, Behan PO, Dinan TG, Gray CE, O'Keane V. Possible upregulation of hypothalamic 5-hydroxytryptamine receptors in patients with postviral fatigue syndrome. BMJ 1992;304:1010–2.

[79] Cleare AJ, Bearn J, Allain T, McGregor A, Wessely S, Murray RM, et al. Contrasting neuroendocrine responses in depression and chronic fatigue syndrome. J Affect Disord 1995;34:283–9.

[80] Portenoy RK, Itri LM. Cancer-related fatigue: guidelines for evaluation and management. Oncologist 1999;4:1–10.

[81] Stone P, Hardy J, Broadley K, Tookman AJ, Kurowska A, A'Hern R. Fatigue in advanced cancer: a prospective controlled cross-sectional study. Br J Cancer 1999;79: 1479–86.

[82] Mendoza TR, Wang XS, Cleeland CS, Morrissey M, Johnson BA, Wendt JK, et al. The rapid assessment of fatigue severity in cancer patients: use of the Brief Fatigue Inventory. Cancer 1999;85:1186–96.

[83] Chalder T, Berelowitz G, Pawlikowska T, Watts L, Wessely S, Wright D, et al. Development of a fatigue scale. J Psychosom Res 1993;37:147–53.

[84] Loge JH, Ekeberg O, Kaasa S. Fatigue in the general Norwegian population: normative data and associations. J Psychosom Res 1998;45:53–65.

[85] Hann DM, Jacobsen PB, Azzarello LM, Martin SC, Curran SL, Fields KK, et al. Measurement of fatigue in cancer patients: development and validation of the Fatigue Symptom Inventory. Qual Life Res 1998;7:301–10.

[86] Smets EM, Garssen B, Bonke B, De Haes JC. The Multidimensional Fatigue Inventory (MFI) psychometric qualities of an instrument to assess fatigue. J Psychosom Res 1995;39: 315–25.

[87] Piper BF, Dibble SL, Dodd MJ, Weiss MC, Slaughter RE, Paul SM. The revised Piper Fatigue Scale: psychometric evaluation in women with breast cancer. Oncol Nurs Forum 1998;25:677–84.

[88] Schwartz JE, Jandorf L, Krupp LB. The measurement of fatigue: a new instrument. J Psychosom Res 1993;37:753–62.

[89] Mock V, Atkinson A, Barsevick A, Cella D, Cimprich B, Cleeland C, et al. NCCN practice guidelines for cancer-related fatigue. Oncology (Huntingt) 2000;14:151–61.

[90] Breitbart W, Mermelstein H. Pemoline: an alternative psychostimulant for the management of depressive disorders in cancer patients. Psychosomatics 1992;33:352–6.

[91] Fernandez F, Adams F, Levy JK, Holmes VF, Neidhart M, Mansell PW. Cognitive impairment due to AIDS-related complex and its response to psychostimulants. Psychosomatics 1988;29:38–46.

[92] Katon W, Raskind M. Treatment of depression in the medically ill elderly with methylphenidate. Am J Psychiatry 1980;137:963–5.

[93] US Preventive Servies Task Force. Exercise counseling: guide to clinical preventive services. An assessment of the effectiveness of 169 interventions. Baltimore: Williams & Wilkins; 1989.

[94] Kasch FW, Boyer JL, Van Camp SP, Verity LS, Wallace JP. Effect of exercise on cardiovascular ageing. Age Ageing 1993;22:5–10.

[95] McArdle WD, Katch FI, Katch VL. Enhancement of energy capacity. In: McArdle WD, editor. Exercise physiology: energy, nutrition and human performance. Philadelphia: Lea & Febiger; 1991. p. 423–51.

[96] Nied RJ, Franklin B. Promoting and prescribing exercise for the elderly. Am Fam Physician 2002;65:419–26.

[97] Balady GJ, Berra KA, Golding LA, Gordon NF, Mahler DA, Myers JN, et al. ACSMs guidelines for exercise testing and prescription. 6th edition. Baltimore: Lippincott Williams & Wilkins; 2000.

[98] Buchner DM, Coleman EA. Exercise consideration in older adults: intensity, fall prevention, and safety. Phys Med Rehabil Clin N Am 1994;5:357–75.

[99] Liao S, Ferrell BA. Fatigue in an older population. J Am Geriatr Soc 2000;48:426–30.

[100] Glader EL, Stegmayr B, Asplund K. Poststroke fatigue: a 2-year follow-up study of stroke patients in Sweden. Stroke 2002;33:1327–33.

[101] Stone P, Richards M, A'Hern R, Hardy J. A study to investigate the prevalence, severity and correlates of fatigue among patients with cancer in comparison with a control group of volunteers without cancer. Ann Oncol 2000;11:561–7.

[102] Fuhrer R, Wessely S. The epidemiology of fatigue and depression: a French primary-care study. Psychol Med 1995;25:895–905.

[103] Fisk JD, Pontefract A, Ritvo PG, Archibald CJ, Murray TJ. The impact of fatigue on patients with multiple sclerosis. Can J Neurol Sci 1994;21:9–14.

ELSEVIER
SAUNDERS

Phys Med Rehabil Clin N Am
16 (2005) 109–128

PHYSICAL MEDICINE
AND REHABILITATION
CLINICS OF
NORTH AMERICA

Falls in the elderly population

Julie T. Lin, MD[a,b,*], Joseph M. Lane, MD[c]

[a]*Department of Physiatry, Hospital for Special Surgery, The New York-Presbyterian Hospital, Weill Medical College of Cornell University, New York, NY 10021, USA*
[b]*Department of Rehabilitation Medicine, The New York-Presbyterian Hospital, Weill Medical College of Cornell University, New York, NY 10021, USA*
[c]*Department of Orthopedic Surgery, Hospital for Special Surgery The New York-Presbyterian Hospital, Weill Medical College of Cornell University, New York, NY 10021, USA*

Falls represent a common and significant problem, especially in the elderly population. Falls may often be falsely perceived as a "normal" part of aging [1] by patients and physicians, minimizing the seriousness of falls and their consequences. There are many potentially deleterious consequences of falls, including low-energy fracture in patients with osteoporosis and serious and life-threatening injuries to the brain. Falls can be reflective of underlying pathology and should not be viewed as an independent disease entity [1]. Treatment of falls can be challenging because falls are often multifactorial in nature and because optimal treatment plans incorporate a multimodal approach that addresses all contributing factors.

The risk factors for falling are many and include intrinsic and extrinsic factors [2]. Intrinsic issues include muscle weakness, gait and balance dysfunction, visual impairment, cognitive impairment, depression, functional decline, medications [3], syncope, and postural hypotension. Extrinsic factors consist poor lighting, clutter, environmental obstacles, and ill-footing footwear.

Specific subgroups of patients often require special attention because they frequently have numerous risks for falls. Patients with chronic and disabling medical conditions such as osteoporosis, spinal cord injury, stroke, traumatic brain injury, and amputation are some of the special subpopulations of patients who may be at increased risk for falls. These subgroups are discussed later in this article.

---

* Corresponding author: Hospital for Special Surgery, 535 East 70th Street, New York, NY 10021.

E-mail address: linj@has.edu (J.T. Lin).

1047-9651/05/$ - see front matter © 2004 Elsevier Inc. All rights reserved.
doi:10.1016/j.pmr.2004.06.005

Epidemiology

Falling is the leading cause of death in women and the fourth leading cause of death in men between 65 and 85 years of age and is the leading cause of death for men and women older than 85 years [4]. Two thirds of all accidents among persons older than 65 years of age are due to falls [5]. Less than one fall in 10 results in fracture, but one fall in five requires medical attention [6]. Falls are responsible for serious chronic injuries in the elderly population, such as spinal cord injuries including central cord syndrome [7] and traumatic brain injury; these conditions can increase the risk for more falls. Fall-induced spinal cord injuries secondary to fracture, especially in the elderly population, are on the rise. In Finnish older adults admitted to hospitals from 1 January 1970 through 31 December 1995, the number of spinal cord injuries increased 24% annually, from 60 in 1970 to 419 in 1995 [8].

Falls are the leading mechanism leading to osteoporotic fractures [9], with hip fractures representing one of the most devastating consequences of falls. Falls are strongly associated with hip fractures [10,11], and women with decreased bone mineral density who fall are at highest risk for hip fracture. Women who fall onto their hips have a more than twofold increased risk for fracture for each standard deviation decrease in bone density at the hip [10]. The incidence of hip fractures is increasing 1% to 3% per year in most parts of the world [12]. In 1990, there were 1.7 million hip fractures worldwide [13]; by the year 2050, it is estimated that there will be 6.26 million hip fractures annually [13]. The estimated lifetime risk of hip fracture is 14% in postmenopausal women and 6% in elderly men [14]. Ten to thirteen percent of those who sustain one hip fracture will have another hip fracture [15]. The sequelae of hip fractures can be devastating, with increases in mortality within 6 months of fracture noted [16]. Men have a 31% mortality rate 1 year after fracture, and women have a 10% mortality rate [17]. There is a 20% increased mortality 5 years after hip fracture [18,19]. One year after hip fracture, 40% of patients cannot ambulate independently, 60% have difficulty with at least one essential activity of daily living, 80% are restricted in other activities such as driving, and 27% enter a nursing home for the first time [18].

The consequences of falls are enormous economically and emotionally. Total costs for falls in 1995 are estimated at $37.3 billion, with the costs estimated to be $85.37 billion in 2020 [20]. Economic costs related to osteoporosis treatment in the United States have been estimated at almost $14 billion annually [21]. Less tangible and often underestimated costs to society resulting from osteoporosis include negative impact on quality of life secondary to loss of independence, loss of self-esteem, social isolation, and resulting depression [21,22]. Fear of falling, or "fallophobia" [2], can be debilitating. Formal measures to assess quality of life are needed to highlight the often overlooked deleterious effects of osteoporosis.

Community dwellers versus institutionalized patients

One third of community dwellers older than 65 years of age sustain a fall each year, with 5% of falls resulting in fracture and 5% to 10% resulting in other serious injuries [23]. Fifty percent of elderly institutionalized patients experience falls annually [24]. In nursing homes, the mean incidence of falls is 1.5 falls per bed per year [25]. Risk factors for hip fracture include fall risk, type of fall, type of impact, energy absorption, and bone strength [14]. Specific information on falls in specific subgroups of patients with disabilities including spinal cord injury, traumatic brain injury, multiple sclerosis, Parkinson disease and cerebral palsy is presented later in this article.

Risk factors for falls

Multiple risk factors for falls in the institutionalized frail elderly population have been identified. Intrinsic factors, such as poor vision and peripheral neuropathy, and extrinsic factors, such as environmental factors, have been implicated [26]. In one study involving 181 elderly subjects in three institutions, extrinsic factors were responsible for two thirds of falls, and intrinsic factors were responsible for the remaining one third of falls [27]. Kron et al [28] identified short-term memory loss, transfer assistance, urinary incontinence, positive fall history, and use of trunk restraints as predictors of falls in 472 long-term care residents with a mean age of 84 years. In addition, depressive symptoms, transfer assistance, urinary incontinence, and positive fall history were associated with frequent falls.

Balance deficits are secondary to many causes. Factors including peripheral neuropathy, hypovitaminosis D, and vitamin B12 deficiency are some of the etiologies contributing to poor balance. Patients with osteoporosis and kyphosis have increased postural sway [29].

Peripheral neuropathy in the elderly population is common and is associated with increased falls risk [30,31]. The etiologies of peripheral neuropathy include hereditary disorders such as hereditary motor sensory neuropathies, diabetes mellitus, alcohol, organophosphate poisoning, lead, and the use of medications such as vincristine and dapsone [32].

Hypovitaminosis D affects at least 72% of patients in a falls clinical population [33]. A cross-sectional study correlated the relationship between vitamin D, functional performance, and psychomotor function in elderly people and found that those with the lowest levels of serum 25-hydroxyvitamin D (<12 μg/L) had the greatest degree of postural sway and weakest quadriceps strength [34]. Vitamin D deficiency is often associated with malabsorption syndromes [35] or anorexia nervosa [36]. Therefore, weakness can be secondary to general malnutrition. Vitamin D supplementation in vitamin D-deficient elderly people can improve muscle strength, walking distance, and functional ability and results in decreased falls and nonvertebral fractures [37].

Vitamin B12 deficiency can result in peripheral neuropathy, spinal cord degeneration, and altered mental status [38]. Vitamin B12 deficiency may primarily affect the central nervous system [39]. Vitamin B12 deficiency among elderly outpatients has a reported high prevalence. Yao et al [40] demonstrated that 16% of geriatric patients had cobalamin levels of 200 pg/mL or below, with 21% of patients having levels between 201 and 299 pg/mL; these prevalences are higher than reported previously in other studies.

Sleep problems [41,42] and insomnia are significant risk factors for falls resulting in major injury [31]. Medications used for insomnia, especially the longer-acting benzodiazepine receptor agonists, are associated with increased risk of falls and hip fracture in the elderly population [43].

The use of multiple medications is a risk factor for falls. In particular, psychotropic medications such as antidepressants, narcotic pain killers, and anti-convulsants are associated with increased falls risk [44–46]. Furthermore, there is increased risk of any nonspine fracture in elderly women taking narcotic and antidepressant medication, with a 1.7-fold increase in the risk for hip fracture in those taking anti-depressant medications [47].

Vision impairments are a prominent risk factor for falls. Visual function measurements such as visual acuity, contrast sensitivity, and depth perception may provide valuable information in identifying patients at greatest risk for falls [48,49]. These visual impairments are potentially reversible in at least 70% of patients [50]. Multifocal glasses limit depth perception and edge-contrast sensitivity at critical distances for perceiving environmental obstacles and thus increase falls risk [51].

Inappropriate footwear may increase fall risk [52]. Ill-fitting footwear or footwear that does not adequately support the foot (eg, high heels) can increase the likelihood for falls. In addition, slippery soles can increase the risk of slipping. One study [53] found that the most common type of footwear worn at the time of falls were slippers (22%), followed by walking shoes (17%) and sandals (8%). Seventy-five percent of patients in the study wore shoes that were deficient in some way, including excessively flexible heel counters and excessively flexible soles.

Sarcopenia, or age-related loss in skeletal muscle, is associated with aging and is a risk factor for falls [54]. Sarcopenia also has adverse effects on bone density [55].

Spasticity may be present in any disease states involving upper motor neurons, such as multiple sclerosis, traumatic brain injury, stroke, and spinal cord injury. Spasticity of the lower extremities can make supporting one's body impossible; similarly, spasticity of the upper extremities can contribute to instability by making it difficult to hold onto grab bars and assistive devices. Increased body sway has been noted with increasing age [56,57], contributing to falls risk.

Postural changes, such as in kyphosis, scoliosis, and leg length discrepancies, can alter one's center of gravity and impair balance. For example, patients with osteoporotic vertebral fracture and resulting kyphosis have postural changes that make it difficult to maintain their centers of gravity. Furthermore, patients who have had limb injuries or who have diseases such as cerebrovascular accident have alterations in their posture that can make affect maintaining balance.

Dementia is an independent risk factor for fall. Van Doorn et al [58] performed a study in nursing home residents with and without dementia and found that residents with dementia fall more often than their residents without dementia. Traumatic brain injury resulting in altered cognition and impulsiveness can be assumed to similarly increase falls risk.

Mechanisms of injury

Syncope

Etiologies of syncope include cardiac and neurogenic causes. Cardiac causes include atrial fibrillation, atrioventricular blocks, sick sinus syndrome, and carotid sinus syndromes [59,60]. Neurogenic causes of syncope include orthostasis secondary to orthostatic hypotension, autonomic disturbances, and the vasovagal reaction [61,62].

Dizziness

Dizziness is common in elderly patients and can be divided into four subtypes: vertigo, pre-syncopal lightheadedness, disequilibrium, and other dizziness [63]. Its etiologies are typically multifactorial, including causes such as vestibular etiologies (eg, benign positional vertigo). Hypoglycemia in diabetic patients can cause autonomic and neuroglycopenic symptoms, including altered cognitive functioning and increased anxiety [64], both of which may increase the likelihood of fall.

Accidents related to transfers and wheelchair/prosthetics and orthotics use

There are many mechanisms of injury in falls, with unique considerations in specific subgroups of patients. For example, in the spinal cord injury population, wheelchair-related falls represent a significant risk. In a retrospective review of 45 medical records of patients with spinal cord injuries who sustained fractures, there were 31 fractures sustained in 27 fall episodes in 24 subjects. Contributing factors included loss of balance, equipment failure, muscle spasm, excessive speed, not wearing protective straps, and narcolepsy. Amputees also have special fall risks because they often have significant fear of falling and falls: in one study, 52.4% reported falling in the past year, and 49.2% reported a fear of falling [65]. Amputees can have increased risk of falls during transfers [66] and wheelchair transfers, especially with difficulty with brakes [67]. The specific incidence of falls related to the use of prosthetics and orthotics has not been reported in the literature.

Poor vision

Impaired vision is a risk factor for falls [25,68]. Poor vision can hinder perception of one's surroundings, thus increasing the likelihood for tripping and slipping over obstacles and hindering one's protective responses of finding objects to hold on to for support.

Environmental hazards

Environmental hazards are risk factor for falls [3,52]. Slippery floors, throw rugs, and clutter can contribute to falls. In addition, poor lighting and inadequate structural supports, such as the lack of grab bars in a bathroom, can compound these risks.

Diagnosis

History

A thorough history involving review of the risk factors can provide key information. The mnemonic "SPLATT" [69], which stands for Symptoms, Previous Falls, Location, Activity, Time, and Trauma, can be used to document the key components of the fall history.

Physical examination

Assessing gait, including heel, toe, and tandem gait, can help to identify specific muscle group deficiencies and unsafe gait patterns. The need for assistive devices such as walkers or canes can be evaluated at this time. Traditional neurologic screening tools used during physical examination can help to assess patients at risk for falls. Sensory deficits seen in stroke patients or those with peripheral neuropathy may be assessed with the use of light touch, pinprick, vibration, proprioception, and neurofilament testing. Proprioception may also be assessed by performing the Romberg [26]. Cerebellar deficits can be assessed with heel-to-shin and rapid alternating movements. Gross visual deficits can be detected by using eye charts to assess overall visual acuity with more detailed testing as needed performed by an ophthalmologist. Manual muscle strength testing can identify focal or gross muscular weaknesses.

Several neuromuscular assessments may be used in evaluating an elderly patient at risk for falls. These add useful clinical information because standard physical assessments have been found to be insufficient to detect functional deficits [70]. The "get up and go" test [71,72] involves recording the amount of time it takes a patient to arise from a chair, walk several meters, and return to the chair. Patients should be able to perform single limb stance for at least 12 seconds. The 6-minute walk, in which the distance walked in six minutes is measured, has also been identified as a powerful functional tool in osteoporotic patients (JT Lin, unpublished observation). The functional reach test, a measure of flexibility and balance, may also be easily performed in the office. Using a fixed base of support, the difference between arm's length and maximal forward reach is documented. This test is a good approximator of stability and is useful in designing modified environments in impaired elderly persons [73,74]. In nonambulatory patients, such as those with amputations spinal cord injury, traumatic brain injury, multiple sclerosis, and Parkinson disease, performance of these functional tests may be impossible. Assessing how these patients transfer or ambulate short distances may provide all the information that is needed. Evaluation of patients with amputations should include inspection of their prostheses and assessment of their gait. The soft tissues around the amputated site should be inspected for evidence of skin breakdown.

Postural hypotension may be monitored with the use of blood pressure and pulse monitoring, especially when changing positions, such as supine to sitting or sitting to standing. Conditions such as benign positional vertigo can be identified with the use of a rapid position change from the sitting to head-hanging position in the presence of nystagmus and electronystagmography [75]. More detailed assessments of the middle ear can be provided by an otolaryngologist.

Laboratory studies to detect potentially reversible medical conditions such as vitamin D deficiency, vitamin B12 deficiency, and diabetes mellitus should be performed. Diagnostic imaging including radiographs, MRI, and CT can rule out new serious medical conditions such as cerebrovascular accident, spinal cord injury, or traumatic brain injury secondary to recurrent falls. Nerve conduction studies/electromyography testing should be considered an extension of the physical examination and can help provide additional information in the assessment of peripheral neuropathy, radiculopathy, myopathies, focal compression neuropathies, and diseases of the neuromuscular junction. Somatosensory-evoked potentials can help to detect vitamin B12 deficiency [76].

Management of falls

Recurring falls should be managed with a multifaceted treatment approach. First, medical treatment should be initiated for reversible or potentially reversible medical conditions such as nutritional deficiencies, diabetes mellitus, visual impairments, and underlying cardiac diseases. Interventions in elderly patients in the community and nursing home setting include multifaceted treatment approaches. Interventions likely to be beneficial in reducing falls include programs of muscle strengthening and balance retraining; a 15-week Tai Chi exercise intervention; home hazard assessment and modification; withdrawal of psychotropic medication; and a multidisciplinary, multifactorial, health/environmental risk factor screening and intervention program [6]. Stevens et al [77] showed that interventions consisting of home hazard assessments; education strategies on fall hazard reduction and methods to reduce home hazards; and free installation of safety devices including grab rails, nonslip stripping on steps, and double-sided tape for floor rugs and mats resulted in a reduction in the mean number of hazards per house. Simple interventions in the nursing home setting including environmental modifications, increased staffing, and restorative activity programs can decrease the number of falls [78]. Repositioning furniture, adding an additional staff member during the peak incidence of falls, and adding a program in situations of high falls incidence resulted in a 38% reduction in the number of falls and a 50% reduction in the total number of fractures [78]. A cluster randomized, nonblinded controlled trial involving nine residential facilities evaluated the effectiveness of a multifactorial fall and injury prevention program in older people [79]. This program included staff education, environmental adjustment exercise, drug review, aids, hip protectors, and postfall problem-solving conferences. The authors found a significant reduction of falls in the intervention group involving patients with higher Mini-Mental Status Examination versus those with lower scores, suggesting that cognition plays a significant role in a fall prevention program.

Exercise programs

Exercise programs including Tai Chi Chuan and medically supervised, goal-directed rehabilitation programs are important for the patient who is at increased falls risk. A comprehensive physical therapy program should be tailored to the needs of the patient but should generally include balance training, gait training with appropriate assistive devices, strengthening exercises of the upper and lower extremities, transfer training, energy conservation techniques, safety awareness, and a home exercise program. Adaptive equipment such as grab bars should be provided.

Tai Chi Chuan, a Chinese martial art, is one of the most efficacious exercises in fall risk reduction and has been shown to decrease the risk of multiple falls by nearly 50% [80]. Similarly, Tae Kwon Do, a Korean martial art, can increase balance time on each foot and may similarly reduce falls risk [81].

Vestibular therapy

Various maneuvers such as the Epley and Semont maneuvers can help to serve diagnostic and therapeutic roles [82–85] and can be performed by appropriately trained clinicians. The Epley maneuver, a treatment for canalithiasis [86,87], starts with the Dix-Hillpike manuever, turning the head to the opposite side before sitting up, waiting 6 to 13 seconds between position changes [88]. The Semont maneuver, a treatment for cupulothiasis [89], involves facing the head away from the involved side. The head is tilted backward and toward the involved side, then tilted nose-downward toward the uninvolved side while facing away from the involved side. The patient sits up for 2 to 3 minutes between position changes [89].

Hip protectors

Hip protectors, which are orthoses comprised of undergarments with hip pads placed over the trochanters, are indicated in the elderly patient with fall risk. Many different types of hip protectors are available, and they have been shown to be inexpensive, simple, and efficacious. A randomized controlled trial demonstrated that the use of external hip protectors resulted in reduction in falls risk in elderly community dwellers [90]. Cameron et al [90] demonstrated that in 600 women 74 years of age or older, the risk of hip fracture when falling while wearing hip protectors compared with a fall with no hip protector in place was significantly reduced (relative risk 0.23). Numerous studies have demonstrated that hip protector use is cost-effective. Waldegger et al [91] performed a meta-analysis investigating the cost-effectiveness of hip protectors in an elderly population living in institutions. They found that hip protectors compared with controls resulted in a relative risk of hip fracture of 0.40. The use of hip protectors can help to increase self-esteem, which is an important issue in patients who have experienced falls in the past. Often, these patients fear that fall is imminent. Cameron et al [92] noted that those who wore hip protectors had improved self-efficacy or the belief in their ability to avoid falling. The main drawback to hip protector use is their low compliance. Patients typically cite discomfort, bulkiness of the hip protectors, and difficulty dressing with the hip protectors as their main criticisms.

Safety floor

A safety floor made of a padded material that absorbs impact and cushions falls has been suggested but has not been manufactured for distribution.

Environmental modifications

A home environmental assessment by an experienced physical therapist to identify environmental hazards in the home, such as throw rugs, slippery floors, poor furniture layout, and obstacles, can minimize fall risk. Assessments by caretakers may also be made using the general guidelines outlined in Table 1. For institutionalized patients, a similar assessment can provide useful information.

Table 1
Home modifications pearls room by room [69,104]

Room	Problem	Correction
Kitchen	Wet or waxed floor	Place rubber mat in sink area; use nonslip wax; wear rubber-soled shoes in kitchen; use nonslip strips on floor
	Cabinets and shelves too high	Keep common items at waist level; install shelves at lower level; use hand-held reacher
Bathroom	Slippery tub floor	Use rubber mat or nonslip strips; use shower shoes or bath seat
	Toilet seat too low	Use elevated toilet seat
	Inadequate wall supports	Install grab rails
Bedroom	Slippery throw rugs	Attach adhesive strips to rugs
	Frayed carpet or rugs	Repair or replace worn rugs or carpeting
	Inadequate lighting	Provide adequate lighting, especially if patient gets up frequently in the middle of night
	Excessive clutter	Avoid obstacles in the bedroom
	Inadequate supports	Ensure adequate grab rails and objects to be held for support

Physical restraints

Physical restraints are often used in rehabilitation facilities to help prevent falls, especially for patients with history of prior fall or risk factors such as impulsivity. Their use has not been shown to prevent the risk of falls [93], and therefore they are not a recommended modality in fall prevention. Some studies have suggested that they may increase falls risk and associated injuries [94].

Medication management

Medications should be reviewed and assessed for need, fall potential, and potential interactions. Unnecessary or redundant medications that can increase falls risk should be eliminated. Review of medications should be performed regularly, with patients encouraged to keep track of all medications prescribed by their various practitioners.

Monitoring devices for falls and syncope

Devices including quantitative measures of postural sway, blood pressure monitoring using a noninvasive digital photoplethysmographic device, and long-term ECG monitoring can be useful in the assessment of patients who fall [95]. Alarm devices, which are attached to a bed, chair, or wheelchair, are used for patients at falls risk who are attempting dangerous bed or chair transfers. These alarms allow residents to maintain a free movement zone but alarm if residents leave their chair or bed [96] and may be a superior alternative to physical restraints in the nursing home setting. One case-controlled study involving 70 patients at falls risk demonstrated that the alarm devices were an acceptable method of preventing falls [97].

Case study

WL is an 83-year-old man with a past medical history of diabetes mellitus and recurrent falls. He has had an increasing number of falls recently, which began with one specific fall 1.5 years ago. Since then, it has been "all downhill" according to the patient and his wife, and they are depressed about his lack of function. They live in a duplex apartment in Manhattan, which they admit is not fall friendly. Recently, they both fell down a flight of stairs. The patient sustained rib fractures, and his wife sustained vertebral compression fractures. The patient relates his falls occasionally to turning his head. The patient ambulates with a straight cane. He has been receiving physical therapy at home for several months.

Past medical history is positive for poorly controlled diabetes mellitus for 30 years. The patient was recently admitted to the hospital after a fall. According to the patient, he had a number of tests performed, all of which were negative. He mentions something about the diagnosis of "hypotension." Although the patient is aware that he should keep his blood sugars low, he states that he "feels better" when his blood sugar is kept in a slightly higher range, close to the 200s. He has been maintaining his blood sugars in this range for many years. He states that he does not have an internist who is coordinating his medical care. The patient and his wife have some difficulty communicating the issues at hand, including the names of their physicians and the various testing that has been performed. The wife is noted to be generally frail, complains of back pain secondary to vertebral compression fractures sustained during the fall, and is noted to doze off several times during the interview.

Physical examination reveals an elderly man with slightly depressed affect who ambulates with a slow, unsteady, and shuffling gait without the use of his rolling walker. He has difficulty performing heel gait. He is noted to have a mild thoracic kyphosis. His lower extremities are discolored. Sensation is diminished to light touch in a stocking glove distribution in his lower extremities. Manual muscle strength (MMS) testing reveals mild weakness in the bilateral hamstrings, left dorsiflexors, and bilateral hip abductors (MMS 4+). When the patient changes position from supine to sitting to standing, he reports some dizziness.

Recommendations for this patient include an environmental assessment and modification by the physical therapist; nerve conduction studies/electromyography to determine the presence of peripheral neuropathy; hip protectors to be worn as tolerated; physical therapy for tilt table exercises, balance exercises, and continued strengthening exercises of the bilateral lower extremities; vestibular therapy for benign positional vertigo; hip protectors; bone mineral density testing to determine the presence of osteopenia or osteoporosis; consideration of a lumbosacral MRI to workup the weakness in the L5 myotome; referral to an internist for general medical care; and a prescription for a wheelchair to be used when the patient wants to be mobile for prolonged time periods. In addition, the patient was advised to discuss with his internist the importance of adequate blood sugar control. A request for prior laboratory studies, including those performed during his most recent hospital stay, was made. Monitoring of the patient's depressed mood was to be performed, with appropriate referral for psychiatric evaluation as needed. Nerve conduction studies/electromyography demonstrated severe axonal sensorimotor peripheral neuropathy. The patient has also continued to receive physical therapy at home but has had difficulties with transportation to vestibular therapy. He wishes to defer the use of hip protectors, bone mineral density testing, and referral to psychiatrist. He has an appointment to see an internist in the near future. Review of the requested medical records demonstrates documentation of "autonomic hypotension" secondary to his diabetes mellitus. He continues to be counseled on the importance of addressing all of the suggested recommendations; he states he will slowly fulfill these recommendations.

This case study demonstrates the complexity of issues in an elderly patient with history of recurrent falls. In this patient, multiple factors contributing to falls include the presence of severe axonal sensorimotor peripheral neuropathy that was diagnosed on nerve conduction studies/electromyography, the presence of autonomic hypotension secondary to diabetes, weakness in the bilateral lower extremities, thoracic kyphosis (which alters the patient's center of gravity), environmental hazards in the home (including a slippery floor and the lack of grab bars), benign positional vertigo, and somewhat compromised cognition. In addition, the patient's wife had physical impairments secondary to overall frailty and the recent vertebral compression fractures resulting from fall. The patient deferred undergoing the bone mineral density testing secondary to difficulty with transportation. The approach to this patient requires perseverance and dedication on the part of the physician, patient, and family members. This patient has some limitations due to the overall frailty and mild cognitive deficits that he and his wife possess. Continued reinforcement and close follow-up with the physician are needed to ensure that the risks of fall in this patient are minimized.

Advice for caretakers and families

Many older patients may not accept recommendations to minimize falls risk, a concern that must be addressed appropriately. Cumming et al [98] demonstrated that in 121 homes revisited after 12 months, 419 home modifications had been recommended, and 52% were met with partial or complete adherence. Predictors of adherence were a belief that home modifications can prevent falls and having help at home from relatives.

Encouragement by caretakers and families to use the discussed treatment measures, including exercise programs and the use of hip protectors, can help to increase compliance. Poor compliance [99,100] remains a major drawback to the successful implementation of hip protectors.

Caregivers of patients with disabilities or patients who are wheelchair bound should pay special attention to transfers and to the condition of the wheelchair, including functioning and easily accessible brakes. Caregivers should be aware of proper body mechanics and their own physical limitations in providing support to patients.

Recognition of the psychologic aspects of recurrent falls, especially "fallophobia" [2], is important because patients who have an overwhelming fear of falling may turn this fear into a self-fulfilling prophecy. Fear of falling can lead to low self-esteem, social isolation, and depression as patients limit their activities and remain largely housebound. Psychologic counseling may prove beneficial in reducing these fears.

In addition, caretakers and family members should understand that recurrent falls are usually multifactorial in nature, with factors such as sarcopenia, psychotropic medications, and environmental hazards. Therefore, a multifaceted approach can best serve the patient. Addressing each of the contributing factors can be a laborious and difficult task for the physician, caregiver, and patient, but patience and perseverance can help to minimize fall risks for the patient. In a nursing home setting, the use of a multidisciplinary team that addresses risk may best suit the patient [101].

Future areas of inquiry and research

Future areas of research include identifying the most efficacious screening tests for identifying those at highest risk for falls. For example, a questionnaire that includes physical examination findings may best identify those at highest risk for falls, with broad implementation enabling physicians to identify those at highest risk for falls.

Additional areas of research include the identification minimalization of patient objections to hip protectors and assistive devices. The cost effectiveness, in terms of economic and quality of life measures, of the widespread development of "Fall Clinics" and similar geriatrics clinics specializing in falls remains an unanswered question to the problem of falls in the elderly population.

Summary

Falls among elderly persons remain a difficult problem with few easy solutions. Falls are symptomatic of underlying clinical deficits, and a multidisciplinary approach is essential in identifying the risk factors and appropriate treatments for these patients. Patients with chronic medical conditions, such as spinal cord injury, traumatic brain injury, and amputations, possess additional unique risk factors that must be addressed.

Interventions include treatment of potentially reversible medical conditions such as B12 and vitamin D deficiencies and home modifications, balance and exercise training programs, medication modification, hip protectors, and monitoring devices.

Physicians, patients, family members, and caretakers should be reminded that minimizing falls risk requires persistence, patience, and dedication. Progress may not be noted overnight, but adherence to recommendations correcting intrinsic and extrinsic factors can help to minimize falls and their potentially devastating complications (see Appendix 1 and 2).

Appendix 1

Key resources for clinicians and family members

General information

1. National Institute of Arthritis and Musculoskeletal and Skin Diseases (www.nih.gov/niams). Address: Information Clearinghouse National Institutes of Health, 1 AMS Circle, Bethesda, MD 20892-3675. Phone: (301) 495-4484 or (877) 22-NIAMS (toll free); TTY: (301) 565-2966; fax: (301) 718-6366; e-mail address: niamsinfo@mail.nih.gov
2. National Institute of Neurological Disorders and Stroke (www.ninds.nih.gov). Address: NIH Neurological Institute, P.O. Box 5801, Bethesda, MD 20824. Phone: (800) 352-9424 or (301) 496-5751; TTY: (301) 468-5981.
3. National Osteoporosis Foundation (www.nof.org). Address: National Osteoporosis Foundation, 1232 22nd Street NW, Washington, DC 20037-1292. Phone: (202) 223-2226.
4. American Academy of Physical Medicine and Rehabilitation (www.aapmr.org). Address: American Academy of Physical Medicine and Rehabilitation, One IBM Plaza, Suite 2500, Chicago, IL 60611-3604. Phone: (312) 464-9700.

Products

Hip protectors may be purchased directly through manufacturers (Safehip Hip Protectors [Tytex Group]: www.tytex.com) or through commercial web sites, including www.hipprotector.com and www.epill.com.

Appendix 2

Pearls for prevention of falls in people with disabilities

1. Spinal cord injury

   - Be mindful of wheelchair transfers because these are strongly associated with falls.

2. Traumatic brain injury

   - Patients may require additional supervision due to impaired cognition and impulsivity.

3. Multiple sclerosis

   - Patients with multiple sclerosis can be predicted to have increased falls risk if they have impaired balance, impaired ability to walk, and difficulties using a cane [102].
   - Patients must be careful when performing transfers secondary to weakness and spasticity.

4. Parkinson disease

   - Patients with Parkinson disease have poor postural reflexes, which can result in increased falls risk. This patient population has been shown to have significant fear of falling compared with age-matched control subjects, which, when coupled with poor balance, can increase risk of falls [103]. Therefore, patients with Parkinson disease who possess fear of falling should receive special attention.

5. Amputees

   - Patients must pay special attention to transfers and to the condition of prosthetics/orthotics and wheelchairs.

6. Cerebral palsy

   - Patients must pay special attention to transfers and ambulation secondary to weakness and spasticity. If there is cognitive involvement, impulsivity must be monitored.

References

[1] Tideiksaar R. Falls in the elderly. Bull N Y Acad Med 1988;64:145–63.
[2] Tideiksaar R, Kay AD. What causes falls? A logical diagnostic procedure. Geriatrics 1986; 41:32–50.
[3] Rubenstein LZ, Josephson KR. The epidemiology of falls and syncope. Clin Geriatr Med 2002;18:141–58.
[4] Long L. Fall prevention & intervention in home care. Caring 2003;22:8–10.

[5] Lange M. The challenge of fall prevention in home care: a review of the literature. Home Healthcare Nurse 1996;14:198–206.

[6] Gillespie LD, Gillespie WJ, Robertson MC, Lamb SE, Cumming RG, Rowe BH. Interventions for preventing falls in elderly people. Cochrane Database Syst Rev 2001; CD000340.

[7] Lovasik D. The older patient with a spinal cord injury. Crit Care Nurs Q 1999;22:20–30.

[8] Kannus P, Niemi S, Palvanen M, Parkkari J. Continuously increasing number and incidence of fall-induced, fracture-associated, spinal cord injuries in elderly persons. Arch Intern Med 2000;160:2145–9.

[9] Suh TT, Lyles KW. Osteoporosis considerations in the frail elderly. Curr Opin Rheumatol 2003;15:481–6.

[10] Nevitt MC, Cummings SR. Type of fall and risk of hip and wrist fractures: the study of osteoporotic fractures. The Study of Osteoporotic Fractures Research Group. J Am Geriatr Soc 1993;41:1226–34.

[11] Cummings SR, Nevitt MC. A hypothesis: the causes of hip fractures. J Gerontol 1989;44: M107–11.

[12] Cummings SR, Melton LJ. Epidemiology and outcomes of osteoporotic fractures. Lancet 2002;359:1761–7.

[13] Kannus P, Parkkari J, Sievanen H, Heinonen A, Vuori I, Jarvinen M. Epidemiology of hip fractures. Bone 1996;18(Suppl):57S–63S.

[14] Lauritzen JB. Hip fractures: epidemiology, risk factors, falls, energy absorption, hip protectors, and prevention. Dan Med Bull 1997;44:155–68.

[15] Pearse EO, Redfern DJ, Sinha M, Edge AJ. Outcome following a second hip fracture. Injury 2003;34:518–21.

[16] Magaziner J, Simonsick EM, Kashner TM, Hebel JR, Kenzora JE. Survival experience of aged hip fracture patients. Am J Public Health 1989;79:274–8.

[17] Campion JM, Maricic MJ. Osteoporosis in men. Am Fam Physician 2003;67:1521–6.

[18] Cooper C. The crippling consequences of fractures and their impact on quality of life. Am J Med 1997;103:12S–7S.

[19] Cooper C, Atkinson EJ, Jacobsen SJ, O'Fallon WM, Melton LJ III. Population-based study of survival after osteoporotic fractures. Am J Epidemiol 1993;137:1001–5.

[20] Englander F, Hodson TJ, Terregrossa RA. Economic dimensions of slip and fall injuries. J Forensic Sci 1996;41:733–46.

[21] Iqbal MM. Osteoporosis: epidemiology, diagnosis, and treatment. South Med J 2000;93: 2–18.

[22] Gold DT. The nonskeletal consequences of osteoporotic fractures: psychologic and social outcomes. Rheum Dis Clin North Am 2001;27:255–62.

[23] Dargent-Molina P, Breart G. [Epidemiology of falls and fall-related injuries in the aged]. Rev Epidemiol Sante Publique 1995;43:72–83.

[24] Six P. [Epidemiology of falls and hip fractures]. Schweiz Rundsch Med Prax 1992;81: 1378–82.

[25] Rubenstein LZ, Josephson KR, Osterweil D. Falls and fall prevention in the nursing home. Clin Geriatr Med 1996;12:881–902.

[26] Tideiksaar R. Geriatric falls: assessing the cause, preventing recurrence. Geriatrics 1989;44: 57–61, 64.

[27] Suzuki M, Okamura T, Shimazu Y, Takahashi H, Eguchi K, Kano K, et al. [A study of falls experienced by institutionalized elderly.], Nippon Koshu Eisei Zasshi 1992;39:927–40.

[28] Kron M, Loy S, Sturm E, Nikolaus T, Becker C. Risk indicators for falls in institutionalized frail elderly. Am J Epidemiol 2003;158:645–53.

[29] Lynn SG, Sinaki M, Westerlind KC. Balance characteristics of persons with osteoporosis. Arch Phys Med Rehabil 1997;78:273–7.

[30] Richardson JK, Ashton-Miller JA. Peripheral neuropathy: an often-overlooked cause of falls in the elderly. Postgrad Med 1996;99:161–72.

[31] Koski K, Luukinen H, Laippala P, Kivela SL. Risk factors for major injurious falls among the home-dwelling elderly by functional abilities: a prospective population-based study. Gerontology 1998;44:232–8.

[32] Donofrio PD, Albers JW. AAEM minimonograph #34: polyneuropathy: classification by nerve conduction studies and electromyography. Muscle Nerve 1990;13:889–903.

[33] Dhesi JK, Moniz C, Close JC, Jackson SH, Allain TJ. A rationale for vitamin D prescribing in a falls clinic population. Age Ageing 2002;31:267–71.

[34] Dhesi JK, Bearne LM, Moniz C, Hurley MV, Jackson SH, Swift CG, et al. Neuromuscular and psychomotor function in elderly subjects who fall and the relationship with vitamin D status. J Bone Miner Res 2002;17:891–7.

[35] Basha B, Rao DS, Han ZH, Parfitt AM. Osteomalacia due to vitamin D depletion: a neglected consequence of intestinal malabsorption. Am J Med 2000;108:296–300.

[36] Fonseca VA, D'Souza V, Houlder S, Thomas M, Wakeling A, Dandona P. Vitamin D deficiency and low osteocalcin concentrations in anorexia nervosa. J Clin Pathol 1988;41: 195–7.

[37] Janssen HC, Samson MM, Verhaar HJ. Vitamin D deficiency, muscle function, and falls in elderly people. Am J Clin Nutr 2002;75:611–5.

[38] Roach ES, McLean WT. Neurologic disorders of vitamin B12 deficiency. Am Fam Physician 1982;25:111–5.

[39] Jones SJ, Yu YL, Rudge P, Kriss A, Gilois C, Hirani N, et al. Central and peripheral SEP defects in neurologically symptomatic and asymptomatic subjects with low vitamin B12 levels. J Neurol Sci 1987;82:55–65.

[40] Yao Y, Yao SL, Yao SS, Yao G, Lou W. Prevalence of vitamin B12 deficiency among geriatric outpatients. J Fam Pract 1992;35:524–8.

[41] Brassington GS, King AC, Bliwise DL. Sleep problems as a risk factor for falls in a sample of community-dwelling adults aged 64–99 years. J Am Geriatr Soc 2000;48: 1234–40.

[42] Suzuki M, Okamura T, Shimazu Y, Takahashi H, Eguchi K, Kano K, et al. [A study of falls experienced by institutionalized elderly.] Nippon Koshu Eisei Zasshi 1992;39:927–40.

[43] Ancoli-Israel S. Insomnia in the elderly: a review for the primary care practitioner. Sleep 2000;23(Suppl 1):S23–30.

[44] Cumming RG. Epidemiology of medication-related falls and fractures in the elderly. Drugs Aging 1998;12:43–53.

[45] Monane M, Avorn J. Medications and falls: causation, correlation, and prevention. Clin Geriatr Med 1996;12:847–58.

[46] Kelly KD, Pickett W, Yiannakoulias N, Rowe BH, Schopflocher DP, Svenson L, et al. Medication use and falls in community-dwelling older persons. Age Ageing 2003;32: 503–9.

[47] Ensrud KE, Blackwell T, Mangione CM, Bowman PJ, Bauer DC, Schwartz A, et al. Central nervous system active medications and risk for fractures in older women. Arch Intern Med 2003;163:949–57.

[48] Abdelhafiz AH, Austin CA. Visual factors should be assessed in older people presenting with falls or hip fracture. Age Ageing 2003;32:26–30.

[49] Legood R, Scuffham P, Cryer C. Are we blind to injuries in the visually impaired? A review of the literature. Inj Prev 2002;8:155–60.

[50] Harwood RH. Visual problems and falls. Age Ageing 2001;30(Suppl 4):13–8.

[51] Lord SR, Dayhew J, Howland A. Multifocal glasses impair edge-contrast sensitivity and depth perception and increase the risk of falls in older people. J Am Geriatr Soc 2002;50: 1760–6.

[52] Unsworth J. Falls in older people: the role of assessment in prevention and care. Br J Community Nurs 2003;8:256–62.

[53] Sherrington C, Menz HB. An evaluation of footwear worn at the time of fall-related hip fracture. Age Ageing 2003;32:310–4.

[54] Marcus R. Relationship of age-related decreases in muscle mass and strength to skeletal status. J Gerontol Biol Sci 1995;50A:86–7.

[55] Evans WJ. What is sarcopenia? J Gerontol Biol Sci 1995;50A:5–8.

[56] Peterka RJ, Black FO. Age-related changes in human posture control: motor coordination tests. J Vestib Res 1990;1:87–96.

[57] Peterka RJ, Black FO. Age-related changes in human posture control: sensory organization tests. J Vestib Res 1990;1:73–85.

[58] van Doorn C, Gruber-Baldini AL, Zimmerman S, Hebel JR, Port CL, Baumgarten M, et al. Dementia as a risk factor for falls and fall injuries among nursing home residents. J Am Geriatr Soc 2003;51:1213–8.

[59] Maurer MS, Bloomfield DM. Atrial fibrillation and falls in the elderly. Clin Geriatr Med 2002;18:323–37.

[60] Kenny RA, Richardson DA. Carotid sinus syndrome and falls in older adults. Am J Geriatr Cardiol 2001;10:97–9.

[61] Mathias CJ. To stand on one's own legs. Clin Med 2002;2:237–45.

[62] Masaki Y, Furukawa T, Watanabe M, Ichikawa G. [Effect of adrenaline on vagus nerve reflexes.] Nippon Jibiinkoka Gakkai Kaiho 1999;102:891–7.

[63] Salles N, Kressig RW, Michel JP. Management of chronic dizziness in elderly people. Z Gerontol Geriatr 2003;36:10–5.

[64] Frier BM. Hypoglycaemia and cognitive function in diabetes. Int J Clin Pract Suppl 2001; 123:30–7.

[65] Miller WC, Speechley M, Deathe B. The prevalence and risk factors of falling and fear of falling among lower extremity amputees. Arch Phys Med Rehabil 2001;82:1031–7.

[66] Gonzalez EG, Mathews MM. Femoral fractures in patients with lower extremity amputations. Arch Phys Med Rehabil 1980;61:276–80.

[67] Kirby RL, Smith C. Fall during a wheelchair transfer: a case of mismatched brakes. Am J Phys Med Rehabil 2001;80:302–4.

[68] Rubenstein LZ, Josephson KR, Robbins AS. Falls in the nursing home. Ann Intern Med 1994;121:442–51.

[69] Tideiksaar R. Preventing falls: how to identify risk factors, reduce complications. Geriatrics 1996;51:43–50, 53.

[70] Tinetti ME, Ginter SF. Identifying mobility dysfunctions in elderly patients: a standard neuromuscular examination or direct assessment? JAMA 1988;259:1190–3.

[71] Podsiadlo D, Richardson S. The timed "Up & Go": a test of basic functional mobility for frail elderly persons. J Am Geriatr Soc 1991;39:142–8.

[72] Mathias S, Nayak US, Isaacs B. Balance in elderly patients: the "get-up and go" test. Arch Phys Med Rehabil 1986;67:387–9.

[73] Duncan PW, Weiner DK, Chandler J, Studenski S. Functional reach: a new clinical measure of balance. J Gerontol 1990;45:M192–7.

[74] Weiner DK, Duncan PW, Chandler J, Studenski SA. Functional reach: a marker of physical frailty. J Am Geriatr Soc 1992;40:203–7.

[75] Baloh RW, Honrubia V, Jacobson K. Benign positional vertigo: clinical and oculographic features in 240 cases. Neurology 1987;37:371–8.

[76] Jones SJ, Yu YL, Rudge P, Kriss A, Gilois C, Hirani N, et al. Central and peripheral SEP defects in neurologically symptomatic and asymptomatic subjects with low vitamin B12 levels. J Neurol Sci 1987;82:55–65.

[77] Stevens M, Holman CD, Bennett N. Preventing falls in older people: impact of an intervention to reduce environmental hazards in the home. J Am Geriatr Soc 2001;49: 1442–7.

[78] Hofmann MT, Bankes PF, Javed A, Selhat M. Decreasing the incidence of falls in the nursing home in a cost-conscious environment: a pilot study. J Am Med Dir Assoc 2003;4: 95–7.

[79] Jensen J, Nyberg L, Gustafson Y, Lundin-Olsson L. Fall and injury prevention in residential care: effects in residents with higher and lower levels of cognition. J Am Geriatr Soc 2003;51:627–35.

[80] Wolf SL, Barnhart HX, Kutner NG, McNeely E, Coogler C, Xu T. Selected as the best paper in the 1990s: reducing frailty and falls in older persons: an investigation of tai chi and computerized balance training. J Am Geriatr Soc 2003;51:1794–803.

[81] Brudnak MA, Dundero D, Van Hecke FM. Are the 'hard' martial arts, such as the Korean martial art, TaeKwon-Do, of benefit to senior citizens? Med Hypotheses 2002;59:485–91.

[82] Haynes DS, Resser JR, Labadie RF, Girasole CR, Kovach BT, Scheker LE, et al. Treatment of benign positional vertigo using the semont maneuver: efficacy in patients presenting without nystagmus. Laryngoscope 2002;112:796–801.

[83] Ruckenstein MJ. Therapeutic efficacy of the Epley canalith repositioning maneuver. Laryngoscope 2001;111:940–5.

[84] Dal T, Ozluoglu LN, Ergin NT. The canalith repositioning maneuver in patients with benign positional vertigo. Eur Arch Otorhinolaryngol 2000;257:133–6.

[85] Lempert T, Tiel-Wilck K. A positional maneuver for treatment of horizontal-canal benign positional vertigo. Laryngoscope 1996;106:476–8.

[86] Epley JM. The canalith repositioning procedure: for treatment of benign paroxysmal positional vertigo. Otolaryngol Head Neck Surg 1992;107:399–404.

[87] Epley JM. New dimensions of benign paroxysmal positional vertigo. Otolaryngol Head Neck Surg 1980;88:599–605.

[88] Cohen HS, Jerabek J. Efficacy of treatments for posterior canal benign paroxysmal positional vertigo. Laryngoscope 1999;109:584–90.

[89] Semont A, Freyss G, Vitte E. Curing the BPPV with a liberatory maneuver. Adv Otorhinolaryngol 1988;42:290–3.

[90] Cameron ID, Cumming RG, Kurrle SE, Quine S, Lockwood K, Salkeld G, et al. A randomised trial of hip protector use by frail older women living in their own homes. Inj Prev 2003;9:138–41.

[91] Waldegger L, Cranney A, Man-Son-Hing M, Coyle D. Cost-effectiveness of hip protectors in institutional dwelling elderly. Osteoporos Int 2003;14:243–50.

[92] Cameron ID, Stafford B, Cumming RG, Birks C, Kurrle SE, Lockwood K, et al. Hip protectors improve falls self-efficacy. Age Ageing 2000;29:57–62.

[93] Schleenbaker RE, McDowell SM, Moore RW, Costich JF, Prater G. Restraint use in inpatient rehabilitation: incidence, predictors, and implications. Arch Phys Med Rehabil 1994;75:427–30.

[94] Frank C, Hodgetts G, Puxty J. Safety and efficacy of physical restraints for the elderly: review of the evidence. Can Fam Physician 1996;42:2402–9.

[95] Seifer CM, Parry SW. Monitoring devices for falls and syncope. Clin Geriatr Med 2002;18: 295–306.

[96] Jagella E, Tideiksaar R, Mulvihill M, Neufeld R. Alarm devices instead of restraints? J Am Geriatr Soc 1992;40:191–210.

[97] Tideiksaar R, Feiner CF, Maby J. Falls prevention: the efficacy of a bed alarm system in an acute-care setting. Mt Sinai J Med 1993;60:522–7.

[98] Cumming RG, Thomas M, Szonyi G, Frampton G, Salkeld G, Clemson L. Adherence to occupational therapist recommendations for home modifications for falls prevention. Am J Occup Ther 2001;55:641–8.

[99] Van Schoor NM, Asma G, Smit JH, Bouter LM, Lips P. The Amsterdam Hip Protector Study: compliance and determinants of compliance. Osteoporos Int 2003;14:353–9.

[100] Van Schoor NM, Deville WL, Bouter LM, Lips P. Acceptance and compliance with external hip protectors: a systematic review of the literature. Osteoporos Int 2002;13: 917–24.

[101] Grabowski CJ. Falls: a prelude to litigation. Director 2003;11:50–4.

[102] Cattaneo D, De Nuzzo C, Fascia T, Macalli M, Pisoni I, Cardini R. Risks of falls in subjects with multiple sclerosis. Arch Phys Med Rehabil 2002;83:864–7.
[103] Adkin AL, Frank JS, Jog MS. Fear of falling and postural control in Parkinson's disease. Mov Disord 2003;18:496–502.
[104] Tideiksaar R. Home safe home: practical tips for fall-proofing. Geriatr Nurs 1989;10: 280–4.

ELSEVIER
SAUNDERS

Phys Med Rehabil Clin N Am
16 (2005) 129–161

PHYSICAL MEDICINE
AND REHABILITATION
CLINICS OF
NORTH AMERICA

Aging with spinal cord injury

Jaishree Capoor, MD*, Adam B. Stein, MD

Mount Sinai School of Medicine, 1425 Madison Avenue, New York, NY 10029, USA

Many older people have to make changes in their lifestyle to cope with an inevitable reduction in their physical capacity. In people with spinal cord injury (SCI), the need to make such changes takes place much earlier in life because of the combined effects of their injury and the normal aging process. The rate and effects of normal aging are accelerated in individuals with SCI. SCI-related secondary complications can lead to additional long-term impairments. Because more people with SCI are living longer, there are new challenges for individuals with SCI, their caregivers, and medical providers to facilitate successful aging. The ability to cope with these challenges and with the loss of independence is a major determinant of the quality of later life in persons with SCI.

Biologic capacity plateaus and aging may begin when an able-bodied person is about 25 years old. Aging is not the same as being aged. Although organ systems begin to lose about 1% of their function per year in able-bodied persons with aging, physical illnesses do not show a rapid increase in prevalence until after age 70 because organ systems have large reserve capacities [1]. Clinicians with experience in treating SCI patients have noted evidence of premature aging [2] similar to what has been described in polio survivors and persons with other chronically disabling conditions [3,4]. Factors that can affect the speed and extent of aging with SCI include level, extent, and duration of injury; age at injury; weight; premorbid health history; medical comorbidity; gender; ethnicity; and the success of rehabilitation at the time of injury [5]. Aging is also determined by the complex interaction of genetic factors, lifestyle, adaptation to stress and social roles, alterations in living situation and family structure, and potential depletion of social and economic resources [3,6].

Recent research has helped us to predict the susceptibility to functional change as persons with SCI age and has helped guide interventions. There

---

* Corresponding author.
E-mail address: jc1058@columbia.edu (J. Capoor).

1047-9651/05/$ - see front matter © 2004 Elsevier Inc. All rights reserved.
doi:10.1016/j.pmr.2004.06.016

have been only a few reports of aging-related morbidity in SCI that have separated the effects of aging with SCI from the effects of aging in general, before and after an SCI, and from treatment era and survivor effects [7]. Not all the aging studies that are cited in this article were designed to separate out these effects. Longitudinal research is critical to identify whether changes attributed to aging are inherent in living with an SCI or whether there are modifiable risk factors that can be affected to minimize future problems.

Maintenance of health, maximal functioning, and quality of life (QOL) constitute three major rehabilitation goals for persons aging with SCI. To reduce the impact of aging, it is important that clinicians understand the processes of aging associated with SCI and its impact on physical and psychosocial health. This article provides basic information about some of the medical and psychosocial complications in the individual aging with SCI.

Mortality and life expectancy

Until the mid 20th century, the life expectancy of newly injured persons with SCI was generally felt to be several years, with death commonly occurring as a result of renal failure and infection. Urinary tract complications have markedly declined as a cause of death in persons with SCI over the past 25 years, now accounting for only 2.3% of the deaths reported [8]. Improved survival has resulted from the introduction of antibiotics, advances in long-term health interventions, and the availability of preventative care at specialized treatment centers. There has been a 2000% increase in the post-SCI life expectancy in the past 50 years, in comparison to a 30% increase in life expectancy for the nondisabled population [9]. Life expectancy after SCI is approximately 85% to 90% of normal, depending on the degree of neurologic impairment (ie, level and completeness of injury) and age at onset of injury [10]. Individuals with high tetraplegia are least likely to have a long life. About 40% of persons with SCI now living are over 45 years of age, and one in four has lived 20 or more years with the disability [11]. A shift in mortality to one that increasingly resembles those of the general population results in individuals with SCI having a greater risk for the consequences of normal aging. In recent years, respiratory complications have been the leading cause of death in tetraplegia, and heart disease and cancer are the leading causes of mortality in paraplegia. Cancer as a cause of death has been slowly rising in importance in individuals with SCI [8].

Premature aging

Although SCI was once considered a fairly stable medical condition unaffected by the passage of time, it is now viewed as a dynamic condition in which patients' needs, abilities, and limitations constantly change. These changes may be hastened or intensified by cumulative stresses imposed by years or decades of repetitive activity performed in the course of daily living [12]. Because of SCI-related physical impairments, daily activities such as pushing a wheelchair or performing transfers require more strength and stamina, resulting in more wear and tear and earlier degeneration of the upper limbs, which were primarily designed for prehensile activities.

Although strength, endurance, flexibility, and coordination diminish with normal aging, the body's organ systems have a large functional capacity. In contrast, individuals with SCI are typically young at the time of injury and experience an immediate reduction of some functional reserves and capacities. Thus, for a person with SCI, the consequences of even a small change can have a life-altering impact on independence. As fatigue, pain, weakness, and joint deterioration appear, the performance of locomotion, transfers, weight shifts, and other activities of daily living (ADLs) first mastered after injury may again become challenging [12–15]. Work and leisure activities may be sacrificed to conserve energy for basic ADLs. Losses in function often result in increasing needs for personal assistance, equipment, and medical and ongoing rehabilitation services. It is important to rapidly determine the causes of functional decline, treat the underlying problems, minimize loss of function, and plan for changes that are unavoidable.

Several investigations have identified symptom patterns that herald the onset of a functional impairment syndrome in persons aging with SCI [6,16]. Nonactivity-dependent fatigue is reported by 61%, new pain by 36%, and new weakness by 31% [16]. These symptoms occur in the older nondisabled population but generally have a substantially lower prevalence and occur at older ages than reported in the SCI population [17]. Increased age at injury, higher neurologic level of injury, and longer duration since injury are related to early functional decline and a need for increased assistance [11,16,18]. Although most older adults without disability can expect to remain independent in their ADLs well into their 70s [3,16], the average age of persons with SCI reporting functional decline is 45 years, and their average duration of injury is 18 years [16]. Although individuals injured during or before adolescence enjoy a maintenance phase of 20 years before experiencing functional decline, individuals who are 55 years or older at the onset of SCI have 5 to 7 years of relatively stable functioning before experiencing a decline [5,16]. The level of injury is also related to the timing of functional changes. Tetraplegic patients are likely to require additional assistance at an earlier time postinjury compared with persons with paraplegia. Additional help with transfers is most commonly reported, followed by assistance with dressing and mobility [3]. In a study by Gerhart [11], the average age when additional assistance was first needed was 49 years for those with tetraplegia and 54 years for those with paraplegia. This suggests that a limited reserve or lower tolerance for change in function may exist for older individuals and those with higher levels of injury.

Although a higher level of injury has been shown to be related to earlier functional decline, greater sparing of neurologic function after SCI may predispose to overuse injury with time. Persons with incomplete injuries may have more fatigue, pain, new muscle weakness, and lower endurance than those with complete injuries [16]. Although SCI patients are prone to the same rheumatologic and orthopedic disorders as able-bodied persons as they age, overuse injuries of the upper extremities are more common than in the general population [19]. Fatigue is discussed elsewhere in this issue.

Neuromusculoskeletal changes

There is considerable variability across studies examining predictors of pain after SCI [20]. Pain in aging persons with SCI is often musculoskeletal in nature, resulting from injury to the joints and muscles because of unique physical stresses. This musculoskeletal pain is usually aggravated by movement and may be associated with local swelling, tenderness, loss of joint motion, and instability. If pain is not mechanical in nature, then other causes should be investigated, such as tumor or referred pain from a radiculopathy or syringomyelia.

Upper extremity (UE) pain is common in long-term SCI (30% to 70% prevalence rate) and most frequently affects the shoulder and wrist [14,16,19,21–24]. The prevalence and severity of UE pain generally increases with duration of injury [14,17,19,22,24–26] and age [13,27]. It is unclear whether these findings are independent of treatment era effects or might be affected by environmental changes in accessibility, changing mobility technology (eg, lightweight, ergonomic wheelchairs), and changing re-habilitation practices [7].

UE pain, weakness, and limitations of motion may signal the onset of overuse syndrome of the shoulder, elbow, wrist, and hand or of acromio-clavicular joint deterioration, anterior instability, scapular pain, rotator cuff impingement, tendonitis/tears, subacromial bursitis, osteolysis of the distal clavicle, and adhesive capsulitis. Elbow, wrist, and hand pain may result from carpal tunnel syndrome (CTS) and cubital tunnel syndrome, ulnar nerve entrapment at the wrist, olecranon bursitis, medial and lateral epicondylitis, carpal instability, dorsal radiocarpal impingement, scaphoid impaction syndrome, de Quervain tenosynovitis, osteoarthritis, and stress fractures [23,28].

The most common causes of upper extremity pain are transfers, wheelchair propulsion, and pressure relief maneuvers. Repetitive upper limb weight bearing leads to upward humeral migration, glenohumeral laxity, articular wear, and rotator cuff pathology. Repetitive overhead reaching, leaning, bending, or walking with crutches may contribute. Although most studies attribute shoulder pain and degeneration to overuse, a review of radiographs of persons with long-term SCI demonstrated that moderate joint activity may protect the shoulders from degeneration [29].

Wheelchair athletes do not seem to be more affected by CTS than sedentary paraplegics, suggesting that transfer and wheelchair propulsion technique may be more important than duration of propulsion [30].

Preliminary evidence has linked MRI and radiographic shoulder abnormalities to wheelchair propulsion biomechanics [19]. Extreme humeral internal rotation and extension during wheelchair propulsion increases impingement of the rotator cuff tendons under the acromion. This may be compounded by a muscle imbalance, especially in those with midcervical injuries, that causes relative weakness of the rotator cuff muscles that normally depress the humeral head and minimize impingement [31]. Muscle imbalance that contributes to shoulder pain may result from the original SCI or from the compensatory mechanisms needed to meet new daily demands. Many paraplegic patients with shoulder pain have a muscular imbalance across the glenohumeral joint with overstrengthening/tightness of anterior shoulder muscles and overstretching/weakness of posterior shoulder muscles. A higher prevalence of rotator cuff disorders is found in paraplegics with higher levels of injury, which are associated with decreased trunk control [32]. Midcervical tetraplegic patients often have a muscle imbalance that results in relatively increased scapular retractor and posterior shoulder girdle strength, leading to abnormal scapulothoracic motion, capsulitis, and scapular pain syndrome [33].

Postural issues may contribute to myofascial pain, often characterized by trigger points associated with radiating pain along sclerotomes, or numbness. Postural problems may include forward head lean, increased cervical lordosis, scapulothoracic protraction, kyphosis, and scoliosis [34]. Kyphosis and scoliosis did not progress with increased duration of injury and were not associated with pain in Boninger's cross-sectional study of relatively young individuals with tetraplegia [35]. Spasticity, heterotopic ossification [28,36], and excessive vibration related to inappropriate seating during wheelchair propulsion [19] may contribute to neck, shoulder, or back pain after SCI.

As patients with SCI lead more active lifestyles longer, the potential for late neurologic changes increases. Late-onset muscle weakness or sensory loss has been reported by almost 20% of a large sample of people with chronic SCI [37]. New weakness is most commonly attributed to peripheral nerve injury due to age-related anterior horn cell dropout and loss of myelinated tracts, median or ulnar nerve entrapment, cervical stenosis, or radiculopathy. Atypical demands of SCI, such as prolonged periods of exaggerated cervical extension and rotation to look overhead while seated or to compensate for gait deviations, may contribute to spondylosis and spinal stenosis. Loss of intervertebral motion at fused segments, along with hypermobility adjacent to fused segments, may result in instability, kyphotic deformity, and pain. Repetitive loading of tissue deprived of protective sensory feedback may result in vertebral collapse due to Charcot spondyloarthropathy, which may be characterized by increased spine pain, weakness, new onset autonomic dysreflexia, and loss of sitting balance in persons with long-standing SCI [38,39]. Because the evaluation of spine pain can be difficult, a comparison of findings with past examinations and radiographs is helpful in many cases. Periodic assessment of motor and sensory function and appropriate electrodiagnostic testing and imaging studies are indicated in the presence of signs or symptoms of neurologic deterioration.

If late-onset pain, weakness, dissociated sensory loss (especially pain/temperature sensation), loss of reflexes, changes in spasticity, dysreflexia, a positional Horner syndrome, and functional decline progress rapidly in a patient with chronic SCI, it is imperative to rule out syringomyelia, which can progress cephalad to include the respiratory centers and brainstem. This post-traumatic cystic myelopathy most commonly occurs within the first 5 to 10 years after injury in about 5% of chronic SCI survivors [3]. The diagnosis is suggested by history and physical examination and is confirmed by MRI. Surgical interventions to arrest deterioration should not be postponed when the diagnosis is made in the setting of severe intractable pain or neurologic decline.

Prevention, management, and treatment of neuromusculoskeletal problems

In able-bodied persons with UE pain due to overuse, the usual treatment includes a course of rest for the involved extremity. Because many individuals with SCI depend on their upper extremities for mobility, stability, and weight bearing, treatment for pain and weakness is more effective if it is started early, before the problem becomes chronic. Prevention and conservative management of overuse problems begins with an assessment of the mechanics of ADLs, mobility activities, and functional demands at home and work to identify underlying sources of repetitive trauma and modifiable risk factors. Once the initial evaluation has been completed, acute pain relief may require oral or topical analgesics, trigger point or corticosteroid injections, or physical modalities including ultrasound, transcutaneous electrical stimulation, and manual therapy. Acupuncture has been reported to be an effective treatment for musculoskeletal shoulder pain and other conditions in chronic SCI [40–43]. Rehabilitation includes gentle range of motion, balanced strengthening, endurance training, postural re-education, joint protection techniques, adaptive equipment, and activity modification.

The majority of individuals with SCI who report upper-extremity pain are dissatisfied with the results of recommended treatments [44]. Chronic pain has been reported to affect as many as 94% of persons with SCI [36,45]. The presence of chronic pain has been associated with greater disability, poorer mobility, and greater perceived psychologic stress [45]. If pain becomes chronic, it is best managed with a multidimensional approach, although few studies have addressed chronic pain and neurogenic pain related to aging after SCI [7]. Gabapentin has been shown to be an effective first-line treatment for the management of chronic neuropathic pain after SCI [46].

Activity modifications to preserve upper extremity function may include weight bearing with a neutral wrist position instead of an extended wrist and performing side-to-side or forward lean pressure reliefs instead of wheelchair pushups [47]. Temporary splinting may result in less repetitive trauma or extremes of wrist or elbow motion, causing resolution of symptoms in some cases. The use of adaptive equipment such as overhead reachers and sliding boards can minimize shoulder impingement positions. Adapting the wheelchair with flex rims and using gel-padded gloves may provide shock absorption from repetitive wheel contact and a better grip on the push rim [48]. Suboptimal posture that contributes to neck and shoulder pain may be amenable to wheelchair seating system modifications such as increasing vertical alignment by changing the seat versus axle position, avoiding sling upholstery, and using specialized cushions and arm and back supports. Maintenance of equipment is another important factor because low tire pressure, malaligned wheels, and poor maintenance contribute to increased rolling resistance [49]. Instruction in energy conservation techniques, pacing with rest periods, and changing the environment/workstation can help minimize strain. Management of spondyloarthropathy may include spinal orthotics, rest, analgesics, activity modification, or surgical stabilization [23].

Encouraging weight loss and exercise can help minimize the effect of age-related physiologic changes on daily life. It is important to individualize therapy and to keep most exercises below shoulder height to avoid positions of impingement. An exercise program designed to rebalance the posterior shoulder girdle and restore optimal glenohumeral geometric relationships in paraplegic patients includes stretching the internal rotators and the anterior capsule, pectoral, and biceps muscles and strengthening external rotators, adductors, and scapular retractors [31]. Rowing and backward wheeling can strengthen the posterior scapular retractor muscles [50]. It is important to avoid overstretching soft tissues because instability may result [51]. Curtis et al [31] reported a 40% improvement in Wheelchair User's Shoulder Pain Index scores after a 6-month selective strengthening program, even though there was a transient increase in shoulder pain during the first 2 months of exercise. They recommend that such a program be initiated as part of standard treatment and patient education for all wheelchair users. Boninger et al [49] report that push rim forces and median nerve function were related to body weight, suggesting that maintaining an ideal weight and retraining individuals to incorporate smooth, low-impact strokes during wheelchair propulsion may reduce the chance of median nerve injury.

If pain and weakness are irreversible with conservative therapy, additional equipment may be required to conserve upper extremity function. Push rim-activated power assist wheels, which reduce the physiologic demand of wheelchair propulsion, can often be refitted to a manual wheelchair to offload the upper extremity without causing some of the difficulties associated with switching to a power chair [52,53]. If a power wheelchair is necessary, a van for transportation may be needed. Mechanical aids to lift the chair into the car, hoists, and boards can help with transfers. Because functional decline is accelerated in patients injured at older ages, this subset of individuals should be prescribed a power wheelchair even when the level of injury indicates the need for a manual wheelchair [16].

Needs for new equipment may not be well recognized by the person with SCI. In a study of outpatients with chronic SCI, 78% of 54 individuals presenting with functional decline had new equipment needs identified by a therapist, whereas only 10% of the patients had identified these needs before assessment [16]. This underscores that a proper assessment to identify changing needs and the resources to acquire the appropriate equipment are critical. This can be provided during regularly scheduled patient evaluations.

When conservative treatments fail to provide long-lasting relief of shoulder and wrist symptoms, surgical intervention may provide a successful outcome, although results are mixed [54,55]. Postoperative rehabilitation may be difficult and prolonged, and disability may increase substantially in the immediate postoperative period. The percutaneous endoscopic approach is preferred over surgical release of the transverse carpal ligament to significantly reduce the duration of postoperative activity restriction and the need for a temporary increase in personal care assistance in persons with CTS [3].

People aging with SCI may require an increased level of personal care. Increasing age is a significant predictor of negative reactions to receiving assistance, particularly in those who were previously independent [21]. Delegating to caregivers activities that are most time consuming, difficult, or tedious (eg, dressing, tub transfers, or bowel programs) enables persons with SCI to preserve their energy and use it to engage in more gratifying activities [21]. Because spousal support is an important contributing factor to the ongoing well-being of aging SCI survivors [56], early detection of caregiver stress, especially among aging caregiving spouses, and appropriate interventions (eg, occasional home health aide assistance) can help families attend to issues other than caregiving.

Lower extremity changes, osteoporosis, and fractures

Functional loss due to degenerative change is less common in the lower extremity but is important. Reports of lower extremity pain increase with age in patients with incomplete SCI, rising from only a third of those younger than 30 years of age to nearly 80% of those more than 45 years of age [3]. This is likely related to increased wear and tear during ambulation in these individuals with functionally useful motor sparing in their legs.

Although biomechanical problems are routinely considered when bracing individuals, alignment problems leading to chronic pathomechanical deformities are frequently overlooked. Patients fitted with a posterior leaf-spring orthosis (PLO) may have adequate clearance of their foot during swing phase, but the PLO may not provide adequate support of the subtalar joint during stance phase, leading to excess subtalar eversion, midtarsal pronation, and forefoot abduction. Thus, it is important to consider skeletal alignment and stability in this population in which muscle loss and imbalance are common [57]. Hip flexion and hamstring and plantar flexion contractures are particularly disabling for persons in whom walking is a realistic goal. In persons with chronic SCI, contractures may result from uncontrolled spasticity, heterotopic ossification, or muscle imbalance. Contractures may also affect posture, seating, dressing, skin care, and hygiene. Prevention of lower extremity contractures begins with patient education about proper wheelchair positioning and prone lying and may include stretching and the use of orthotics. Overstretching of hamstring muscles should be avoided because they aid pelvic stabilization in sitting [23,58].

One common complication of SCI is osteoporosis below the level of the lesion. The primary mechanism behind SCI-induced osteoporosis is disuse, resulting in bone hyper-resorption, most severe in the acute phase of the injury. A new homeostasis is thought to be reached by about 16 months with a bone mass at two thirds of the original bone mass, near fracture threshold [59]. Few studies assess bone mass in long-term SCI. Upper-extremity bone seems to respond negatively to paralysis in tetraplegia and positively to overloading in paraplegia [59,60]. Individuals with incomplete motor SCI demonstrate greater bone mineral density (BMD) at the areas of greater lower extremity muscle strength [61]. The amount of demineralization in the lower extremity is related to the completeness and duration of injury [62–64]. In a study by Bauman and Spungen [64] of identical male twins, one of whom had paraplegia, the depletion of bone density seemed to be progressive over decades of disuse after injury, independent of age effects. Demineralization in chronically nonweightbearing areas may be balanced by an increase in bone density in regions of the body where weight bearing has resumed, such as the lumbar spine during wheelchair sitting [63]. However, neuropathic spondyloarthropathy, which may obscure underlying osteoporosis in older patients with SCI, has been proposed to contribute to the observed increase in vertebral bone density [65]. One study used quantitative computed tomography to evaluate vertebral bone density and identified significant cancellous bone loss that was not observed on a DEXA scan [66].

Accelerated osteoporosis is the major underlying risk factor for pathologic fractures after SCI. SCI Model Systems data indicate a nearly 40% incidence of extremity fractures in individuals with long-term SCI [63]. The true incidence is probably higher because not all fractures are recognized or reported. The majority of fractures after SCI occur in the lower extremity, especially around the knee [62,67,68]. Lower BMD around the knee may predict the risk for future fractures at other locations [62,68]. However, no consensus guidelines exist for predicting the fracture risk in this population from specific bone mass values [60,62]. Although most fractures are due to falls during transfers, in patients who are severely osteoporotic, fractures can result from minor stresses such as range of motion exercises or lower extremity dressing. Paraplegic patients are at greater risk because of their higher level of mobility and participation in physical activities. Fracture rates are also higher in persons with complete injuries, in women with increased duration of injury [69], and in those with flaccid rather than spastic paralysis [60].

The goals of fracture care are to minimize complications, to allow for bone healing with satisfactory alignment, and to preserve pre-fracture function. Treatment of fractures is usually nonoperative, with callous formation typically reported in 3 to 4 weeks. The patient should be re-mobilized in a wheelchair within a few days. Because abnormal fracture healing can have significant functional consequences, it is important to maintain a functional position for healing, with the legs flexed at the hip and knee with feet flat on the footrests. Soft-padded splints or knee immobilizers are recommended as preferable to casts in femoral shaft and distal lower extremity fractures. If a circular cast is used after the period of edema, it should be bivalved and well padded. Immobilization can usually be discontinued in 6 to 8 weeks, at which time range of motion exercises can be initiated, although weight bearing (eg, tilt-table, standing, and stand-pivot transfers) should be delayed for longer periods. Femoral neck fractures may be mobilized without lower extremity immobilization because splinting is considered ineffective. Generally, successful bony union is achieved; some degree of angulation and shortening commonly occurs, which is acceptable in full-time wheelchair users. Displaced fractures of the femoral neck and subtrochanteric region may require open reduction and internal fixation [23]. Increased spasticity, edema, deep venous thrombosis (DVT), and skin compromise can complicate fracture management and must be attended to. Increased spasmolytic medications, DVT prophylaxis, and special mattresses or cushions are often necessary to prevent fracture-related complications. It is important to evaluate the functional implications of immobilization and home and community accessibility before the patient is discharged home. The patient may need inpatient rehabilitation for functional retraining, an alternative wheelchair, or wheelchair modifications.

Because no treatment has been shown to provide long-term prevention of osteoporosis in patients with SCI, prevention of fractures is the best treatment method. Patients should be educated about modifiable risk factors such as caffeine, smoking, and alcohol use. They should be taught to transfer with proper leg position, to avoid lateral transfers [47], and to observe for subtle signs of fracture, such as localized swelling, hematoma, crepitus, low-grade fever, or increased spasticity. Extra precautions to prevent trauma during wheelchair sports include the use of lap belts and fall prevention education.

Although early mobilization, weight-bearing exercise (eg, standing), or functional electrical stimulation (FES)-induced lower extremity cycling may be effective in preventing osteoporosis when started within 6 weeks of injury, they are ineffective in increasing bone mass in the chronic SCI population who already have lost significant bone mass. Recently there have been promising accounts of osteoporosis prevention from long-duration FES and from the use of intravenous pamidronate in the acute stage of motor incomplete injury [70]. It is important to obtain a radiograph of the lower extremity before initiating standing or FES in patients who have been chronically non-weightbearing. Because calcium deficiency, vitamin D deprivation and secondary hyperparathyroidism may also contribute to osteoporosis in chronic SCI, supplemental vitamin D and calcium are recommended to reduce bone turnover [63,71,72].

Cardiovascular and endocrine changes

Studies have demonstrated that people with SCI are at increased risk of developing premature coronary heart disease at an earlier age than the general population [2]. Heart disease has steadily risen to be one of the leading causes of death in long-term SCI [34,73–75], causing more than 20% of deaths in patients enrolled in the National Spinal Cord Injury Database from 1993 through 1998 [8]. Cardiovascular disease may also contribute to fatigue and weakness, which may affect QOL.

A number of studies have reported multiple risk factors for the development of cardiovascular in the aging SCI population [2,76–78]. Individuals with SCI have increased prevalence of a pattern of metabolic alteration that is atherogenic, with low high-density lipoprotein (HDL) level in men [2,79,80], glucose intolerance [81], insulin resistance, and a reduction in metabolic rate [76,77,82,83]. Almost 40% of individuals with SCI have significantly reduced HDL, with levels of <35 mg/dL up to four times more common than in the general population [84]. Complete tetraplegics have the lowest HDL values [80] and the highest risk for cardiovascular disease [75,78]. Glucose abnormalities generally increase with advancing age after SCI [81].

A high prevalence of muscle weakness linked to sarcopenia, or loss of lean body mass, has been strongly associated with disability in the aging non-SCI population [16]. The rate of sarcopenia is 3.2% in SCI versus 1% per decade in able-bodied men [76]. Premature body composition changes, such as sarcopenia and adiposity, have been linked to cardiovascular deconditioning, insulin resistance, and increased risk of diabetes, which has been reported to be four times more common in men with SCI than in men without SCI [2,76]. In addition to reduced activity, abnormally low levels of endogenous anabolic hormones (human growth hormone and testosterone) may be partially responsible for premature deleterious body composition changes in subsets of men with SCI [85]. Lower insulin-like growth factor in persons with SCI may be related to reductions in muscle mass, strength, and, hence, functional capacity. Patients taking baclofen, a frequently prescribed antispasticity agent, have been reported to have normal serum insulin-like growth factor I levels, presumably related to central mechanisms [76].

Although tetraplegics have low cardiac output and are somewhat protected from the development of hypertension by sympathetic underactivity, there is an increased incidence of hypertension in paraplegic men that is related to inactivity and obesity [86]. Higher resting catecholamine levels and exaggerated responses to physical work have been reported in paraplegics with mid-thoracic cord injuries [83]. Individuals with SCI may have a reduced exercise tolerance because of the combination of somatic impairment that limits muscle mass available for activation and autonomic impairment that limits the cardiovascular system's ability to respond to the demands of exercise [87,88].

Prevention and management of cardiovascular disease, fitness, and pharmacotherapy

Strategies to reduce the risk of cardiovascular disease include periodic evaluation of modifiable risk factors such as serum lipids [89], oral glucose tolerance, weight, blood pressure, dietary habits, smoking, activity level, and alcohol consumption. Annual EKG screening is important in aging SCI patients because those with higher levels of injury or diabetes may not be able to feel the typical symptoms of angina.

Despite evidence from cross-sectional [90] and longitudinal [91,92] studies that regular physical activity is effective in improving physical fitness and psychologic well-being in the SCI population [93], physical limitations and environmental barriers result in fewer options for exercise in persons with SCI. Nearly 25% of healthy young persons with paraplegia fail to achieve levels of oxygen consumption on an arm exercise test sufficient to perform many essential ADLs [94]. Janssen [95] found that physical strain was inversely related to parameters of physical capacity. Evidence suggests that glucose metabolism [96,97] and HDL [92] can be modified through increased physical activity, but there is controversy regarding the amount and intensity required to achieve these beneficial effects [98]. Circuit resistance training may improve lipid profiles in chronic paraplegics [99]. Long-term benefits of exercise, such as larger cardiac dimensions [100], higher maximal work rate [90], and decreased breathlessness [101], vary according to level of injury, training, and gender and may contribute to functional performance and adaptation in many life activities [87,102]. More research on the effects of conditioning exercise is needed to better examine health and functional changes resulting from physical activity as persons age with SCI.

Because the consequences of poorly planned exercise are more serious than those experienced by persons without disability, it is important to identify effective exercises that improve fitness but do not increase injury risk. Exercise recommendations for the individual with SCI must be highly individualized, taking into account the treatment goals and the level of injury, range of motion, strength, risk of overuse, fatigue, thermal instability, autonomic dysfunction, balance, trunk control, risk of falls and fractures, spasticity, and tolerance of aerobic activity [12,87]. Because suddenly increasing the workload on the cardiovascular system can have catastrophic consequences, exercise tolerance testing can be done in paraplegics with arm crank ergometry. Persantine-thallium scanning is considered a better technique to assess risk for ischemia in those with tetraplegia and high paraplegia because of the prevalence of silent heart disease [78].

Pharmacologic therapy of hypertension and hyperlipidemia should be individualized, taking into consideration autonomic and thermal dysfunction, lowered plasma proteins, edema, anemia, organ denervation, abnormal gastric emptying, and liver and renal dysfunction, which may be associated with chronic SCI. Persons with SCI are at increased risk for drug interactions and adverse affects because of altered pharmacokinetic parameters of drug absorption, distribution, metabolism, and excretion [103,104]. Although special dosing requirements for pediatric and geriatric patients are available, the changes needed for SCI patients are not.

Nutrition and integument

With aging, SCI patients are at increased risk for nutritional problems. Adiposity is related to inactivity, whereas the risk for malnutrition increases with the reduced ability to buy food, inability to feed oneself, caretaker abuse, or increased catabolism related to illness. Hypoalbuminemia is a strong predictor of mortality in bacteremic patients with chronic SCI [105]. A recent weight loss or gain of 10 pounds or more should prompt a search for a cause [86]. Weight management and the functional consequences of being overweight should be incorporated into nutritional and exercise counseling because obesity can have a significant impact on cardiovascular disease, the musculoskeletal system, and the integument. Ideal weight determination for persons with SCI requires adjustments to the general population standards because of alterations in body composition that occur after injury. Paraplegics should aim for a weight that is 10 to 15 pounds below the general population standards, whereas tetraplegic persons should weigh 15 to 20 pounds less. For many individuals, this may be a difficult standard to meet because of limitations on caloric expenditure through exercise [3]. Research on early caloric restriction is an example of an environmental manipulation that has proven to dramatically postpone mouse aging, and this research may have implications on the rejuvenation of humans [106].

Patients should be encouraged to get most of their calories from grains, fruits, and vegetables. A high-fiber, low-fat, low-cholesterol diet along with lean meats and low salt and sugar intake may reduce the risk of diabetes, heart disease, and cancer. Although it has been shown that moderate alcohol consumption may have a beneficial effect on serum HDL, persons with SCI should be aware of the potential weight gain associated with routine alcohol intake. Intake should be limited to one drink per day for women and no more than two for men [3].

Because aging skin loses elasticity, firmness, thickness, moisture, sensitivity, and vascularity, persons with SCI have greater susceptibility to pressure ulcers with aging. The incidence of pressure ulcers increases with completeness and duration of injury, from 15% at 1 year to nearly 30% at 20 years of follow-up [69]. Chronic open skin sores of long duration have been associated with the development of Marjolin ulcers and of squamous cell carcinoma [107]. Although pressure sores are the most common secondary complication of long-term SCI, there are no studies in the literature that specifically address aging-related changes or morbidity in the skin of the individual aging with SCI [7].

Respiratory system changes

Restrictive impairment that occurs at onset of SCI is related to respiratory muscle paralysis and higher level and completeness of injury [21,69]. The early development of kyphosis, scoliosis [35], or increasing spasticity may cause further restrictive disease. Reduced lung and chest wall compliance, ineffective cough, and inability to breathe deeply after SCI may lead to atelectasis and pneumonia, which is the most common cause of death in all age groups and in all post SCI time periods [8]. A British study of 834 persons followed at least 20 years after injury [34] and US Model Systems data [69] suggest that the incidence of pneumonia and atelectasis increases with age rather than with duration of injury. However, recent cross-sectional studies indicate that respiratory function declines with duration of injury independent of age even in paraplegics, and smoking exacerbates the decline in forced vital capacity [7,108,109].

Patients with injuries above T7 display bronchial hyperreactivity resulting in bronchoconstriction and airway obstruction [110,111]. Bronchial hyperreactivity in patients with chronic tetraplegia is possibly related to the loss of sympathetic innervation, reduced baseline airway caliber, and altered mechanical properties of the lungs [110–112]. A high incidence of sleep apnea syndrome (SAS) in tetraplegic men with long-term SCI [113] has been associated with a large neck circumference, long-standing SCI, supine sleep posture, and the use of antihypertensive and antiarrhythmic cardiac medications [114]. The increased use of cardiac medications in tetraplegic patients with SAS may implicate a link between SAS and cardiovascular morbidity, one of the leading causes of death in tetraplegia [114].

Management of respiratory changes with aging

An appreciation of the respiratory risk in aging SCI patients should lead to increased surveillance for changes in function, especially in patients with high-level tetraplegia. Signs and symptoms of late-onset ventilatory failure may include tachypnea, dyspnea, daytime drowsiness, fluctuating mental alertness, unexplained erythrocytosis, increased positional influences on breathing, and respiratory muscle fatigue [115]. Periodic assessments should include measurement of vital capacity, nocturnal oximetry, and chest x-ray. Persons with a vital capacity below 2 liters are at greatest risk for late-onset ventilatory failure and may benefit from oxygen supplementation and assisted ventilation during periods of respiratory compromise [115,116]. Persons with higher-level SCI should be taught a preventive home program of daily incentive spirometry, postural drainage, assisted coughing, and breathing exercises. Regular resistive inspiratory muscle training in individuals with chronic cervical SCI may result in decreased restrictive impairment and dyspnea when performing ADLs [117]. Although the training apparatus is complex, strength training of the pectoralis major and magnetic stimulation of abdominal muscles may produce dynamic compression of the airways and improve cough efficiency and expiratory function in tetraplegic patients [118–120]. Mechanical insufflation-exsufflation, a portable noninvasive method of improving peak expiratory flow, has been effectively used by patients with chronic SCI during episodes of respiratory congestion [121].

Immunization is probably the most cost-effective health measure provided for SCI patients. Although there have been no prospective studies that have examined the clinical benefit of vaccination, persons with SCI develop a favorable immune response to pneumococcal vaccination [122]. Persons with SCI and respiratory susceptibility should receive pneumococcal vaccination every 5 years and yearly influenza immunization. Smoking cessation programs should be offered to decrease the incidence of mucus production and respiratory complications. Effective interventions in the general population include repeated counseling, telephone quitlines, nicotine gum, transdermal patches, and bupropion.

Genitourinary changes

In the general population, urinary tract changes associated with aging include decreased bladder capacity and compliance, an increase in involuntary bladder contractions, and a gradual decline in kidney function related to a loss of functional glomeruli. Increased numbers of urinary tract infections (UTIs) may be related to a decline in immune function, postmenopausal skin changes in women, and the effects of prostatism [21].

Although urinary tract complications have significantly declined as a cause of death after SCI over the past 25 years [8], renal insufficiency in long-standing SCI may result from chronic pyelonephritis, urinary tract calculi, chronic detrusor sphincter dyssynergia, vesicourethral reflux, and amyloidosis [123]. Persons with SCI and proteinuria have more impaired renal function and increased mortality compared with SCI patients without proteinuria [124]. SCI Model Systems data suggest that abnormal renal function testing increases with age and duration of injury, is more common in male patients over the age of 60 in patients with greater neurologic impairment, and increases with indwelling catheter use [69]. Age and gender are not significant factors in the development of stone disease according to Model Systems analysis [69]. However, in Krause's cross-sectional study, individuals younger than 18 years of age at injury onset had over 30 times the odds of having kidney stones than those who were injured at 40 years of age or older [125]. The most important predisposing factors for the development of stones are recurrent UTI caused by urease-producing organisms, urinary stasis, and indwelling catheter use [69,123].

UTIs remain a common complication in long-term SCI, with patients averaging from 1.6 to 2.2 infections per year throughout 20 years of follow-up [18]. UTIs are frequently perpetuated by modifiable risk factors such as impaired urinary drainage, the presence of calculi, or the use of indwelling catheters. A British study of persons with SCI of more than 20 years duration showed a dramatic increase in UTIs among those aged 60 and older but only a slight increase in the frequency of infections between the tenth and thirtieth postinjury years [34]. Signs and symptoms of UTI may be subtle in elderly persons with SCI, who may present with confusion or lethargy rather than common signs such as dysuria, frequency, malodorous/cloudy urine, urinary incontinence, increased spasticity, hematuria, fever, chills, and leukocytosis. Bladder cancer incidence and mortality are significantly higher after SCI. A fourfold higher risk of developing bladder cancer is strongly associated with long-term indwelling catheter use [126], although the cumulative effects of recurrent UTIs, cigarette smoking, and urinary tract stones may contribute [21].

Erectile dysfunction with chronic SCI may be related to the prevalence of common risk factors such as hypertension, hyperlipidemia, smoking, and diabetes. Decreased testosterone levels with increased duration of injury may be related to hypothalamic-pituitary dysfunction and prolonged sitting and euthermia of the scrotal sac and testis [76]. Furthermore, persons with SCI are often prescribed medications that have been shown to affect pituitary and testicular function in able-bodied persons, such as benzodiazepines, anticholinergics, gamma amino butyric acid, and adrenergic agonists.

Genitourinary management

Long-term urologic care of persons with SCI should include screening for infections, stones, upper-tract deterioration and cancer, and patient education about adequate hydration (at least 2 L/d) and compliance with hygienic bladder management. The goals of long-term neurogenic bladder management are adequate bladder emptying and incontinence prevention in a high-capacity/low-pressure storage system, preserving upper urinary tract function, and providing a socially acceptable method of bladder drainage. A retrospective study of patients with long-term SCI comparing clean intermittent catheterization (CIC), reflex voiding, and indwelling catheters found CIC to be the safest method of bladder management in terms of infections, stones, and urethral erosions [127]. However, an increased risk of strictures and false passages [128], along with age-related decline in hand-eye coordination, cognition, vision, sitting balance, transfer, dressing, and toileting skills may preclude CIC in persons aging with SCI. Hydrophilic catheters may enable the ongoing use of CIC in patients with urethral strictures or prostate hypertrophy and play a role in the prevention of urethral strictures [128]. Some patients who experience functional decline may benefit from adaptive equipment or additional home services. Surgical options for long-term bladder management include urinary diversions to increase bladder capacity and sacral anterior root stimulation [129].

In patients who use an indwelling catheter, routine use of oral anticholinergic medications such as oxybutynin is associated with improved bladder compliance, lower leak-point pressures, less hydronephrosis, and possibly fewer febrile UTIs [130]. However, anticholinergic agents frequently cause constipation, which could lead to fecal impaction, especially in elderly persons. Intravesical instillation of oxybutynin has fewer systemic side effects (eg, dry mouth, blurry vision, tachycardia, and drowsiness) but may complicate the performance of IC [131]. Care in using a small-caliber catheter, preventing overdistension of leg bags, and using a thigh holder to decrease traction on the catheter may decrease the frequency of urethral erosions, which are common in women using indwelling catheters [132]. Indwelling catheters should be changed biweekly or monthly.

Routine antibiotic prophylaxis may increase the risk of bacterial resistance and is not recommended for asymptomatic bacteriuria in patients with SCI [128,133]. UTI prevention strategies include neomycin and polymyxin bladder irrigation, introducer tip catheters that bypass the colonized distal urethra [134], and bacterial interference with intravesical inoculation of benign organisms [132]. Functional foods, such as cranberry juice, have been shown to alter the bacterial biofilm load in the bladder and may help reduce the risk of UTI in this highly susceptible population [135].

There are no studies that clearly show which screening method is best for monitoring the upper tracts. Although most institutions use annual renal ultrasound to assess size and morphology of the kidneys as their initial method of screening, the renal scan has been used as a sensitive modality to monitor renal function [131]. Annual evaluations typically include urodynamic studies, kidney/ureter/bladder x-ray, 24-hour urine collection for creatinine clearance, urinalysis, and postvoid residual measurement if the patient voids [136].

There is a general agreement that patients with an indwelling suprapubic or urethral catheter for more than 5 to 10 years should undergo annual cystoscopy to screen for bladder cancer [131,136], which most commonly presents with nonspecific hematuria but may be asymptomatic. Most centers perform annual cystoscopy on patients with an indwelling catheter to remove eggshell calculi and debris in the bladder [131]. Calculi that are growing or that are located in the renal pelvis should be treated before they pass into the ureter and cause obstruction [69]. Although there does not seem to be an association between chronic prostatitis and prostate cancer [21], men aging with SCI should be provided with age-specific prostate cancer screening.

There are many mechanical and pharmacologic interventions, such as sildenafil, for the treatment of erectile dysfunction after SCI [137,138]. Testosterone therapy may be considered in older men with SCI [139], perhaps to enhance libido, after screening for prostate cancer, dyslipidemia, and other potential complications of therapy.

Gastrointestinal issues: neurogenic bowel and aging

In able-bodied individuals, aging is accompanied by decreased secretion of digestive juices, diminished emptying of fluid meals in the stomach, increased intestinal transit times, and diminished gut motility, with an increase in water resorption in the colon, leading to hard stool and an increased risk of rectal fissures, hemorrhoids, and diverticular disease [21].

The effects of aging on the colon are compounded by neurogenic bowel dysfunction, which depends on the level of SCI. The lower motor neuron (LMN) or areflexic bowel syndrome produces segmental peristalsis, prolonged rectosigmoid transit times, and constipation, with a high risk of frequent incontinence because of a flaccid external sphincter mechanism. Upper motor neuron (UMN) bowel dysfunction results in abnormalities involving the entire colon, with markedly delayed colon and rectal transit times, which produces constipation with fecal retention behind a spastic anal sphincter [140,141]. Persons with UMN SCI also have lower basal colonic activity than spinally intact individuals and have a suboptimal postprandial colonic response. It is believed that autonomic dysfunction alters modulation of the intact enteric nervous system after SCI [142].

Although prevalence varies, approximately half of long-term SCI survivors report constipation, incomplete evacuation, and intermittent abdominal distension, whereas approximately one third report gastrointestinal pain and fecal incontinence [143–146]. Diarrhea alternating with constipation is often related to fecal impaction, which may be caused by reduction in activity, diet, inadequate fluid intake, inefficient or infrequent bowel routine, stress, and potentially constipating medications prescribed for pain, depression, spasticity, and detrusor hyperreflexia. Even though constipation and rectal bleeding are reported to decrease with increased duration of injury [18], persons with chronic SCI spend a considerable amount of time on bowel care [145]. More than one third of subjects with SCI rank neurogenic bowel dysfunction as one of their major life-limiting problems. Fear of incontinent episodes is a commonly stated reason why persons with SCI do not engage in social activities outside the home [140].

Bowel management after spinal cord injury

The goals of long-term neurogenic bowel management are to achieve predictable, complete bowel evacuation and to prevent incontinence, chronic constipation, and related complications such as hemorrhoids, fissures, rectal prolapse, and proctitis. In addition to diet, fluid intake, activity level, and medications, neurogenic bowel management is affected by age-related functional decline, the availability of caregiver assistance, the need for and use of adaptive equipment that optimizes positioning and independence, and home accessibility. An effective bowel program should consider cultural, social, and vocational issues.

Management of LMN bowel may require frequent digital evacuation of stool from the rectum. UMN bowel often requires the combination of oral stool softeners, stimulant laxatives, and a chemical or mechanical trigger for defecation. There is no convincing evidence that increased dietary fiber results in improved bowel function after SCI. An increase in dietary fiber, which increases stool bulk, may delay left colonic transit in persons with SCI [141]. Activities such as turning, transferring, and pressure relief may promote peristalsis. Increasing intra-abdominal pressures with an abdominal belt during bowel care may facilitate defecation [147].

When a patient's bowel program is ineffective, changing only one element at a time and maintaining the change for three to five bowel care cycles is recommended [132]. Following a regular schedule of bowel evacuation should be encouraged because missed bowel evacuation sessions promote stasis of stool and colonic dilatation. Fecal impaction can be observed on plain radiographs and requires complete evacuation of the bowel. The mistaken use of antidiarrheal agents in the setting of impaction can exacerbate the condition. Elective colostomy may help improve QOL in select patients with excessively long duration of bowel routine and frequent fecal incontinence [148].

Long-term use of enemas and stimulant laxatives should be avoided. Cathartic colon, which presents with a progressive decrease in responsiveness to stimulant laxatives, may lead to a dilated atonic bowel. Saline enemas can result in electrolyte imbalances, especially in elderly persons.

For ongoing use, hyperosmolar laxatives such as lactulose are preferred because neither organ damage nor tolerance develops, although some individuals may experience flatulence and cramping [140]. Because hemorrhoids may be more common in individuals who primarily use suppositories and enemas for bowel care [146], their use should be adjunctive to digital stimulation and evacuation. Minimizing trauma and supporting the pelvic floor with a gel or air cushion to distribute pressure over the entire perineal surface may help prevent enlargement of hemorrhoids and help maintain closure of the anal sphincter. If topical hemorrhoid therapy fails, elastic band ligation, sclerotherapy, or hemorrhoidectomy may be necessary for severe refractory cases with recurrent bleeding or autonomic dysreflexia [140].

Persons with SCI are considered to be at equal risk with the general population for colorectal cancer, but symptoms such as constipation are more difficult to interpret. Persons with SCI at normal risk should be screened according to national guidelines with an annual digital rectal examination and tested for occult blood beginning at 40 years of age [140]. The frequent presence of hemorrhoids and other rectal pathology in SCI patients may produce minor bleeding. Because fecal occult blood may not be a reliable screening tool, SCI patients should be screened periodically by sigmoidoscopy or colonoscopy, which is recommended every 5 years beginning at 50 years of age [140].

Other gastrointestinal complications with chronic spinal cord injury

Symptoms of reflux esophagitis are reported by 45% of persons with chronic SCI [149]. An increased risk of high-grade gastroesophageal reflux disease in persons with chronic SCI may result from delayed diagnosis because the classic symptomatology may be absent or less reliable in tetraplegics and in patients with injuries above T7. Nonpharmacologic therapy includes lifestyle modifications, such as reducing the intake of caffeine, chocolate, peppermint, and alcohol and smoking cessation. Staying upright after meals and avoiding meals immediately before bedtime may improve symptoms. Pharmacologic therapy is directed toward acid suppression and improvement of gut motility and includes H2 blockers and proton pump inhibitors.

There is a significantly higher prevalence of gallstones with long-term SCI, independent of age or duration of injury. However, prophylactic cholecystectomy is not warranted because the risk for biliary complications is not of sufficient magnitude [150]. Annual ultrasound surveillance has been suggested because the typical symptoms of cholelithiasis may be absent in patients with tetraplegics [149]. Persons with SCI are higher risk for late presentation of abdominal emergencies. Although laparoscopic cholecystectomy has decreased the convalescent time, postlaparotomy mobilization may be prolonged because of impaired abdominal wall support. Progression to independent transfers may require 3 to 6 weeks [149].

Psychosocial aspects of spinal cord injury and aging

In addition to physical and functional changes, aging with SCI is often associated with alterations in psychologic functioning, living and economic situation, social support, community integration, environmental barriers, employment, and life satisfaction. Early identification and interventions can delay, modify, or eliminate potential negative consequences of age-related psychosocial changes.

Most people with SCI consider the ability to control and manage their personal care and daily activities to be essential to their QOL. A change in the level of independence with aging has been related to stress, depression, and declining QOL in the general population and in people with SCI [9]. There is a tendency for stress and depression to be greater for people with SCI compared with what is reported in the general population [9,155]. Depression is often underdiagnosed and undertreated, particularly when depressive symptoms may be attributable to other medical problems or to cognitive decline with aging. People with SCI who are depressed may neglect their health and lose interest in social activities and work. They may turn to substance abuse or suicide [151,152]. The suicide rate in individuals with SCI is two to six times greater than able-bodied persons [9,188]. An association between depression, adverse lipid profiles, and adiposity may compound the risk for cardiovascular disease in persons with paraplegia [153]. Most depression is readily treated with psychotherapy and medicines. Caution should be exercised with prescription of tricyclic antidepressants in patients with SCI because of their anticholinergic effects. Annual screening for depression is recommended [154].

Despite reports of greater physical impairment and depression with long-term SCI [155], life satisfaction and self-reported QOL improve with increased duration of injury [9,156–159]. Care must be taken in interpreting longitudinal studies because they reflect survivors who are more likely to be better adjusted. A meta-analysis of over 25 studies concerning life satisfaction and well-being in SCI concluded that QOL was unrelated to severity of impairment and was minimally related to level of disability in ADLs, whereas greater handicap did affect well-being [160]. Thus, participation in enjoyable activities and the feeling of contributing to society and fulfilling one's potential can be as important to a healthy later life as physical well-being [156].

A social support system and good coping skills enable patients to contend with age-related changes in health and functioning, and facilitate adjustment to disability [9,56,161,162]. In one study of patients with SCI, the more social support individuals perceived to be present, the fewer problems they reported [163]. This may be attributed to increased involvement in self-care and health maintenance behaviors. Recent research suggests that perceived QOL at one point may predict later stress, depression, and psychologic well-being [164]. The need to identify the multitude of underlying factors that contribute to declines in perceived QOL, increased stress, or depressive symptoms is underscored by a study of priority shifting among men with SCI that revealed that younger men placed a high focus on health, employment, learning, and family, whereas older men placed higher priority on socializing or spending time in passive leisure activities [21]. Persons with SCI and ventilator-assisted breathing report high life satisfaction [157], comparable with able-bodied subjects, even though staff consistently rate the QOL of patients less than the patients report [102].

Because access to the environment is an important predictor of life satisfaction and QOL [165], it is recommended that review of perceived and real environmental barriers be included as part of long-term follow-up. Physical inaccessibility, attitudes of professionals, inadequate expertise about disability, insufficient insurance coverage for preventative services, and inadequate transportation are frequently mentioned barriers to access to primary and preventative health services in persons aging with SCI [132,166,167]. Although employment is associated with younger onset of injury [168,169], enhanced QOL [170], and longer survival after SCI [171,172], individuals who return to work after SCI retire earlier than their non-SCI peers [156,173], possibly because of changes in health and functioning. Job-site accommodations, modification of job roles, the availability of transportation, and assistive technology to increase efficiency and safety may help preserve employment. Further research is needed to elucidate the effect of environmental factors (eg, employer attitudes, financial disincentives against part-time employment, and public policy) and to discover meaningful alternatives to gainful employment.

Although home and job modifications, the availability of a power wheelchair, and an accessible van or computer may minimize the impact of barriers and significantly improve independence and QOL, the prohibitive costs may necessitate additional financial resources to facilitate community re-entry. The estimated direct lifetime costs of an individual injured at age 25 ranges from $600,000 to $2.7 million, varying according to severity of injury [174,175]. Because aging frequently coincides with a fall in income combined with greater equipment and care expenses, life care planning, which projects the estimated lifetime costs of needed goods and services, may help increase QOL while controlling costs for future medical care [102,176].

Issues of women aging with spinal cord injury

It is estimated that over 40,000 women with SCI are living in the United States, and 18.5% of people enrolled in the National SCI database are female [177]. Because women are more likely to be injured at older ages than men, women may be adjusting to the original injury when age-related difficulties begin [166,178]. Women with SCI experience more pain [179], fatigue, depression, and transportation problems than men [155,180]. Skin problems, increased spasticity, and autonomic dysreflexia may accompany menopause [180,181].

Women with SCI report profound feelings of isolation and perceptions of being overlooked by the health care and social service system. They report that continuity of care by physicians who validate their concerns and collaborate with them contributes to their health and well-being [167]. It can be a challenge for women with SCI to find a doctor's office with adjustable examination tables to accommodate transfers and positioning for mammograms and gynecologic examinations [181]. Screening for cervical cancer is recommended every 3 years until the age of 65 in those with previously normal smears, unless high-risk behavior occurs. Because some women with SCI have limited use of their hands precluding breast self-examination, it is even more important to have regular breast examinations. Annual mammograms are recommended for women between the ages of 50 and 69 and should be initiated in the early 40s if there is a family history of breast cancer [21]. Although lower extremity fracture risk increases with duration of injury [69,181], vertebral fractures are rare, and BMD of the spine does not seem to decrease with increased duration of injury in women with long-term SCI, unlike able-bodied women, with age [182].

Summary

The years after SCI may be associated with acceleration of the aging process because of diminished physiologic reserves and increased demands on functioning body systems [11,125,183]. Clinicians with expertise in the treatment and prevention of SCI-specific secondary complications need to collaborate with gerontologists and primary care specialists and need to invest in the training of future physicians to ensure a continuum of accessible, cost-effective, and high-quality care that meets the changing needs of the SCI population (Table 1). Managed care payers often do not adequately cover long-term disability needs to prevent secondary SCI-specific complications. In this era of increasing accountability, evidence-based clinical practice guidelines are needed to document scientific evidence and professional consensus to effectively diagnose, treat, and manage clinical conditions; to reduce unnecessary testing and procedures; and to improve patient outcomes. Longitudinal research is needed to minimize cohort effects that contribute to misinterpretation of cross-sectional findings as representative of long-term changes in health and functioning. However, longitudinal studies confound chronologic age, time since injury, and environmental change. Thus, time-sequential research, which controls for such confounding effects, is essential, as is research on the effects of gender, culture, and ethnicity [184–186].

If we consider how much progress has been made over the past 50 years with respect to SCI mortality related to infectious disease, we can expect to achieve even greater progress against the effects of aging in the next 50 years.

Table 1
Follow-up guidelines for healthy spinal cord injury survivors

General health maintenance	SCI-specific

Things to do monthly
  Women: breast self-examination
  Men: testicular self-examination
	Things to do daily
	  Self-skin checks

Things to do every year
  Check-up with health care provider
  Gynecologic exam and Pap smear[a]
  Clinical breast cancer exam, beginning at age 40[a]
  Mammography, beginning at age 40–50[b]
  Digital rectal exam, beginning at age 40
  Digital prostate exam and PSA, beginning at age 50[c]
  Fecal occult blood, beginning at age 50
	Things to do every year
	  Check weight and blood pressure
	  Flu immunization, especially T8 and higher-level injuries

Things to do every 2–3 y
  Complete blood count with biochemistry survey
  Cardiac risk assessment, beginning at age 40
	Things to do at least every 2–3 y with SCI specialist/team[d]
	  Full history and physical review with physician[d]
	  Urologic assessment—upper and lower tracts[d,e]
	  Assess equipment and posture[d]
	  Assess range of motion, contractures, and functional status[d]
	  Full skin evaluation[d]

Things to do every 5 y
  Vital capacity (lung test)
  Lipid panel (cholesterol)
  Eye evaluation, beginning at age 40
  Screening sigmoidoscopy or colonoscopy, after age 50
	Things to do at least every 5 y with SCI specialist/team
	  Motor and sensory testing
	  Review changes in life situation, including coping, adjustment, life satisfaction

Things to do every 10 y
  Tetanus booster
	Things to do every 10 y
	  Pneumococcal pneumonia vaccination at earliest opportunity, especially for T8 and higher-level injuries

Abbreviation: SCI, spinal cord injury.

[a] In woman.

[b] In addition to baseline mammogram between age 30 and 40 or between age 40 and 50. (Note: A number of guidelines conflict on the age at which yearly mammography should begin, with some specifying age 40 and others age 50)

[c] In men. Age 40 if black, or if grandfather, father, or brother has or had prostate cancer.

[d] Assessments done annually for the first 3–5 y after injury, until health established.

[e] Do annually for the first 3 y after any major change in urologic management.

Data from Charlifue SW, Lammertse DP. Aging in spinal cord injury. In: Kirshblum S, Campagnolo D, DeLisa J, editors. Spinal cord medicine. Philadelphia: Lippincott, Williams and Wilkins; 2002. p. 409–23.

Recent developments in molecular biology regarding growth and neuro-trophic factors are bringing us closer to the goal of repairing the damaged spinal cord [187]. The challenge remains for rehabilitation professionals to provide the most comprehensive and holistic approach to long-term follow-up, with an emphasis on health promotion and disease prevention, to postpone functional decline and enhance QOL.

Acknowledgments

We thank Raj Laxmi Capoor, William Bauman, Ann Spungen, Marvin Lesser, Marcel Dijkers, Jill Wecht, Greg Schilero, Mark Korsten, Jonathan Vapnek, and Jerry Weissman for their honest input, help, and guidance and Adrian Cristian for making this opportunity possible.

References

[1] Isaacson Kailes J. Aging with disability. Available at: http://www.jik.com/awdrtcawd. html. Accessed February 2, 2001.
[2] Bauman WA, Spungen AM. Disorders of carbohydrate and lipid metabolism in veterans with paraplegia or quadriplegia: a model of premature aging. Metabolism 1994;43:749–56.
[3] Lammertse DP. Maintaining health long-term with spinal cord injury. Top Spinal Cord Inj Rehabil 2001;6:1–21.
[4] Agre JC, Rodriguez AA. Postpolio syndrome. In: Kirshblum S, Campagnolo D, DeLisa J, editors. Spinal cord medicine. Philadelphia: Lippincott, Williams and Wilkins; 2002. p. 553–64.
[5] Winkler T. Spinal cord injury and aging. eMed J June 14, 2002; 3.
[6] Pentland W, McColl MA, Rosenthal C. The effect of aging and duration of disability on longterm health outcomes following spinal cord injury. Paraplegia 1995;33:367–73.
[7] Adkins RA. Research and interpretation perspectives on aging related physical morbidity with spinal cord injury and brief review of systems. NeuroRehabilitation 2004;19:3–13.
[8] DeVivo MJ, Krause JS, Lammertse DP. Recent trends in mortality and causes of death among persons with spinal cord injury. Arch Phys Med Rehabil 1999;80:1411–9.
[9] Kemp BJ, Krause JS. Depression and life satisfaction among people aging with post-polio and spinal cord injury. Disabil Rehabil 1999;21:241–9.
[10] Kemp B, Adkins RH. Foreward. Top Spinal Cord Inj Rehabil 2001;6:vii.
[11] Gerhart KA, Bergstrom E, Charlifue SW, Menter RR, Whiteneck GG. Longterm spinal cord injury: functional changes over time. Arch Phys Med Rehabil 1993;74:1030–4.
[12] Jacobs PL, Nash MS. Modes, benefits, and risks of voluntary and electrically induced exercise in persons with spinal cord injury. J Spinal Cord Med 2001;24:10–7.
[13] Curtis KA, Drysdale GA, Lanza D, Kolber M, Vitolo RS, West R. Shoulder pain in wheelchair users with tetraplegia and paraplegia. Arch Phys Med Rehabil 1999;80:453–7.
[14] Sie IH, Waters RL, Adkins RH, Gellman H. Upper extremity pain in the postrehabilitation spinal cord injured patient. Arch Phys Med Rehabil 1992;73:44–8.
[15] Dalyan M, Cardenas DD, Gerard B. Upper extremity pain during spinal cord injury. Spinal Cord 1999;37:191–5.
[16] Thompson L, Yakura J. Aging related functional changes in persons with spinal cord injury. Top Spinal Cord Inj Rehabil 2001;6:69–82.
[17] Pentland WE, Twomey LT. Upper limb function in persons with long-term paraplegia and implications for independence: part II. Paraplegia 1994;32:219–24.

[18] Charlifue SW, Weitzenkamp DA, Whiteneck GG. Longitudinal outcomes in spinal cord injury: aging, secondary conditions and well-being. Arch Phys Med Rehabil 1999;80: 1429–34.

[19] Boninger ML, Cooper RA, Fay B. Musculoskeletal pain and overuse injuries. In: Lin V, Cardenas D, Cutter NC, et al, editors. Spinal cord medicine principles and practice. New York: Demos; 2003. p. 527–34.

[20] Putzke JD, Richards JS, Hicken BL. Interference due to pain following spinal cord injury: important predictors and impact on quality of life. Pain 2002;100:231–42.

[21] Charlifue S, Lammertse DP. Aging in spinal cord injury. In: Kirshblum S, Campagnolo D, DeLisa J, editors. Spinal cord medicine. Philadelphia: Lippincott, Williams and Wilkins; 2002. p. 409–23.

[22] Waters RL, Sie IH. Upper extremity changes with SCI contrasted to common aging in the musculoskeletal system. Top Spinal Cord Inj Rehabil 2001;6:61–8.

[23] Little JW, Burns SP. Neuromusculoskeletal complications of spinal cord injury. In: Kirshblum S, Campagnolo D, DeLisa J, editors. Spinal cord medicine. Philadelphia: Lippincott, Williams and Wilkins; 2002. p. 241–53.

[24] Pentland WE, Twomey LT. Upper limb function in persons with long-term paraplegia and implications for independence:part I. Paraplegia 1994;32:211–8.

[25] Gellman H, Sie I, Waters RL. Late complications of the weight-bearing upper extremity in the paraplegic patient. Clin Orthoped Related Res 1988;233:132–5.

[26] Ballinger DA, Rintala DH, Hart KA. The relation of shoulder pain and range of motion problems to functional limitations, disability and perceived health of men with spinal cord injury: a multifaceted longitudinal study. Arch Phys Med Rehabil 2000;81: 1575–81.

[27] Nichols PJR, Norman PA, Ennis JR. Wheelchair user's shoulder? Shoulder pain in persons with spinal cord lesions. Scand J Rehab Med 1979;11:29–32.

[28] Goldstein B. Musculoskeletal conditions after spinal cord injury. Phys Med Rehabil Clin North Am 2000;11:91–107.

[29] Wylie EJ, Chakera TMH. Degenerative joint abnormalities in paraplegia of duration greater than 20 years. Paraplegia 1988;26:101–6.

[30] Boninger ML, Robertson RN, Wolff M, Cooper RA. Upper limb entrapments in elite wheelchair racers. Am J Phys Med Rehabil 1996;75:170–6.

[31] Curtis KA, Tyner TM, Zachary L, Lentell G, Brink D, Didyk T, et al. Effect of a standard exercise protocol on shoulder pain in long-term wheelchair users. Spinal Cord 1999;37: 421–9.

[32] Sinnott KA, Milburn P, McNaughton H. Factors associated with thoracic spinal cord injury, lesion level and rotator cuff disorders. Spinal Cord 2000;38:748–53.

[33] Silfverskiold J, Waters RL. Shoulder pain and functional disability in spinal cord injury patients. Clin Orth 1991;272:141–5.

[34] Whiteneck GG, Charlifue SW, Frankel HL, Fraser MH, Gardner MA, Gerhart MS, et al. Mortality, morbidity, and psychosocial outcomes of persons spinal cord injured more than 20 years ago. Paraplegia 1992;30:617–30.

[35] Boninger ML, Saur T, Trefler E, Hobson DA, Burdett R, Cooper RA. Postural changes with aging in tetraplegia: effects on life satisfaction and pain. Arch Phys Med Rehabil 1998; 79:1577–81.

[36] Bockenek WL, Stewart PJB. Pain in patients with spinal cord injury. In: Kirshblum S, Campagnolo D, DeLisa J, editors. Spinal cord medicine. Philadelphia: Lippincott, Williams and Wilkins; 2002. p. 389–408.

[37] Bursell JP, Little JW, Steins SA. Electrodiagnosis in spinal cord injury persons with new weakness or sensory loss: central and peripheral etiologies. Arch Phys Med Rehabil 1999;80:904–9.

[38] Selmi F, Frankel HL, Kumaraguru AP. Charcot joint of the spine, a cause of autonomic dysreflexia in spinal cord injury patients. Spinal Cord 2002;40:481–3.

[39] Abel R, Cerrel Bazo HA, Kluger PJ. Management of degenerative changes and stenosis of the lumbar spinal canal secondary to cervical spinal cord injury. Spinal Cord 2003; 41:211–9.

[40] Nayak S, Shiflett SC, Schoenberger NE. Is acupuncture effective in treating chronic pain after spinal cord injury? Arch Phys Med Rehabil 2001;82:1578–86.

[41] Dyson-Hudson TA, Shiflett SC, Kirshblum SC. Acupuncture and Trager Psychosocial Integration in the treatment of wheelchair user's shoulder pain in individuals with spinal cord injury. Arch Phys Med Rehabil 2001;82:1038–46.

[42] Wong JY, Rapson LM. Acupuncture in the management of pain of musculoskeletal and neurologic origin. Phys Med Rehabil Clin North Am 1999;10:531–45.

[43] Paola FA, Arnold M. Acupuncture and spinal cord medicine. J Spinal Cord Med 2003; 26:12–20.

[44] Murphy D, Reid DB. Pain treatment satisfaction in spinal cord injury. Spinal Cord 2001; 39:44–6.

[45] Rintala D, Loubser PG, Castro J, Hart KA, Fuhrer MJ. Chronic Pain in a community-based sample of men with spinal cord injury: prevalence, severity, and relationship with impairment, disability, handicap and subjective well-being. Arch Phys Med Rehabil 1998; 79:604–14.

[46] Levendoglu F, Ogun CO, Ozerbil O, Ogun TC, Ugurlu H. Gabapentin is a first line drug for treatment of neuropathic pain in spinal cord injury. Spine 2004;29:743–51.

[47] Nyland J, Quigley C, Lloyd J, Harrow J, Nelson A. Preserving transfer independence among individuals with spinal cord injury. Spinal Cord 2000;38:649–57.

[48] Deltombe T, Theys S, Jamart J. Protective effect of glove on median nerve compression in the carpal tunnel. Spinal Cord 2001;39:215–22.

[49] Boninger ML, Cooper RA, Baldwin MA. Wheelchair pushrim kinetics: body weight and median nerve function. Arch Phys Med Rehabil 1999;80:910–5.

[50] Olenik LM, Laskin JJ, Burnham R, Wheeler GD, Steadward RD. Efficacy of rowing, backward wheeling and isolated scapular retractor exercise as remedial strength activities for wheelchair users: application of electromyography. Paraplegia 1995;33:148–52.

[51] Campbell CC, Koris MJ. Etiologies of shoulder pain in cervical spinal cord injury. Clin Orthop Related Res 1996;322:140–5.

[52] Cooper R, Boninger ML, Cooper R, Thorman T. Wheelchairs and seating. In: Lin V, Cardenas D, Cutter NC, et al, editors. Spinal cord medicine principles and practice. New York: Demos; 2003. p. 635–54.

[53] Corfman TA, Cooper RA, Boninger ML, Koontz AM, Fitzgerald SG. Range of motion and stroke frequency differences between manual wheelchair propulsion and pushrim-activated power-assisted wheelchair propulsion. J Spinal Cord Med 2003;26:135–40.

[54] Robinson MD, Hussey RW. Surgical decompression of impingement in the weightbearing shoulder. Arch Phys Med Rehabil 1993;74:324–7.

[55] Goldstein B, Young J, Escobedo EM. Rotator cuff repairs in individuals with paraplegia. Am J Phys Med Rehabil 1997;76:316–22.

[56] Holicky R, Charlifue S. Ageing with spinal cord injury: the impact of spousal support. Disabil Rehabil 1999;21:250–7.

[57] Yumane A. Lower limb orthoses and rehabilitation. In: Lin V, Cardenas D, Cutter NC, et al, editors. Spinal cord medicine principles and practice. New York: Demos; 2003. p. 675–89.

[58] Harvey LA, Herbert RD. Muscle stretching for treatment and prevention of contracture in people with spinal cord injury. Spinal Cord 2002;40:1–9.

[59] Garland DE, Stewart CA, Adkins RH. Osteoporosis after spinal cord injury. J Orthop Res 1992;10:371–8.

[60] Kiratli B. Bone loss and osteoporosis following spinal cord injury. In: Lin V, Cardenas D, Cutter NC, et al. Spinal cord medicine principles and practice. New York: Demos; 2003. p. 539–48.

[61] Garland DE, Foulkes GD, Adkins RH. Regional osteoporosis following incomplete spinal cord injury. Contemp Orthop 1994;28:134–9.

[62] Garland DE, Adkins RH. Bone loss at the knee in SCI. Top Spinal Cord Inj Rehabil 2001;6:37–46.

[63] Garland DE, Adkins RH, Rah A, Stewart CA. Bone loss with aging and the impact of SCI. Top Spinal Cord Inj Rehabil 2001;6:47–60.

[64] Bauman WA, Spungen AM. Continuous loss of bone during chronic immobilization: a monozygotic twin study. Osteoporos Int 1999;10:123–7.

[65] Jaovisidha S, Sartoris DJ, Martin EM. Influence of spondyloarthropathy on bone density using dual energy x-ray absorptiometry. Calcif Tissue Int 1997;60:424–9.

[66] Liu CC, Theodorou SJ, Theodorou MP, Andre MP, Sartoris SM, Szollar SM. Quantitative computed tomography in the evaluation of spinal osteoporosis following spinal cord injury. Osteoporos Int 2000;11:889–96.

[67] Ragnarsson KT, Sell H. Lower extremity fractures after spinal cord injury: a retrospective study. Arch Phys Med Rehabil 1980;61:139–42.

[68] Garland DE, Maric Z, Adkins RH. Bone mineral density about the knee in spinal cord injured patients with pathologic fractures. Contemp Orthop 1993;26:375–9.

[69] McKinley WO, Jackson AB, Cardenas DD, DeVivo MJ. Long-term medical complications after traumatic spinal cord injury: a regional model system analysis. Arch Phys Med Rehabil 1999;80:1402–10.

[70] Nance PW, Schryvers O, Leslie W. Intravenous pamidronate attenuates bone density loss after acute spinal cord injury. Arch Phys Med Rehabil 1999;80:243–51.

[71] Bauman WA, Zhong Y, Schwartz E. Vitamin D deficiency in veterans with chronic spinal cord injury. Metabolism 1995;44:1612–6.

[72] Stewart AF, Adler M, Byers CM. Calcium homeostasis in immobilization: an example of resorptive hypercalciuria. N Engl J Med 1982;306:1136–40.

[73] DeVivo MJ, Black KJ, Stover SL. Causes of death during the first 12 years after spinal cord injury. Arch Phys Med Rehabil 1993;74:248–54.

[74] Frankel HL, Coll JR, Charlifue SW, Whiteneck GG, Gardner BP, Jamous MA, et al. Long term survival in spinal cord injury: a fifty year investigation. Spinal Cord 1998;36: 266–74.

[75] Groah SL, Weitzenkamp D, Sett P, Soni B, Savic G. The relationship between neurological level of injury and symptomatic cardiovascular disease in the aging spinal injured patient. Spinal Cord 2001;39:1310–7.

[76] Bauman WA, Spungen AM. Body composition in aging: adverse changes in able-bodies persons and in those with spinal cord injury. Top Spinal Cord Inj Rehabil 2001;6: 22–36.

[77] Bauman WA, Spungen AM. Carbohydrate and lipid metabolism in chronic spinal cord injury. J Spinal Cord Med 2001;24:266–77.

[78] Bauman WA, Raza M, Chayes Z, Machac J. Tomographic Thallium-201 myocardial perfusion imaging after intravenous dipyridamole in asymptomatic subjects with tetraplegia. Arch Phys Med Rehabil 1993;74:740–4.

[79] Bauman WA, Adkins RH, Spungen AM, Herbert R, Schechter C, Smith DD, et al. Is immobilization associated with an abnormal lipoprotein profile? Observations from a diverse cohort. Spinal Cord 1999;37:485–93.

[80] Bauman WA, Adkins RH, Spungen AM, Kemp BJ, Waters RL. The effect of residual neurologic deficit on serum lipoproteins in individuals with chronic spinal cord injury. Spinal Cord 1998;36:13–7.

[81] Bauman WA, Adkins RH, Spungen AM, Waters RL. The effect of residual neurologic deficit on oral glucose tolerance in persons with chronic spinal cord injury. Spinal Cord 1999;37:765–71.

[82] Bauman WA. Carbohydrate and lipid metabolism in individuals after spinal cord injury. Top Spinal Cord Inj Rehabil 1997;2:1–22.

[83] Bauman WA. Risk factors for atherogenesis and cardiovascular autonomic function in persons with spinal cord injury. Spinal Cord 1999;37:601–16.

[84] Bauman WA, Spungen AM, Zhong YG, Rothstein JL, Petry C, Gordon SK. Depressed serum high density lipoprotein cholesterol levels in veterans with spinal cord injury. Paraplegia 1992;30:697–703.

[85] Bauman WA. Growth hormone response to intravenous arginine in subjects with a spinal cord injury. Horm Metab Res 1994;26:149–53.

[86] Schmitt JK, James J, Midha M, Armstrong B, McGurl J. Primary care for persons with spinal cord injury. In: Lin V, Cardenas D, Cutter NC, et al. Spinal cord medicine principles and practice. New York: Demos; 2003. p. 237–46.

[87] Glaser RM, Janssen TWJ, Suryaprasad AG, Gupta SC, Mathews T. The physiology of exercise. In: Apple DF. Physical fitness: a guide for individuals with spinal cord injury. Baltimore: Department of Veterans Affairs; 1996. p. 3–23.

[88] Davis GM. Exercise capacity of individuals with paraplegia. Med Sci Sports Exerc 1993;25:423–32.

[89] Szlachcic Y, Adkins RH, Adal T, Yee F, Bauman W, Waters RL. The effect of dietary intervention on lipid profiles on individuals with spinal cord injury. J Spinal Cord Med 2001;24:26–9.

[90] Davis GM, Shephard RJ. Cardiorespiratory fitness in highly active versus inactive paraplegics. Med Sci Sports Exerc 1988;20:463–8.

[91] DiCarlo SE, Supp MD, Taylor HC. Effect of arm ergometry on physical work capacity of individuals with spinal cord injuries. Phys Ther 1983;63:1104–7.

[92] Hooker SP, Wells CL. Effects of low and moderate intensity training in spinal cord-injured persons. Med Sci Sports Exerc 1989;21:18–22.

[93] Hicks AL, Martin KA, Ditor DS, Latimer AE, Craven C, Bugaresti J, et al. Long-term exercise training in persons with spinal cord injury: effects on strength, arm ergometry performance and psychological well-being. Spinal Cord 2003;41:34–43.

[94] Noreau L, Shephard RJ, Simard C, Pare G, Pomerleau P. Relationship of impairment and functional ability to habitual activity and fitness following spinal cord injury. Int J Rehabil Res 1993;16:265–75.

[95] Janssen TWJ, van Oers JM, Veeger HEJ, Hollander AP, van der Woude LHV, Rozendal RH. Relationship between physical strain during standardized ADL tasks and physical capacity in men with spinal cord injuries. Paraplegia 1994;32:844–59.

[96] Hjeltnes N, Galuska D, Bjornholm M, Aksnes A, Lannem A, Zierath JR, et al. Exercise-induced overexpression of key regulatory proteins involved in glucose uptake and metabolism in tetraplegic persons: molecular mechanism for improved glucose homeostasis. FASEB J 1998;12:1701–12.

[97] Jeon JY, Weiss CB, Steadward RD, Ryan E, Burnham RS, Bell G, et al. Improved glucose tolerance and insulin sensitivity after electrical stimulation-assisted cycling in people with spinal cord injury. Spinal Cord 2000;40:110–7.

[98] Washburn RA, Figoni SF. High density lipoprotein cholesterol in individuals with spinal cord injury: the potential role of physical activity. Spinal Cord 1999;37:685–95.

[99] Nash MS, Jacobs PL, Mendez AJ, Goldberg RB. Circuit resistance training improves atherogenic lipid profiles of persons with chronic paraplegia. J Spinal Cord Med 2001;24:2–9.

[100] Huonker M, Schmid A, Sorichter S, Schmidt-Trucksab A, Mrosek P, Keul J. Cardiovascular differences between sedentary and wheelchair-trained subjects with paraplegia. Med Sci Sports Exerc 1998;30:609–13.

[101] Ayas N, Garshick E, Lieberman SL, Wien M, Tun C, Brown R. Breathlessness in spinal cord injury depends on injury level. J Spinal Cord Med 1999;22:97–101.

[102] Steins SA, Kirshblum SC, Groah SL, McKinley WO, Gittler MS. Spinal cord injury medicine: 4. Optimal participation in life after spinal cord injury: physical, psychosocial,

and economic reintegration into the environment. Arch Phys Med Rehabil 2002; 83(Suppl 1):S72–81.

[103] Richardson JS, Segal JL. Spinal cord injury: the role of pharmacokinetics in optimizing drug therapy. In: Lin V, Cardenas D, Cutter NC, et al, editors. Spinal cord medicine principles and practice. New York: Demos; 2003. p. 247–56.

[104] Segal JL, Rosenzweig IB. Therapeutic drug monitoring and treatment of spinal cord injury. Ther Drug Monitor Toxicol 2000;21:37–48.

[105] Wall BM, Mangold T, Huch KM, Corbett C, Cooke CR. Bacteremia in the chronic spinal cord injury population: risk factors for mortality. J Spinal Cord Med 2003;26:248–53.

[106] de Grey AD, Baynes JW, Berd D, Heward CB, Pawelec G, Stock G. Is human aging still mysterious enough to be left only to scientists? Bioessays 2002;24:667–76.

[107] Eltorai IM, Montroy RE, Kobayashi M, Jakowitz J, Gutierrez P. Marjolin's ulcer in patients with spinal cord injury. J Spinal Cord Med 2002;25:191–6.

[108] Linn WS, Spungen AM, Gong H. Forced vital capacity in two large outpatient populations with chronic spinal cord injury. Spinal Cord 2001;39:263–8.

[109] Linn WS, Adkins RH, Gong H Jr. Pulmonary function in chronic spinal cord injury: cross sectional survey of 222 Southern California outpatients. Arch Phys Med Rehabil 2000;81:757–63.

[110] Dicipinigaitis PV, Spungen AM, Bauman WA. Bronchial hyperresponsiveness after cervical spinal cord injury. Chest 1994;105:1073–6.

[111] Singas E, Lesser M, Spungen AM. Airway hyperresponsiveness to methacholine in subjects with spinal cord injury. Chest 1996;110:911–5.

[112] Grimm DR, Chandy D, Almenoff Pl. Airway hyperreactivity in subjects with tetraplegia is associated with reduced baseline airway caliber. Chest 2000;118:1397–404.

[113] Burns SP, Kapur V, Yin KS, Buhrer R. Factors associated with sleep apnea in men with spinal cord injury: a population based case-control study. Spinal Cord 2001;39: 15–22.

[114] Stockhammer E, Tobon A, Michel F, Scheuler W, Bauer W, Baumberger M. Characteristics of sleep apnea syndrome in tetraplegic patients. Spinal Cord 2002;40:286–94.

[115] Little JW. Pulmonary system. In: Medical care of persons with SCI. Washington, DC: Department of Veterans Affairs; 1998. p. 35–41.

[116] Peterson P, Kirshblum S. Pulmonary management of spinal cord injury. In: Kirshblum S, Campagnolo D, DeLisa J, editors. Spinal cord medicine. Philadelphia: Lippincott, Williams and Wilkins; 2002. p. 136–55.

[117] Rutchik A, Weissman AR, Almenoff PL. Resistive inspiratory muscle training in subjects with chronic cervical spinal cord injury. Arch Phys Med Rehabil 1998;79:2293–7.

[118] De Troyer A, Estenne M, Heilporn A. Mechanism of active expiration in tetraplegic subjects. N Engl J Med 1986;314:740–4.

[119] Estenne M, Pinet C, De Troyer A. Abdominal muscle strength in patients with tetraplegia. Am J Respir Crit Care Med 2000;161:707–12.

[120] Estenne M, Knoop C, Vanvaerenbergh J, Heilporn A, De Troyer A. The effect of pectoralis muscle training in tetraplegic subjects. Am Rev Respir Dis 1989;139:1218–22.

[121] Bach JR. Mechanical insufflation-exsufflation. Chest 1993;104:1553–62.

[122] Waites KB, Canupp KC, Edwards K, Palmer P, Gray BM, De Vivo MJ. Immunogenicity of pneumococcal vaccine in persons with spinal cord injury. Arch Phys Med Rehabil 1981;62:418–23.

[123] Barton CH, Vaziri ND. Renal insufficiency in patients with spinal cord injury. In: Lin V, Cardenas D, Cutter NC, et al, editors. Spinal cord medicine principles and practice. New York: Demos; 2003. p. 623–35.

[124] Wall BM, Huch KM, Mangold T, Steere EL, Cooke CR. Risk factors for the development of proteinuria in chronic spinal cord injury. Am J Kidney Dis 1999;33:899–903.

[125] Krause JS. Aging after spinal cord injury: an exploratory study. Spinal Cord 2000;38: 77–83.

[126] Groah S, Weitzenkamp D, Lammertse DP, Whiteneck GG, Lezotte DC, Hamman RF. Excess risk of bladder cancer in spinal cord injury: evidence of an association between indwelling catheter use and bladder cancer. Arch Phys Med Rehabil 2002;83:346–51.

[127] Weld KJ, Dmochowski R. Effects of bladder management on urological complications in spinal cord injured patients. J Urol 2000;163:768–72.

[128] Wyndaele JJ. Complications of intermittent catheterization: their prevention and treatment. Spinal Cord 2002;40:536–41.

[129] Vastenholt JM, Snoek GJ, Buschman HPJ, van der Aa HE, Alleman ERJ, Ijzerman MJ. A 7 year follow-up of sacral anterior root stimulation for bladder control in patients with spinal cord injury: quality of life and users' experiences. Spinal Cord 2003;41:397–402.

[130] Kim YH, Bird ET, Priebe M, Boone TB. The role of oxybutynin in spinal cord injured patients with indwelling catheters. J Urol 1997;158:2083–6.

[131] Linsenmeyer TA. Neurogenic bladder following spinal cord injury. In: Kirshblum S, Campagnolo D, DeLisa J, editors. Spinal cord medicine. Philadelphia: Lippincott, Williams and Wilkins; 2002. p. 181–206.

[132] Groah SL, Stiens SA, Gittler MS, Kirshblum SC, McKinley WO. Spinal cord injury medicine: 5. Preserving wellness and independence of the aging patient with spinal cord injury: a primary care approach for the rehabilitation medicine specialist. Arch Phys Med Rehabil 2002;83(Suppl 1):S82–9.

[133] Lightner DJ. Contemporary urologic management of persons with spinal cord injury. Mayo Clin Proc 1998;73:434–8.

[134] Bennett CJ, Young MN, Razi SS, Adkins R, Diaz F, McCrary A. The effect of urethral introducer tip catheters on the incidence of urinary tract infection outcomes in spinal cord injured patients. J Urol 1997;158:519–21.

[135] Reid G, Hsieh J, Potter P, Mighton J, Lam D, Warren D, et al. Cranberry juice consumption may reduce biofilms on uroepithelial cells: pilot study in spinal cord injury patients. Spinal Cord 2001;39:26–30.

[136] Goetz L, Little J. Genitourinary system. In: Medical care of the person with SCI. Washington, DC: Department of Veterans Affairs; 2001. p. 64–73.

[137] Elliot S. Sexual dysfunction and infertility in men with spinal cord disorders. In: Lin V, Cardenas D, Cutter NC, et al. Spinal cord medicine principles and practice. New York: Demos; 2003. p. 349–65.

[138] Gans WH, Zaslau S, Wheeler S, Galea G, Vapnek JM. Efficacy and safety of oral sildenafil in men with erectile dysfunction and spinal cord injury. J Spinal Cord Med 2001;24:35–9.

[139] Schmitt JK, Schroeder DL. Endocrine and metabolic consequences of spinal cord injuries. In: Lin V, Cardenas D, Cutter NC, et al, editors. Spinal cord medicine principles and practice. New York: Demos; 2003. p. 221–35.

[140] Steins S, Bergman S, Goetz L. Neurogenic bowel dysfunction after spinal cord injury: clinical evaluation and rehabilitative management. Arch Phys Med Rehabil 1997;78:S-86.

[141] Lynch AC, Antony A, Dobbs BR, Frizelle FA. Bowel dysfunction following spinal cord injury. Spinal Cord 2001;39:193–203.

[142] Fajardo NR, Pasiliao R, Modeste-Duncan R. Decreased colonic motility in persons with chronic spinal cord injury. Am J Gastroenterol 2003;98:128–34.

[143] Kirshblum SC, Gualti M, O'Connor KC, Voorman SJ. Bowel care practices in chronic spinal cord injury. Arch Phys Med Rehabil 1998;79:20–3.

[144] De Looze D, Van Laere M, De Muynck M, Beke R, Elewaut A. Constipation and other chronic gastrointestinal problems in spinal cord injury patients. Spinal Cord 1998;36:63–6.

[145] Harari D, Sarkarati M, Gurwitz JH, McGlinchey-Berroth G, Minaker KL. Constipation-related symptoms and bowel program concerning individuals with spinal cord injury. Spinal Cord 1997;35:394–401.

[146] Menter R, Weitzenkamp D, Cooper D, Bingley J, Charlifue S, Whiteneck G. Bowel management outcomes in individuals with long-term spinal cord injuries. Spinal Cord 1997;35:608–12.

[147] Korsten MA, Fajardo NR, Rosman AS, Creasey GH, Spungen AM, Bauman WA. Difficulty with evacuation after spinal cord injury: colonic motility during sleep and effects of abdominal wall stimulation. J Rehabil Res Dev 2004;41:95–100.

[148] Rosito O, Nino-Murcia M, Wolfe V, Kiratli J, Perkash I. The effects of colostomy on quality of life in patients with spinal cord injury: a retrospective analysis. J Spinal Cord Med 2002;25:174–83.

[149] Stiens S. Gastrointestinal system. In: Medical care of the person with SCI. Washington, DC: Department of Veterans Affairs; 2001. p. 52–63.

[150] Rotter KP, Larrain CG. Gallstones in SCI: a late medical complication. Spinal Cord 2003;41:105–8.

[151] Heinemann AW, Doll MD, Armstrong KJ, Schnoll S, Yarkony GM. Substance use and receipt of treatment by persons with long-term spinal cord injuries. Arch Phys Med Rehabil 1991;72:482–7.

[152] Raditz CL, Tirch D. Substance misuse in individuals with spinal cord injury. Int J Addict 1995;30:1117–40.

[153] Kemp BJ, Spungen AM, Adkins RH, Krause JS, Bauman WA. The relationships among serum lipid levels, adiposity, and depressive symptomology in persons aging with spinal cord injury. J Spinal Cord Med 2001;24:216–20.

[154] Consortium for Spinal Cord Medicine. Depression following spinal cord injury: a clinical practice guideline for primary care physicians. Washington, DC: Paralyzed Veterans of America; 1998.

[155] Krause JS, Kemp B, Coker J. Depression after spinal cord injury: relation to gender, ethnicity, aging and socioeconomic factors. Arch Phys Med Rehabil 2000;81:1099–109.

[156] Kemp B, Ettelson D. Quality of life while living and aging with a spinal cord injury and other impairments. Top Spinal Cord Inj Rehabil 2001;6:116–27.

[157] Hall KM, Knudsen ST, Wright J, Charlifue SW, Graves DE. Follow-up study of individuals with high tetraplegia (C1–C4) 14 to 24 years postinjury. Arch Phys Med Rehabil 1999;80:1507–13.

[158] Dowler M, Richards JS, Putzke JD, Gordon W, Tate D. Impact of demographic and medical factors on satisfaction with life after spinal cord injury: a normative study. J Spinal Cord Med 2001;24:87–93.

[159] Duggan CH, Dijkers M. Quality of life after spinal cord injury: a qualitative study. Rehabil Psychol 2001;46:3–27.

[160] Dijkers M. Quality of life after spinal cord injury: a meta analysis of the effects of disablement components. Spinal Cord 1997;35:829–40.

[161] Elfstrom ML, Kreuter M, Ryden A, Persson L-O, Sullivan M. Effects of coping on psychological outcome when controlling for background variables: a study of traumatically spinal cord lesioned persons. Spinal Cord 2002;40:408–15.

[162] Heinemann AW. Spinal cord injury. In: Goreczny AJ, editor. Handbook of health and rehabilitation psychology. New York: Plenum Press; 1995. p. 341–58.

[163] McColl MA, Arnold R, Charlifue S, Gerhart K. Social support and aging with a spinal cord injury: Canadian and British experiences. Top Spinal Cord Inj Rehabil 2001;6:83–101.

[164] Charlifue S, Gerhart K. Changing psychosocial morbidity in people aging with spinal cord injury. NeuroRehabilitation 2004;19:15–23.

[165] Richards JS, Bombardier CH, Tate D, Dijkers M, Gordon W, Shewchuk R, et al. Access to the environment and life satisfaction after spinal cord injury. Arch Phys Med Rehabil 1999;80:1501–6.

[166] McColl MA. A house of cards: women, aging and spinal cord injury. Spinal Cord 2002; 40:371–3.

[167] Pentland W, Walker J, Minnes P, Tremblay M, Brouwer B, Gould M. Women with SCI and impact of aging. Spinal Cord 2002;40:374–87.

[168] Anderson CJ, Vogel LC. Employment outcomes of adults who sustained spinal cord injuries as children or adolescents. Arch Phys Med Rehabil 2002;83:791–801.

[169] Krause JS, Kewman D, DeVivo MJ, Maynard F, Coker J, Roach MJ, et al. Employment after spinal cord injury: an analysis of cases from the model spinal cord injury. Arch Phys Med Rehabil 1999;80:1492–500.

[170] Francescchini M, Di Clemente B, Rampello A, Nora M, Spizzichino L. Longitudinal outcome 6 years after spinal cord injury. Spinal Cord 2003;41:280–5.

[171] Tate DG, Haig AJ, Krause JS. Vocational aspects of spinal cord injury. In: Kirshblum S, Campagnolo D, DeLisa J, editors. Spinal cord medicine. Philadelphia: Lippincott, Williams and Wilkins; 2002. p. 312–21.

[172] Krause JS, Kjorsvig JM. Mortality after spinal cord injury: a four year prospective study. Arch Phys Med Rehabil 1992;73:558–63.

[173] Krause JS. Aging and self-reported barriers to employment after spinal cord injury. Top Spinal Cord Inj Rehabil 2001;6:102–15.

[174] Spinal Cord Injury Information Network. Available at: www.spinalcord.uab.edu. Accessed August 2004.

[175] Berkowitz M. The costs of spinal cord injury. In: Lin V, Cardenas D, Cutter NC, et al, editors. Spinal cord medicine principles and practice. New York: Demos; 2003. p. 949–53.

[176] Weed R. Life care planning development. Top Spinal Cord Inj Rehabil 2002;7:5–20.

[177] Jackson A. Women's health challenges after spinal cord injury. In: Lin V, Cardenas D, Cutter NC, et al, editors. Spinal cord medicine principles and practice. New York: Demos; 2003. p. 839–50.

[178] Nobunaga AI, Go BK, Karunas RB. Recent demographic and injury trends in people served by the model spinal cord injury care systems. Arch Phys Med Rehabil 1999;80: 1372–82.

[179] Budh CN, Lund I, Hultling C. Gender related differences in pain in spinal cord injured individuals. Spinal Cord 2003;41:122–8.

[180] McColl MA, Charlifue S, Glass C, Lawson N, Savic G. Aging, gender and spinal cord injury. Arch Phys Med Rehabil 2004;84:363–7.

[181] Jackson AB, Wadley V. A multicenter study of women's self-reported reproductive health after spinal cord injury. Arch Phys Med Rehabil 1999;80:1420–8.

[182] Garland DE, Adkins RH, Stewart CA, Ashford R, Vigil D. Regional osteoporosis in women who have a complete spinal cord injury. J Bone Joint Surg 2001;83-A:1195–200.

[183] Putzke JD, Barrett JJ, Richards JS, DeVivo MJ. Age and spinal cord injury: an emphasis on outcomes among the elderly. J Spinal Cord Med 2003;26:37–44.

[184] Krause JS, Crewe NM. Chronologic age, time since injury and time of measurement: effect of adjustment after spinal cord injury. Arch Phys Med Rehabil 1991;72:91–100.

[185] Krause JS. Aging and life adjustment after spinal cord injury. Spinal Cord 1998;36:320–8.

[186] Weitzenkamp DA, Jones RH, Whiteneck GG, Young DA. Aging with spinal cord injury: cross-sectional and longitudinal effects. Spinal Cord 2001;39:301–9.

[187] Cheng H, Lee Y. Spinal cord repair strategies. In: Lin V, Cardenas D, Cutter NC, et al, editors. Spinal cord medicine principles and practice. New York: Demos; 2003. p. 801–11.

[188] Fichtenbaum J, Kirshblum S. Psychologic adaptation to spinal cord injury. In: Kirshblum S, Campagnolo D, DeLisa J, editors. Spinal cord medicine. Philadelphia: Lippincott, Williams and Wilkins; 2002. p. 299–311.

ELSEVIER
SAUNDERS

Phys Med Rehabil Clin N Am
16 (2005) 163–177

PHYSICAL MEDICINE
AND REHABILITATION
CLINICS OF
NORTH AMERICA

The impact of age on traumatic brain injury

Steven R. Flanagan, MD*, Mary R. Hibbard, PhD,
Wayne A. Gordon, PhD

*Department of Rehabilitation Medicine, Box 1240, Mount Sinai School of Medicine,
1425 Madison Avenue, New York, NY 10029, USA*

Advancing age predisposes individuals to many health care problems. Although some disease states primarily afflict the elderly population (eg, Alzheimer disease), others are adversely affected by old age; this is the case with traumatic brain injury (TBI). Although the greatest incidence of TBI occurs in young adults, a second peak incidence occurs in the elderly population. The associated physical, emotional, and cognitive manifestations are typically more pronounced in elderly TBI patients. As more individuals with TBI survive, the prevalence of TBI will grow, which is becoming increasingly important as the population ages. The United States Census Bureau reported that the fastest growing portion of the population is comprised of individuals over 65 years of age, with the number expected to increase by 53.2% by 2020. Therefore, the number of older adult survivors of TBI and elderly persons with new-onset TBI will increase dramatically. Clinicians and policy makers must prepare for the impact this will have on society and medicine.

TBI is affected by age in many ways. The epidemiology, pathophysiology, outcomes, and comorbidities after TBI vary with the age of onset, which may be due to difference in age-related comorbidities, limited regenerative capacity, and genetics. Regardless of the age-related variations in the manifestations of TBI, good outcomes are often achievable, albeit at greater costs and longer hospitalizations for elderly patients. The financial concerns involved in more intensive service delivery may become a significant barrier to providing adequate care to elderly individuals with TBI who require

This work was partly supported by The National Institute on Disability and Rehabilitation Research Grant H1333A021918.

* Corresponding author.
E-mail address: steve.flanagan@mssm.edu (S.R. Flanagan).

intensive rehabilitation services. This article reviews what is known about the impact of aging on TBI and identifies areas of needed investigation.

Epidemiology

At least 1.5 million Americans sustain TBI each year. Of these individuals, more than 250,000 require hospitalization [1]. TBI is one of the leading causes of death and disability in adults, accounting for 20 times more hospital admissions than traumatic spinal cord injury [2] and having an estimated prevalence of 5.3 million [3]. The prevalence is an underestimate of the true incidence of TBI because only 15% of individuals with TBI are known to the medical system secondary to being hospitalized after moderate to severe TBI [4]. The remaining 85% experience mild TBI. These individuals often do not seek medical attention, and thus the TBI of these individuals remains unidentified to the medical community and to the injured person. These individuals may have sequelae of having had a TBI but may not link the blow to the head to their symptoms. The physical, cognitive, and emotional impairments secondary to TBI are extensive and negatively affect successful community reintegration. For example, it has been reported that one third of individuals who are hospitalized for moderate to severe TBI require the assistance of another person for the completion of activities of daily living 1 year after hospital discharge [5]. Despite the prevalence of TBI and the scope of its functional consequences, it remains a "silent" epidemic because many afflicted individuals seem to be physically well yet have significant impairments in cognition, behavioral control, and mood that impede their full participation in desired activities. These issues are compounded for elderly persons who experience TBI because they are more likely to experience poorer functional outcomes than younger individuals who experience TBI.

Incidence rates, gender, race, etiology of injury, length of hospitalization, hospital discharge disposition, complications, functional outcomes, and mortality statistics are associated with age at the time of injury. TBI has a bimodal age distribution, affecting mostly young adults and elderly persons, with the highest incidence occurring in those 15 to 19 years of age and ≥65 years of age [6]. The age-adjusted rate of TBI in males is approximately twice that for females [6]; however, in elderly men and women, the rates of TBI are equal. This latter finding may reflect the fact that women live longer than men [7,8], which affords them increased opportunity to sustain a TBI, and the fact that men and women are equally likely to fall, which is the leading cause of TBI in the elderly population. Although individuals from minority backgrounds, including American Indians/Alaskan Natives and African Americans, have the highest incidence of TBI, whites have the highest rates among those ≥65 years of age. Although motor vehicle traffic-related incidents, falls, and assaults are the leading causes of TBI, age-based variability exists. Motor vehicle traffic-related events account for the greatest numbers of TBI discharges nationwide and are the leading cause of TBI for those between 5 and 64 years of age. Falls are the leading cause of TBI in individuals <5 and ≥65 years of age. Comorbidity varies by age: Older adults are more likely to experience complicated TBIs, to have longer hospitalizations, to be transferred to a nursing facility at hospital discharge, and to be more severely disabled at the time of discharge than younger individuals with TBI [6]. Finally, mortality varies by age in that older adults have higher mortality than younger adults across all levels of TBI severity.

Pathophysiology

Although the pathophysiologic changes associated with TBI can occur in any age group, advanced age at onset of injury predisposes to particular findings. In general, pathologic findings can be broadly categorized into focal versus diffuse changes and immediate versus delayed changes.

Lesions occurring at the time of injury are considered an immediate result of trauma. These include focal lesions such as contusions, lacerations, and focal hemorrhages. Contusions occur when the brain strikes the sharp, rigid inner surface of the skull. The shape and contour of the skull predispose the inferior frontal lobes and the anterior tips of the temporal lobes to become contused. Penetrating wounds and depressed skull fractures often result in focal brain lacerations at the point where the dura is violated. Focal injury may also result when deep penetrating arteries are sheared during trauma, causing small hemorrhages within deeper brain structures such as the basal ganglia. Focal ischemic lesions result from vasospasm or arterial compression and create localized areas of infarction. Infarctions typically occur at some period after the initial traumatic event and are therefore considered secondary brain injuries.

Extra-axial bleeding resulting from trauma may result in focal or diffuse lesions and includes subarachnoid, epidural, and subdural hemorrhages. Traumatic subarachnoid hemorrhages have been associated with poorer outcomes after TBI [9] and predispose the individual to arterial vasospasm and subsequent focal ischemic lesions, potentially worsening injury severity and outcomes. Epidural hemorrhages arise from ruptured meningeal blood vessels typically injured secondary to a skull fracture. Subdural hemorrhages arise from shearing of the bridging veins, which may result in large hemorrhages because the subdural space is not limited by dural binding to the skull. The risk of subdural hematomas is greater in elderly persons than in younger adults because the bridging veins become more susceptible to shearing forces as the brain naturally atrophies with age [10,11]. Subdural hemorrhages may enlarge quickly, resulting in a rapid neurologic deterioration shortly after trauma, or they may expand slowly, resulting in a more insidious loss of mental abilities and physical agility over the course of several weeks or months post trauma. This slow deterioration is more commonly observed in elderly patients as a result of the natural enlargement of the subdural space that occurs with advancing age. This increased space allows a relatively large volume of fluid to accumulate before causing significant mass effect on the brain. Subdural hemorrhages can also expand over many weeks secondary to re-bleeding resulting from abnormal and dilated blood vessels [12,13], increased fibrinolytic activity, and abnormal coagulation [11]. Unlike younger individuals with TBI in whom subdural hemorrhages are typically observed immediately after a blow to the head, elderly individuals may experience a subdural hemorrhage after a seemingly trivial injury, with many patients unable to recall the inciting event. More typically, the subdural is the result of indirect trauma, occurring from a fall but without direct blunt trauma to the head [14,15]. Common clinical presentations of chronic subdural hematomas include changes in mental state [16,17], focal neurologic deficits [17], and increased frequency of falls, which increases the risk for re-bleeding [18].

Diffuse injuries result from acceleration-deceleration injuries, poor cerebral perfusion, and systemic hypoxia. Acceleration-deceleration injuries cause the brain to contort and torque, resulting in axonal stretching. This stretching may result in neuronal dysfunction by disrupting cytoskeletal integrity and axonal transport [19]. This process, known as diffuse axonal injury (DAI), may cause exopathy or complete axonal disruption and accounts for significant cognitive and behavioral impairments typically seen after TBI [19]. Although the initiating cause of DAI is the traumatic event, animal models indicate that ultimate axopathy may occur days later, with only the most severe injuries resulting in immediate axopathy [20]. Conventional neuroimaging techniques are insensitive in detecting DAI [21,22], so many individuals with significant physical, cognitive, or emotional challenges post-TBI have "normal" neuroimaging studies.

Poor arterial perfusion causes additional pathology at a point after the initial trauma and is another source of secondary brain injury. Intracranial pressure (ICP) often increases after trauma due to such factors as intracranial hemorrhages and edema. As ICP increases, cerebral perfusion may decrease unless there is a compensatory increase in mean arterial pressure (MAP). A goal of the trauma team treating individuals with severe TBI is to maintain adequate cerebral perfusion by lowering ICP and maintaining MAP. Caution is needed to prevent excessive elevation in MAP, which may cause other systemic injuries and worsen overall outcomes [23]. Similarly, systemic hypoxemia, which may result from concomitant pulmonary or other airway lesions, leads to diffuse secondary injury, adversely affecting outcomes post-TBI [24,25].

Outcomes

Outcomes after TBI are viewed in diverse ways. They may be assessed in terms of mortality and morbidity rates, extent of functional disability, nature of hospital disposition, quality of life, degree of community integration, and employability. As a result, assessment tools vary widely, with no uniform outcome measure used. Regardless of the outcome instrument used, elderly persons with TBI have poorer outcomes than their younger counterparts across all injury severity levels. This raises important medical, legal, ethical, and social issues regarding the care provided to elderly persons with severe TBI, particularly as the population ages. Multiple attempts have been made to predict outcomes, using demographics (eg, age) and severity markers (eg, pupillary response, GCS, and adequacy of cerebral perfusion). Intense research and considerable advancements have been made on this topic, but accurate prediction of outcomes remains elusive.

Mortality

Overall TBI-related mortality declined during the 1990s because of a significant reduction in motor vehicle and assault-related deaths, greater use of seat belts, and improved emergency and acute trauma services. Deaths associated with fall-related TBIs increased 25% during this same period. Falls were the leading cause of TBI-related deaths for individuals ≥75 years of age [26]. The greatest incidence of firearm related TBI deaths occurred in men 20 to 24 years of age and in men ≥75 years of age. Despite the overall decline in mortality rates for those <75 years of age, mortality rates were highest for individuals over the age of 75, representing a 21% increase in elderly TBI-related deaths during this period [26]. Factors that may be related to these findings of an increase in mortality in the elderly population may include better neuroimaging techniques, more detailed coding on death certificates, greater prevalence of falls in the elderly population, or potential medication side-effects in the elderly population, including anti-platelet and other anticoagulant drugs [27–30]. Low-dose aspirin was not associated with an increased risk of intracranial hemorrhages in elderly patients after mild to moderate TBI [31], shedding some doubt on the latter interpretation as a possible cause of increased mortality. The increased mortality cannot be attributable to more severe injuries in the elderly population because higher mortality rates exist for older individuals across all severity levels, including mild TBIs [7]. Given this sharp increase in age-related mortality rates, further investigation of factors associated with the onset of TBI in the elderly is warranted, particularly as the population ages. In addition, prevention programs are needed to help reduce TBI-related risk factors. For example, proactive strategies, such as fall prevention programs, "refresher" driving programs, and monitoring of medication compliance in elderly patients, may be beneficial.

Injury-severity factors, including systemic hypotension, poor cerebral perfusion pressure [32], pupil reactivity, and Glasgow Coma Scale score [33], contribute to the overall mortality risk after TBI. When combined with

GCS, advancing age has been associated with mortality and lower GCS scores [34], although age alone is an independent risk factor [33]. Elderly individuals with less severe injuries (ie, GCS 13–15) have higher than expected mortality rates, reported as 7.3% in one study [35]. Longer-term survivals post-TBI in elderly persons are lower when compared with younger adults [36] or age-matched noninjured control subjects [37]. However, elderly individuals with severe TBI who are discharged from the hospital typically live at least several more years, although minimal neurologic or functional improvement is noted over time [38]. The greater incidence of complications and pre-existing comorbidities [39] and a greater likelihood of dying from secondary organ failure [40] in elderly patients may account for these poorer survival rates.

Short-term outcomes

Outcomes studies post TBI reveal a significant and consistent adverse impact of advancing age on functional skills, cognitive abilities, length of hospitalization, medical charges, and hospital disposition. When interpreting the literature on this topic, it is important to consider several limitations. With rare exceptions, most studies have examined relatively short-term outcomes, looking at the person's status at the time of acute care hospital discharge or several months post discharge. The majority of studies examining functional outcome have used the Glasgow Outcome Scale (Box 1), a measure criticized for its lack of specificity in outcomes. Also, a wide range of abilities can exist within a specific GOS score, which has led to the development of the Extended GOS (Box 2). However, this measure has not been widely used to assess outcomes based on age. Furthermore, most studies do not account for premorbid functional skills or comorbid conditions, which affect a patient's ability to recover from injury and benefit from intensive rehabilitation. Without considering these limitations, the poor prognosis predicted for older adults may lead health care providers to forgo aggressive rehabilitation efforts. Significant functional and cognitive improvements are achievable, and the majority of elderly patients is capable of being discharged to a community setting after intensive rehabilitation [41].

Box 1. Glasgow Outcome Scale [42]

1. Dead
2. Vegetative state
3. Severely disabled
4. Moderately disabled
5. Good recovery

Box 2. Extended Glasgow Outcome Scale [43]

1. Dead
2. Vegetative state
3. Lower severe disability
4. Upper severe disability
5. Lower moderate disability
6. Upper moderate disability
7. Lower good recovery
8. Upper good recovery

There is a consistent association between poorer functional outcomes and advancing age despite the previously mentioned limitations. Studies examining functional (GOS scores 4–5) versus nonfunctional outcomes (GOS scores 1–3) revealed that across all injury severities, elderly patients fared worse than their younger counterparts [7,33,38,44]. This association is strengthened when age is combined with GCS. In one study, all elderly individuals with an admission GCS <11 were discharged in a vegetative or severely disabled state or died in the hospital [35]. For elderly patients who do survive severe TBI, further functional improvement after hospital discharge was found to be unlikely in one study, although the intensity of rehabilitation efforts was not reported [38]. Unexpectedly poor outcomes are also seen after mild injuries, immediately after hospital discharge (where one study found poor outcomes in 27% of elderly patients with admission GCS of 13 to 15 [35]) and at 1 year post injury (where another study found that elderly survivors of mild TBI fared worse than younger adults [45]).

Despite the seemingly poorer prognosis, elderly patients can benefit from aggressive rehabilitation [41,46]. Cifu et al [41] reported that elderly patients benefitted physically and cognitively from intensive inpatient rehabilitation and that the vast majority of these individuals was discharged to a community setting. Although the overall length of stay and hospital charges of the older adults were roughly twice that for their matched younger counterparts, good outcomes were frequently achieved. Potential explanations for the longer length of stay included delayed recovery times due to reduced physical reserve, reduced processing speed and reduced rate of learning new information, higher incidence of medical complications, and lack of pressure from insurance carriers to discharge elderly patients who were generally covered by Medicare [41]. However, the initiation of the Prospective Payment System (PPS) for Medicare beneficiaries beginning in 2002 by the Center for Medicare and Medicaid Services (CMS) may result in limiting the length of acute inpatient rehabilitation stays, thus curtailing the maximal benefits that may be achieved by elderly patients and limiting the outcomes attained. In other words, financial pressure resulting from the initiation of this prospective payment system may lead to a greater percentage of elderly individuals with TBI discharged to skilled nursing facilities rather than to community settings. A recent analysis indicated that the new PPS may reimburse rehabilitation facilities significantly less than their costs for treating individuals with TBI. This may have an adverse impact on how and where elderly patients with TBI receive needed rehabilitation services [47], with aggressive rehabilitation potentially viewed as too costly to provide in many centers. It is unknown what financial and social impact will result if elderly individuals cannot be discharged to their community due to lack of aggressive post-acute care.

Aging with traumatic brain injury

Long-term outcomes after TBI have not been well studied, and little is known regarding how the aging processes is affected by TBI. Decades-long longitudinal studies are difficult to design and expensive to carry through to completion. Few such studies exist, leaving cross-sectional analysis the primary mode of determining long-term outcomes.

Evidence suggests that the cognitive impairments manifested acutely after TBI persist throughout life [48]. The chronicity of TBI impairments is supported by two retrospective studies on veterans who sustained injuries in World War II. One study revealed that personnel who sustained TBI had worse cognitive function than those with peripheral nerve lesions 30 years post injury [49]. The other study found a higher incidence of Alzheimer disease in those who sustained TBI as compared with non-TBI injured control subjects [50]. The association of Alzheimer disease development after TBI is controversial because some studies found an association [51–53], whereas others did not [54–56]. If a link between TBI and Alzheimer disease exists, it may be related to polymorphism of the apolipoprotein E (APOE) gene. APOE has three alleles: ∈2, ∈3, and ∈4. Each allele encodes for a specific protein (E2, E3, and E4 respectively). Possession of the ∈4 allele is associated with an increases risk for Alzheimer disease, which may be related to the beta-amyloid deposition seen in this disease [57]. Poorer cognitive skills in boxers with chronic TBI possessing the ∈4 allele were found in one study as compared with those with ∈2 or ∈3 [58]. Unfavorable short-term outcomes have been found post TBI in individuals carrying the ∈4 allele [59–62]. In a long-term study of 396 subjects with severe TBI assessed 15 to 20 years post injury, there was a trend ($P = 0.08$) for ∈4 carriers to have good outcomes less frequently than noncarriers [63]. Although the results did not reach statistical significance, the authors point out that the relatively youth of the population studied (mean 42 years) was probably too young to manifest age-related cognitive declines, as noted by previous epidemiologic studies that found the age of onset for Alzheimer disease post TBI to be ≥ 70 years [52,53]. This study supported the hypothesis that decline in overall function occurs after TBI because twice as many individuals experienced a deterioration in function as had improved compared with their status 6 months post injury [63]. In contrast to these findings, other studies found no indication of long-term cognitive deterioration or risk of Alzheimer disease after brain injury [54–56,64]. Furthermore, recent evidence raises doubts that the presence of ∈4 increases the risk of Alzheimer disease post TBI [52,65,66]. It has been suggested that reliable data on this issue will require dedicated research over many years [67].

After TBI, the majority of adults experience significant psychiatric disorders, with rates of comorbid psychiatric diagnoses considerably higher than expected in individuals living in the community. The most prevalent psychiatric diagnosis is major depression, with prevalence rates varying between 13% at 1 year post injury [68] to >60% [69] during the first decade post TBI. Anxiety disorders are the next most common psychiatric diagnosis, with frequencies varying between 18% and 60% [69–71]. Of the varied anxiety disorders, the most prevalent post TBI is post-traumatic stress disorder [69,72]. These long-term psychiatric sequelae pose additional challenges to community re-entry and quality of life for individuals post TBI and have been viewed as more seriously handicapping than the cognitive or physical consequences of the TBI [69]. Although age has not been found to be a significant predictor of psychiatric comorbidity post TBI [69,72], a positive history of a psychiatric disorder before TBI was a significant predictor of post TBI psychiatric comorbidity. This latter finding points to the need for detailed history taking in elderly patients to determine if the patient has had prior psychiatric diagnoses and thus is at heightened risk of development of a post-TBI psychiatric disorder. Proactive monitoring of mood in these individuals is strongly recommended, with ongoing psychologic support provided to minimize the severity of psychiatric sequelae post TBI. When indicated, proactive use of antidepressant medications should be implemented.

Behavioral dyscontrol is another common sequelae of TBI, with symptoms most commonly emerging during the period of post-trauma amnesia. Behavioral dyscontrol symptoms include frank agitation, impulsivity, and aggression. Often, these symptoms are precipitated by overstimulation (an environmental challenge in an inpatient hospital setting) or impaired sleep (a known health change in older adults post TBI) [73]. In elderly patients whose TBI remains unidentified, these behaviors can be misinterpreted as indicators of an incipient dementia. Clinicians working with elderly patients must be vigilant in differentiating aggressive symptoms of TBI from dementia because interventions are driven by the diagnosis. Thorough history taking focused on determining the timeline of symptom onset, potential precipitating events of the behavioral change, premorbid functioning, and environmental situations that seem to escalate or minimize these aberrant behaviors are indicated. A neuropsychologic assessment identifies cognitive impairments underlying TBI versus dementia and adds to the certainty of the diagnosis [74]. As is typical of good rehabilitation of all individuals with TBI, elderly patients with agitation due to TBI profit from a combination of behavioral/environmental interventions (eg, low-stimulation environment, constant reorientation, etc.) combined with medications to enhance alertness and cognitive recovery and in-depth cognitive testing and remediation.

Other health-related issues affect individuals with TBI over the course of their lives. Hibbard et al [69] reported that community-dwelling individuals with TBI were more likely to endorse problems related to their neurologic, endocrine, genitourinary, and musculoskeletal systems and to sleep disturbances than noninjured control subjects. Age seemed to have little impact the pattern of their self-reported health problems, with sleep disturbances being the only symptom reported as more commonly occurring among older as compared with younger individuals with TBI [69]. In a follow-up study, Breed et al [75] reported similar findings, with the impact of TBI on self-reported findings being stronger than the effect of age. In this study, sleep disturbances were found to occur more frequently in younger adults. The results of these studies suggest that clinicians treating individuals with TBI need to be aware of multiple health issues that are commonly reported in this population.

Special considerations are required when prescribing treatment to elderly patients, particularly after any central nervous system injury. Pharmacologic effects are often unpredictable or more pronounced in elderly as compared with younger individuals and may predispose the elderly persons to altered mental states, greater fall risk, and additional injury. The axiom "start low and go slow" with drug treatment is important in elderly individuals with TBI, who, as result of their injury, have problems associated with cognition and ambulation in addition to age-related comorbidities. As a result, they are more susceptible to the adverse effects of many pharmacologic agents. Extra consideration is required when planning discharge from the hospital because spouses of elderly individuals with TBI are more likely to be physically or cognitively impaired than those of younger individuals and therefore may not be capable of caring for a disabled loved one. Greater use of home care services is often needed, and if the caretaker is unavailable or unable to provide a safe environment, continued medical and rehabilitation care in appropriate skilled nursing facilities should be sought.

Previous research has documented the benefits of intensive focused rehabilitation interventions for elderly persons with TBI to maximize recovery and increase the probability of older adults being able to return to their homes and communities after TBI [41]. Rehabilitation efforts during acute and post-acute phases of TBI recovery require greater intensity and duration to achieve functional change equivalent to those observed in younger individuals post TBI. Unlike patients with dementia where the prognostic course is one of further cognitive decline, elderly patients with TBI have a relatively stable brain injury with a stable, or slowly improving, cognitive course if provided adequate supports. Elderly individuals can learn and retain new information but typically require additional opportunities to repeat and rehearse newly learned information. Teaching of compensatory strategies is needed with direct application of these techniques within the home and community setting, which is essential to maximize generalization. To achieve this, joint sessions with a family member or caregiver are encouraged so that techniques taught in rehabilitation can be directly applied and reinforced within the home or community setting.

For elderly persons presenting with psychiatric comorbidities post TBI, the combined use of antidepressant/antianxiety medications and individual psychotherapy is indicated to prevent further functional deterioration. Within sessions, issues of mourning cognitive or functional losses in the context of advanced aging need to be addressed. Research has suggested that the most efficacious psychologic interventions are those that use a cognitive behavioral approach embedded within cognitive remediation sessions [76,77].

A high index of suspicion of TBI should be maintained in several situations when treating elderly patients. Progressive loss of cognitive and physical abilities is frequently caused by expanding subdural hemorrhages, often when no obvious history of trauma can be elicited. Patients with a known history of falls should be followed closely and observed for altered cognitive or physical skills that may represent a brain injury. In either case, timely procurement of neuroimaging studies may lead to the correct diagnosis and appropriate treatment. Without this index of suspicion, these individuals may be erroneously diagnosed with dementia rather than with a treatable condition.

Many questions remain unanswered regarding the long-term effects of TBI. Specific issues that should be addressed in research include long-term disposition, causes of mortality many years post-TBI, long-term medical complications in institutionalized and community-dwelling individuals, and the long-term impact on families and caregivers of aging individuals with TBI.

As with all aging individuals, those with TBI require routine primary medical care. After a person sustains TBI, routine preventative care should be provided in addition to the services required as a result of TBI.

Summary

Older individuals with TBI differ from younger adults with TBI in several ways, including their incidence rates, etiology of injury, nature of complications, lengths of hospitalization, functional outcomes, and mortality. Despite the greater likelihood of poorer functional outcomes, older adults with TBI often achieve good functional outcomes and can live in community settings after receiving appropriate rehabilitation services, although at higher costs and longer hospitalizations than younger individuals. The future of rehabilitation care for elderly patients after TBI is uncertain due to financial limitations associated with the implementation of the PPS payment system by

CMS. Little is known regarding the long-term impact of TBI on individuals as they age, but this is an important issue as the population ages.

References

[1] Traumatic brain injury in the United States: a report to Congress. Atlanta (GA): US Department of Health and Human Services, CDC, National Center for Injury Prevention and Control; 1999.

[2] Injury fact book 2001–2002. Atlanta (GA): CDC, National Center for Injury Prevention and Control; 2001.

[3] Thurman DJ, Alverson CA, Dunn KA, Guerrero J, Sniezek JE. Traumatic brain injury in the United States: a public health perspective. J Head Trauma Rehabil 1999;14:602–15.

[4] Krause JF, Arthur DL. Incidence and prevalence of, and cost associated with traumatic brain injury. In: Rosenthal M, Griffith ER, Bond MR, Miller JD, editors. Rehabilitation of the adult and child with traumatic brain injury. 3rd edition. Philadelphia: F.A. Davis Company; 1999. p. 3–18.

[5] Whiteneck G, Mellick D, Brooks CA, Harrison-Felix C, Terrill MS, Noble K. Colorado traumatic brain injury registry and follow up system—databook. Denver (CO): Craig Hospital; 2001.

[6] Langlois JA, Kegler SR, Butler JA, Gotsch KE, Johnson RL, Reichard AA, et al. Traumatic brain injury-related hospital discharges: results from a 14-state surveillance system, 1997. MMWR Surveill Summ 2003;52:1–20.

[7] Susman M, DiRusso SM, Sullivan T, Risucci D, Nealon P, Cuff S, et al. Traumatic brain injury in the elderly: increased mortality and worse functional outcome at discharge despite lower injury severity. J Trauma 2002;53:219–23.

[8] Population Projections Program, Population Division. Washington, DC: US Census Bureau; 2000.

[9] Servadei F, Murray GD, Teasdale GM, Dearden M, Iannotti F, Lapierre F, et al. Traumatic subarachnoid hemorrhage: demographic and clinical study of 750 patients from the European brain injury consortium survey of head injuries. Neurosurgery 2002;50:261–7.

[10] Ellis GL. Subdural hematoma in the elderly. Emerg Med Clin North Am 1990;8:281–94.

[11] Traynelis VC. Chronic subdural hematoms in the elderly. Clin Geriatr Med 1991;7:583–98.

[12] Sato S, Suzuki J. Ultrastructural observations of the capsule of chronic subdural hematoma in various clinical stages. J Neurosurg 1975;43:569–78.

[13] Ito H, Yamamoto S, Saito K, Ikeda K, Hisada K. Quantitative estimation of hemorrhage in chronic subdural hematoma using the ^{51}Cr erythrocyte labeling method. J Neurosurg 1987; 66:862–4.

[14] Feldman RG, Pincus JH, McEntee WJ. Cerebrovascular accident or subdural fluid collection? Arch Intern Med 1963;112:966–76.

[15] Rozzelle CJ, Wofford JL, Branch CL. Predictors of hospital mortality in older patients with subdural hematoma. J Am Geriatr Soc 1995;43:240–4.

[16] Potter JF, Fruin AH. Chronic subdural hematoma: "the great imitator." Geriatrics 1977;32: 61–6.

[17] Luxon LM, Harrison MJG. Chronic subdural hematoma. Q J Med 1979;48: 43–53.

[18] Jones S, Kafetz K. A prospective study of chronic subdural hematomas in elderly patients. Age Ageing 1999;28:519–21.

[19] Gennarelli TA. The spectrum of traumatic axonal injury. Neuropathol Appl Neurobiol 1996;22:509–13.

[20] Povlishock JT. Structural aspects of brain injury. In: Bach-y-Rita P, editor. Comprehensive neurological rehabilitation, vol. 1. New York: Demos Publications; 1989. p. 87–96.

[21] Gale SD, Johnson SC, Bigler ED, Blatter DD. Trauma-induced degenerative changes in brain injury: a morphometric analysis of three patients with pre-injury and post-injury MR scans. J Neurotrauma 1995;12:151–8.

[22] Anderson CV, Wood DG, Bigler ED, Blatter DD. Lesion volume, injury severity, and thalamic integrity following head injury. J Neurotrauma 1996;13:59–65.

[23] Feng H, Huang G, Gao L, Tan H, Liao X. Effect of intracranial pressure and cerebral perfusion pressure on outcome prediction of severe traumatic brain injury. Chin J Traumatol 2000;3:226–30.

[24] Chesnut RM, Marchall LF, Klauber MR, Blunt BA, Baldwin N, Eisenberg KW, et al. The role of secondary brain injury in determining outcome from severe head injury. J Trauma 1993;34:216–22.

[25] Stocchetti N, Furlan A, Volta F. Hypoxemia and arterial hypotension at the accident scene in head injury. J Trauma 1996;40:764–7.

[26] Adekoya N, Thurman DJ, White DD, Webb KW. Surveillance for traumatic brain injury deaths: United States, 1989–1998. MMWR 2002;51:1–14.

[27] Tinetti ME, Doucette J, Claus E, Marottoli R. Risk factors for serious injury during falls by older person in the community. J Am Geriatr Soc 1995;43:1214–21.

[28] Speechley M, Tinetti M. Falls and injuries in frail and vigorous community elderly persons. J Am Geriatr Soc 1991;39:46–52.

[29] Ray WA, Griffin MR, Downey W, Melton LJ III. Long-term use of thiazide diuretics and risk of hip fracture. Lancet 1989;1:687–90.

[30] Thapa PB, Gidean P, Fought RL, Ray WA. Psychotropic drugs and risk of recurrent falls in ambulatory nursing home residents. Am J Epidemiol 1995;142:202–11.

[31] Spektor S, Agus S, Merkin V, Constantini S. Low-dose aspirin prophylaxis and risk of intracranial hemorrhage in patients older than 60 years of age with mild or moderate head injury: a prospective study. J Neurosurg 2003;99:661–5.

[32] Andrews PJ, Sleeman DH, Statham PF, McQuatt A, Corruble V, Jones PA, et al. Predicting recovery in patients suffering from traumatic brain injury by using admission variables and physiological data: a comparison between decision tree analysis and logistic regression. J Neurosurg 2002;97:326–36.

[33] Mosenthal AC, Lavery RF, Addis M, Kaul S, Ross S, Marburger R, et al. Isolated traumatic brain injury: age is an independent predictor of mortality and early outcome. J Trauma 2002; 52:907–11.

[34] Quigley MR, Vidovich D, Cantella D, Wilberger JE, Maroon JC, Diamond D. Defining the limits of survivorship after very sever head injury. J Trauma 1997;42:7–10.

[35] Ritchie PD, Cameron PA, Ugoni A, Kaye AH. A study of the functional outcome and mortality in elderly patients with head injuries. J Clin Neurosci 2000;7:301–4.

[36] Harrison-Felix C, Whiteneck G, DeVivo M, Hammond FM, Jha A. Mortality following rehabilitation in the Traumatic Brain Injury Model Systems of Care. NeuroRehabilitation 2004;19:45–54.

[37] Gubler KD, Davis R, Koepsell T, Soderberg R, Maier RV, Rivara FP. Long-term survival of elderly trauma patients. Arch Surg 1997;132:1010–4.

[38] Kilaru S, Garb J, Emhoff T, Fiallo V, Simon B, Swiencicki T, et al. Long-term functional status and mortality of elderly patients with severe closed head injuries. J Trauma 1996;41: 957–63.

[39] Perdue PW, Watts DD, Kaufman CR, Trask AL. Differences in mortality between elderly and younger adult trauma patients: geriatric status increases risk of delayed death. J Trauma 1998;45:805–10.

[40] Pennings JL, Bachulis BL, Simons CT, Slazinski T. Survival after severe brain injury in the aged. Arch Surg 1993;128:787–93.

[41] Cifu DX, Kreutzer JS, Marwitz JH, Rosenthal M, Englander J, High W. Functional outcomes of older adults with traumatic brain injury: a prospective, multicenter analysis. Arch Phys Med Rehabil 1996;77:883–8.

[42] Jennett B, Bond MR. Assessment of outcome after severe brain damage. Lancet 1975;1:
     480–4.
[43] Jennett B, Snoek J, Bond MR, Brooks N. Disability after severe head injury: observations on
     the use of the Glasgow Outcome Scale. J Neurol Neurosurg Psychiatry 1981;44:285–93.
[44] Hukkelhoven CW, Steyerberg EW, Rampen AJ, Farace E, Habbema JD, Marshall LF, et al.
     Patient age and outcome following severe traumatic brain injury: an analysis of 5600
     patients. J Neurosurg 2003;99:66–73.
[45] Rothweiler B, Temkin NR, Dikmen SS. Aging effect on psychosocial outcome in traumatic
     brain injury. Arch Phys Med Rehabil 1998;79:881–7.
[46] Reeder K, Rosenthal M, Lichtenberg P, Wood D. Impact of age on functional outcome
     following traumatic brain injury. J Head Trauma Rehabil 1996;11:22–31.
[47] Hoffman JM, Doctor JN, Chan L, Whyte J, Jha A, Dikmen S. Potential impact of the new
     Medicare prospective payment system on reimbursement for traumatic brain injury in-
     patient rehabilitation. Arch Phys Med Rehabil 2003;84:1165–72.
[48] Klein M, Houx PJ, Jolles J. Long-term persisting cognitive sequelae of traumatic brain injury
     and the effect of age. J Nerv Ment Dis 1996;184:459–67.
[49] Corkin S, Rosen TJ, Sullivan EV, Clegg RA. Penetrating head injury in young adulthood
     exacerbates cognitive decline in later years. J Neurosci 1989;9:3876–83.
[50] Plassman BL, Havlick RJ, Steffens DC, Helms MJ, Newman TN, Drosdick D, et al.
     Documented head injury in early adulthood and risk of Alzheimer's disease and other
     dementias. Neurology 2000;55:1158–66.
[51] Fleminger S, Oliver DL, Lovestone S, Rabe-Hesketh S, Giora A. Head injury as a risk factor
     for Alzheimer's disease: the evidence 10 years on; a partial replication. J Neurol Neurosurg
     Psychiatry 2003;74:857–62.
[52] Guo Z, Cupples LA, Kurz A, Auerbach SH, Volicer L, Chui H, et al. Head injury and risk of
     AD in the MIRAGE study. Neurology 2000;54:1316–23.
[53] Nemetz PN, Leibson C, Naessens JM, Beard M, Kokmen E, Annegers JF, et al. Traumatic
     brain injury and time to onset of Alzheimer's disease: a population-based study. Am J
     Epidemiol 1999;149:32–40.
[54] Canadian Study of Health and Aging (CSHA). The Canadian Study of Health and Aging:
     risk factors for Alzheimer's disease in Canada. Neurology 1994;44:2073–80.
[55] Katzman R, Aronson M, Fuld P, Kawas C, Brown T, Morgenstern H, et al. Development of
     dementing illnesses in an 80-year-old volunteer cohort. Ann Neurol 1989;25:317–24.
[56] Williams DB, Annegers JF, Kokmen E, O'Brien PC, Kurland LT. Brain injury and
     neurologic sequelae: a cohort study of dementia, parkinsonism, and amyotrophic lateral
     sclerosis. Neurology 1991;41:1554–7.
[57] Nicoll JA, Roberts GW, Graham DI. Apolipoprotein E ∈4 allele is associated with
     deposition of β-amyloid protein following head injury. Nat Med 1995;1:135–7.
[58] Jordan BD, Relkin NR, Ravdin LD, Jacobs AR, Bennett A, Gandy S. Apolipoprotein E
     epsilon4 associated with chronic traumatic brain injury in boxing. JAMA 1997;278:
     136–40.
[59] Teasdale GM, Nicoll JAR, Murray G, Fiddes M. Association of apolipoprotein E
     polymorphism with outcome after head injury. Lancet 1997;350:1069–71.
[60] Sorbi S, Nacmias B, Piacentini S, Replice A, Lattorraca S, Forleo P, et al. ApoE as
     a prognostic factor for post-traumatic coma. Nat Med 1995;1:852.
[61] Friedman G, Froom P, Sazbon L, Grinblatt I, Shochina M, Tsenter J, et al. Apolipoprotein
     E-epsilon4 genotype predicts a poor outcome in survivors of traumatic brain injury.
     Neurology 1999;52:244–8.
[62] Lichtman SW, Seliger G, Tycko B, Marder K. Apolipoprotein E and functional recovery
     from brain injury following postacute rehabilitation. Neurology 2000;55:1536–9.
[63] Millar K, Nicoll JA, Thornhill S, Murray GD, Teasdale GM. Long term neuro-
     psychological outcome after head injury: relation to APOE genotype. J Neurol Neurosurg
     Psychiatry 2003;74:1047–52.

[64] Newcombe F. Very late outcome after local wartime brain wounds. J Clin Exp Neuropsychol 1996;18:1–23.

[65] Jellinger KA, Paulus W, Wrocklage C, Litvan I. Effects if closed traumatic brain injury and genetic factors on the development of Alzheimer's disease. Eur J Neurol 2001;8:707–10.

[66] Jellinger KA, Paulus W, Wrocklage C, Litvan I. Traumatic brain injury as a risk factor for Alzheimer's disease: comparison of two retrospective autopsy cohorts with evaluation of ApoE genotype. BMC Neurol 2001;1:3, Epub July 30, 2001.

[67] Brooks N. Mental deterioration late after head injury: does it happen? J Neurol Neursurg Psychiatry 2003;74:1014.

[68] Deb S, Lyons I, Koutzoukis C, Ali I, McCarthy G. Rate of psychiatric illness 1 year after traumatic brain injury. Am J Psychiatry 1999;156:374–8.

[69] Hibbard MR, Uysal S, Kepler K, Bogdany J, Silver J. Axis I psychopathology in individuals with traumatic brain injury. J Head Trauma Rehabil 1998;13:24–39.

[70] Brooks N, Campsie L, Symington C, Beattie A, McKinlay W. The five year outcome of severe blunt head injury: a relative's view. J Neurol Neurosurg Psychiatry 1986;49:336–44.

[71] Schoenhuber R, Gentilini M. Anxiety and depression after mild head injury: a case control study. J Neurol Neurosurg Psychiatry 1988;51:722–4.

[72] Ashman T, Spielman LA, Hibbard MR, Silver JM, Chandra T, Gordon WA. Psychiatric challenges in the first 6 years after traumatic brain injury: cross-sequential analyses of Axis I disorders. Arch Phys Med Rehabil 2004;85(Suppl 2):S36–42.

[73] Hibbard MR, Uysal S, Sliwinski M, Gordon WA. Undiagnosed health issues in individuals with traumatic brain injury living in the community. J Head Trauma Rehabil 1998;13:47–57.

[74] Bigler ED, Rosa L, Schultz F, Hall S, Harris J. Rey-Auditory Learning and Rey-Osterrieth Complex Figure Design performance in Alzheimer's disease and closed head injury. J Clin Psychol 1989;34:1013.

[75] Breed ST, Flanagan SR, Watson KR. The relationship between age and the self-report of health symptoms in individuals with TBI. Arch Phys Med Rehabil 2004;85(Suppl 2):S61–7.

[76] Hibbard MR, Gordon WA, Egelko S, Langer K. Issues in the assessment and cognitive therapy of depression in brain damaged individuals. In: Freeman A, Greenwood V, editors. Cognitive therapy applications in psychiatric and medical settings. New York: Human Services Press; 1986.

[77] Grober S, Hibbard MR, Gordon WA, Stein, Freeman A. The psychotherapeutic treatment of post stroke depression with cognitive- behavioral therapy. In: Gordon WA, editor. Advances in stroke rehabilitation. Andover (MA): Andover Medical Publishers; 1986.

ELSEVIER
SAUNDERS

Phys Med Rehabil Clin N Am
16 (2005) 179–195

PHYSICAL MEDICINE
AND REHABILITATION
CLINICS OF
NORTH AMERICA

The geriatric amputee

Richard A. Frieden, MD

*Department of Rehabilitation Medicine, Mount Sinai School of Medicine, Mount Sinai
Medical Center, 5 East 98th Street, Box #1240B, New York, NY 10029, USA*

The needs of the person who had a lower limb amputation as a youth and now faces the trials of aging with a disability are unique, as are those of the person who has amputation after age and disability have begun to take their toll. The following exploration of these two areas of rehabilitation medicine is based upon reviewing literature that is primarily anecdotal and descriptive in nature and is derived mainly from retrospective (chart review) or prospective (telephone interviews and surveys) studies. Two review articles that evaluated the geriatrics literature for strength of evidence did not include a discussion of amputation [1,2].

Epidemiology

As the population ages, peripheral vascular disease (PVD) is becoming one of the most prevalent and possibly undertreated chronic illnesses in the United States. The most common form of PVD is caused by the process of atherosclerosis. This usually manifests in the legs as an asymptomatic arterial insufficiency, an exercise-induced pain that is relieved with rest, or as a limb-threatening ischemia that may lead to amputation. Because much of the disease is a silent process, reliance upon history-taking is not enough. Noninvasive testing has revealed a much greater incidence than was previously suspected [3]. Atherosclerosis is a systemic process, so even patients with asymptomatic disease are at risk for cardiovascular [4] and cerebrovascular morbidity and mortality. Furthermore, because people who are symptomatic by intermittent claudication cannot walk enough to participate in an exercise stress test, many people with atherosclerotic involvement of the coronary vessels go undiagnosed [4]. It is expected that early detection and intervention can prevent limb damage and can decrease the risk of other diseases [3].

E-mail address: richard.frieden@mssm.edu

1047-9651/05/$ - see front matter © 2004 Elsevier Inc. All rights reserved.
doi:10.1016/j.pmr.2004.06.004   pmr.theclinics.com

The process of atherosclerosis is accelerated by diabetes mellitus. The incidence of newly diagnosed cases of diabetes rose 33% between 1993 and 2001. More than half of lower-extremity amputations occur in people with diagnosed diabetes [5]. Other risk factors associated with PVD include smoking, hypertension, hyperlipidemia, obesity, an inactive lifestyle, and a family history of vascular or heart disease.

Whereas trauma and neoplasm used to account for most amputations in the younger population, the combination of juvenile obesity and earlier diagnosis of type 2 (adult-onset) diabetes earlier greatly increases the possibility of limb loss in early adulthood [5].

When examining the statistics, it is difficult to compare the numbers because the levels of amputation are usually grouped together. In the early 1980s, there were approximately 30,000 new lower extremity amputations performed annually in the United States [6]. By the mid-1990s, there were approximately 50,000 new major lower limb amputations performed each year in the United States [7]. PVD and diabetes mellitus account for over 90% of these amputations. The majority occurs in patients over 60 years of age, and men outnumber women.

In 1967–1968, it was estimated that 95% of leg amputations for elderly people were due to atherosclerosis, and 50% to 55% died within 5 years after surgery (usually from complications of atherosclerosis) [8,9]. In 1972, it was noted that more than one half of leg amputations due to vascular disease were performed at the transfemoral level [10]. By the 1990s, two thirds of amputations for PVD were at the transtibial level [11]. It has been estimated that between the years 1988 and 1996, there was a 27% increase in the incidence of dysvascular amputations, and amputations for trauma and neoplasm had decreased by approximately one half [12].

There is an increased mortality in the geriatric amputee population over that of the general population that continues for 1 or 2 years after surgery [13], after which the mortality rate returns to approximately that of the general population [14]. In 1994, it was estimated that 5-year survival after amputation is 35% to 40% [15]. The risk of contralateral amputation is 20% within the first 2 years after surgery [15] and is as high as 46% to 66% within 5 years after surgery in diabetic patients [13].

Despite instituting earlier and better screening and prevention methods and despite advances in surgical techniques for revascularization of threatened limbs, the rate of lower limb amputation has not decreased. This is in part due to the fact that, as the population ages, comorbidities arise that may lead to injury and the need for amputation. Thus, the pool of potential amputees continues to increase [16,17]. In addition, the introduction of improved revascularization methods caused a transient decrease in lower-extremity amputations in the late 1980s, but when the hospitals' capacity for performing these procedures reached the maximum, the rate of amputations rose again [16].

Revascularization and limb salvage

Prevention of amputation in the elderly population by revascularization procedures has been widely debated [3,11,17–24]. One discussion concerns the possibility of a more proximal amputation if the bypass fails than if a primary amputation had been performed [20,25]. Revascularization should not be used as a means of obtaining a more distal level of amputation, such as when attempting to save a knee joint [22]. Another factor is comparing the cost of revascularization, a procedure that may have to be revised and that may lead to amputation anyway, with the cost of primary amputation and prosthetic rehabilitation [21]. Primary amputation is associated with fewer postoperative complications than secondary amputation after attempted revascularization [17]. In 1984, it was noted that attempting revascularization would occasionally lead to a delay in amputation while waiting to see whether the bypass would work. This allows more time for complications to arise [25].

Amputation surgery and pre/postoperative care issues

In the area of amputation surgery, there are several important perioperative considerations. Medical stability is a critical factor when contemplating limb amputation. The patient has to withstand metabolic "stress" due to sepsis, anesthesia, and the surgery. The cardiac status and the other comorbidities (especially renal and respiratory) must be brought under control before surgery [26].

Preoperative assessment is critical especially when discussing preserving the knee joint [27,28]. Although it has been recognized that preserving the knee joint is beneficial [7], careful planning of the primary procedure is necessary to avoid the need for revisions and longer patient hospitalizations [29].

Until the early to mid 1970s, the preferred operation was transfemoral amputation because the techniques for transtibial amputation had not been improved upon and had a high failure rate and high re-operation rate [22]. There are several descriptions of surgical technique in the literature [13,28,30,31].

The energy expenditure required by an amputee for ambulation with or without a prosthesis should be considered before surgery. Although exercise tolerance decreases with age, the likelihood of more proximal amputation and the need for a heavier prosthesis increases with age [7]. For example, the increase in energy expenditure required by a transtibial amputee compared with the able-bodied population is much less than that required by a transfemoral amputee. A transfemoral amputee spends more energy in ambulation than does a bilateral transtibial amputee. Because the metabolic demand to walk with crutches (without a prosthesis) is greater than the demand to walk with a prosthesis, it was felt that crutch walking would be a good predictor of the ability to use a prosthesis [32]. This rule is recognized as applying to younger people. As people age and balance declines, a more accurate assessment would be to test ambulation ability with a walker (without a prosthesis) [33]. It is important that cardiac testing, preferably by exercise, be conducted on patients who face amputation and that pulmonary function testing be conducted on people with known respiratory problems [6].

If the other leg is at risk of amputation, should the patient be encouraged to consider prosthetic ambulation after the first amputation? This is not an easy question to answer. If the patient's cardiac status can withstand the effort, the usual answer is to proceed apace with fitting and training [31]. Bear in mind the considerable risks of myocardial infarction and cerebrovascular accident due to atherosclerosis. We want people "up" and functioning optimally as soon as possible and should not deny them that opportunity [34]. Early ambulation has been explored with devices such as the immediate post-operative prosthesis [8,35] or an off-loading device that resembles a hip-knee-ankle-foot orthosis but has a prosthetic foot attached [36]. The risk to the remaining limb is not accelerated by fitting and training to use a prosthesis [32]. The studies that addressed these issues used fewer than 30 patients each and were not randomized.

It is important to assess the patient's level of functioning before the onset of leg ischemia and the need for amputation. This is critical in determining postoperative expectations [37]. For example, if the patient were a fully functional community ambulator, then, barring difficulties encountered during the hospital stay, one would anticipate restoration of that activity level [38]. If the patient were a minimal household ambulator due to arthritis or other conditions, one would not anticipate a higher level of activity after surgery. It is wrong to tell people that they will be "as good as new" after surgery because many people think this means that amputation will cure or solve all of their mobility problems. Remember that prosthesis use is only one part of the rehabilitation process.

Often the amputation is the culmination of months of treatment that leaves the person weak and debilitated. Sometimes the loss of the limb follows a period of general physical and mental decline that had an adverse impact on the amputee and his/her family. Starting rehabilitation quickly prevents further deterioration of the health and stamina of the older patient. For this reason it is important to begin prosthetic fitting as soon as feasible after the amputation. Such early ambulation has been demonstrated to decrease the debilitating effects of prolonged inactivity, allay fears of immobilization and dependency, and improve the quality and length of life for the amputee [32].

Whenever possible, the physiatrist should be called before surgery [39] to help with the preoperative assessment and aid discharge planning. The physiatrist can advise the surgeon about useful length and potential function of the residual limb and the patient overall and can answer questions and clarify for the patient and family what is available for prosthetic replacement.

The postoperative management of patients who have undergone amputation includes the need for support and counseling. The initial lifestyle change is profound. There are a host of self-image and dependency issues that persist beyond the postoperative period. Function, comfort, appearance, social, and economic factors are involved. Some people benefit from a support group, whereas others prefer a one-on-one approach to counseling. Some people are bolstered by a visit from a "successful" amputee, whereas others are helped by friends and family members who facilitate the rehabilitation process. Intensive psychologic support may be needed [40].

Patients must be kept mobile, and complications must be prevented. The initial physical goals during the postoperative period are to relieve pain, prevent medical complications (including pulmonary, GI, and renal problems), and prevent mobility problems (including joint contractures and muscle atrophy). Management of the phantom and avoidance of falls are also important. Later, the rehabilitation team works on balance, self-care, and ambulation skills. The chief goal at that point is to achieve independent function in a patient with only one leg. Information about the home environment is necessary to train the patient to deal with the situation safely. Family members can help with this process.

Rehabilitation issues specific to the geriatric amputee

Management of the older amputee is different from the management of the younger amputee in several ways. First, expectations are different in that more physical activity and more participation in society are anticipated of the younger person. Negative perceptions of elderly people that may adversely influence decision-making include decreased motivation and adaptability, increased psychologic distress, and increased physical limitations [41]. Second, more resources are allotted to the care of the younger population. Third, more research has been conducted using younger subjects than older subjects. Fourth, a widely held view among clinicians is that more advanced prosthetic components are not appropriate for the older person solely because of advanced age, an erroneous opinion that should be discarded in favor of the concept of selection by functional criteria [42,43].

There are several articles that describe similar versions of the general course of the amputation and rehabilitation program [10,14,30,44–47]. Ideally, there would be a continuum of care for the patient undergoing amputation surgery. There was a time when a patient walked into the hospital with an ischemic leg, underwent amputation, stayed until healing was finished, was fitted with a prosthesis, and walked out of the hospital. Those days are largely passed. Now, after a patient has the surgery, he learns the basics of mobility and self-care and then goes home to finish healing. The therapies are pursued at home, at a private facility, or in an outpatient setting.

Age-associated risk factors

The risk of falls is greater for the elderly population [48,49], which leads to the increased risk of limb injury that may lead to amputation and the increased risk of injury to the residual limb that may hamper ambulation with a prosthesis [14]. The risk of sensory disturbance increases with age, making the patient's skin vulnerable to injury [50,51]. Other risks that are greater for the elderly person with or at risk of having an amputation include

- Skin breakdown, with decreased ability to heal well [14,52]
- Development of arthritis in the shoulders from arm weight bearing or in the sound leg from over-reliance on it [14]
- Development of restricted back or hip motion due to arthritis [14]
- The occurrence of systemic and disabling diseases [14,53,54]
- Development of complications such as diabetic retinopathy and neuropathy [37]

Other changes that occur with aging include loss of lean body mass, loss of bone density, loss of vision, poor nutrition, and onset of neurologic diseases [54]. In general, aging affects all organ systems. Exercise can improve strength, endurance, and coordination [55].

Diagnostics

Many of the assessment scales and treatment protocols designed for younger adults cannot be applied to the elderly population because they do not take into account the altered physiology and life circumstances of the older population. For example, gait analysis has shown that older people adopt gait patterns different from younger people [14,56,57]. Gait analysis of older amputees has shown increased use of the nonamputated leg for push-off [58] and a correlation between speed of gait and functional status [59]. One study examined the gait of eight men who had transtibial amputation due to trauma and who wore the same socket and foot designs [58]; another study looked at the gait of 20 men who had transtibial amputation as a result of PVD, all of whom wore the same socket and foot designs [59].

The prosthetic phase

Assuming no complications ensue [60], the next process includes obtaining a prosthesis and training the patient to use it. Patients may be daunted by the appearance of the prosthesis, by the weight of the limb [7], and by the new skills they must learn to walk. Support and education are necessary. The details of this process are beyond the scope of this article.

The process of prosthetic prescription is based upon the physician's awareness of the patient's prior functional status, prior and current medical status, learning ability, and goals for future function [47,61]. There are approximately 12 socket and suspension designs, scores of knee joints, and myriad foot models [42], each with different characteristics that should be considered when writing a prescription [31]. Insurance issues; the cost of components; and the need for clear communication among the physician, therapists, prosthetist, patient, and insurance company representatives further complicate the situation.

When considering lower-limb prosthetic replacement, older amputees should have available to them a wide range of technology and componentry. One may be prescribing for a senior athlete who lost a leg due to vascular disease (who may benefit from a lightweight device with advanced knee and foot mechanisms) or a sedentary older person who may be able to achieve some degree of independence by using a simple prosthesis with a secure suspension. The technical details of the prosthesis should be determined by the specific needs and capacities of each individual amputee, not by an arbitrary prescription based on age or diagnosis alone. The goal should be to improve the quality of life and the degree of independence for the older amputee.

There is little information available about socket designs for the elderly amputee. One article mentioned that newer technologies, such as the use of plastics, can be applied to all age groups but also commented that older people would tend to choose a wooden socket and that younger people are more likely to select a plastic socket but did not offer evidence to confirm this notion [35]. Studies comparing the effect of different prosthetic feet on amputee gait and energy expenditure have not included statistically significant numbers of subjects, nor have they focused exclusively on elderly subjects [58]. Several articles recommended (as clinical guidelines without presenting supporting evidence) prescribing a patellar-tendon bearing or patellar-tendon/supracondylar socket with augmented suspension and a solid-ankle-cushion-heel (SACH) foot for the typical elderly patient who had a transtibial amputation and a quadrilateral nonsuction socket, safety knee or other articulated knee, and SACH foot for the elderly patient who had transfemoral amputation [7,31]. The logic seems to be that relatively sedentary people need lightweight, uncomplicated devices that do not require much maintenance and that more active people would benefit from devices such as hydraulic knees and energy-storing or dynamic-response feet.

In exploring the intertwined topics of predicting function and prescribing a prosthesis, it should first be noted that most insurance companies, including Medicare (the largest financial resource in the United States for prosthetic care), will not pay for a nonfunctional, cosmesis-only leg. When considering functional devices, the patient must be able to learn how to use the device. This process may be impeded by the problem of delirium due to preoperative toxicity and sepsis or mental status changes due to anesthesia. Visual loss, arthritis, and neuropathy of the hands are not contraindications for prosthetic prescription. If necessary, the patient can get adaptations or human assistance to help don the leg and then stand and start walking. Even the use of a prosthesis for ease of transfers is worthwhile.

Some authors advocate giving all amputees a wheelchair because independence in self-care at that level is a worthwhile goal [62]. Ambulation solely at the wheelchair level may be necessary if there is pre-existing cerebrovascular disease or if the patient has bilateral amputations [22]. There is a paucity of research on the subject of powered mobility for the elderly population, but one widely held view is that the factors of lowered endurance due to cardiopulmonary disorders, the need for independent functioning, and the loss of mobility within the home due to arthritis, stroke, amputation, etc. are indications for powered mobility. Early post-operative prostheses have been proposed as a means of testing the functional potential of the amputee [9,15,20,63].

Until recently, Medicare had no standard classification by which to categorize the components and procedures appropriate for each amputation level. The introduction of the five-level or "K-Modifiers" scale helped organize components and amputees' access to them based on the patient's rehabilitation potential as determined by the prosthetist and ordering physician [43]. Criteria considered for assessing the functional level include the patient's past history and current condition including the status of the residual limb, the nature of other medical problems, and the patient's desire to ambulate. Many people feel that the five-level scale is based upon subjective judgments and that an objective rating scale is needed [64].

Predicting functional outcome in a reliable and uniform manner has been a difficult task [64,65]. Assessments of balance, cognition, and the number and type of comorbidities have been suggested [66]. In 1960, being older than 55 years was considered a negative factor predicting against optimal functioning [61]. Age is no longer considered to be an obstacle [33], but the comorbidities that arise with aging must be taken into account [33,67]. The ability to don the prosthesis, the distance walked without a rest break, and the use of minimal assistive devices have been suggested as predictors [68,69]. Level of amputation may play a role [68–70]. However, the choice of level ("site of election") may be influenced by the presence of comorbidities and perceived frailty [71]. In cases of dual disabilities, such as stroke and amputation, some authors have noted that having a stroke before amputation impedes subsequent rehabilitation efforts [71,72], but other investigators have not reached this conclusion [73]. Although people with end-stage renal disease may need a longer rehabilitation hospital stay, they can achieve some degree of improved function [74].

Training to use a prosthesis is usually accomplished outside of the hospital. Sometimes patients are admitted to learn to use a prosthesis if they have a medical condition that should be monitored while they are in training, such as brittle diabetes or labile blood pressure.

Complications that can ensue during training with a prosthesis include skin irritation from materials, skin breakdown, infection, and hip and back pain. Careful, regular monitoring of the situation and education of the patient regarding skin care and prosthetic hygiene are needed [32]. Skin breakdown, ulcerations, and infections are some of the sequelae of wearing an ill-fitting prosthesis [75]. Training should proceed cautiously to avoid rapid progression to less secure assistive devices [45]. As patients become more active, they must be monitored for increased cardiac stress and manifestations of other conditions [76].

Prevention of future limb loss/advice for caregivers and families

After an amputation of one leg, the remaining leg needs even closer scrutiny. The same principles apply as with general screening, including inspection and cleaning, disease modification, shoe fit, and dietary and smoking habits. If the remaining leg is also compromised, the ability of the person to walk will be threatened.

Prevention of future limb loss is a vital area in which the clinician can guide patients and families. This is important in light of the continuing risk of amputation despite therapeutic interventions. It follows, therefore, that risk factor modification is one of the key principles in avoiding amputation [24].

Preventive measures fall into a few basic categories. Patient education and screening on an individual basis in the office and in groups is a vital part of the process. This must be an ongoing activity, as should staff education about the importance of these efforts.

Screening for PVD should be part of routine office visits, starting with obtaining the history and performing the physical examination. Patients with diabetic neuropathy may not report the pain of ischemia [77]. One may note the presence of pulse abnormalities, hair loss, skin discoloration, unusual temperature changes, and ulceration. The feet should be inspected on a regular basis. Footwear needs to be examined as well.

As with many conditions associated with aging, one needs to be aware that the pain of PVD may be mistaken for or dismissed as "arthritis" or "getting old." Symptomatic patients have exercised-induced pain or intermittent claudication usually in the calves if the disease process is distal and in the thighs or even buttocks if the blockage is in more proximal vessels. More severe disease is marked by numbness, rest pain, infection, and tissue damage.

Noninvasive tests are helpful in screening patients. By using a portable Doppler ultrasound device, one can derive the ankle-brachial index (ABI), which is the ratio of the systolic blood pressure at the ankle divided by the systolic blood pressure measured at the arm. The ratio should be equal to or greater than one. As the number declines, the risk of PVD rises.

Other tests are available by consulting with a vascular surgeon, vascular laboratory, or radiology department. These include segmental pressures, pulse volume recordings, duplex and color flow ultrasound, and magnetic resonance angiography.

Teaching patients to care for their feet is a major preventive measure [78]. Patients should be instructed to wash their feet and inspect them daily, stay dry between the toes, avoid exposure to extreme temperatures, avoid walking barefooted, inspect their shoes before donning, avoid crossing their legs, stop smoking, avoid excessive alcohol consumption, avoid cutting corns or calluses, watch for ingrown or misshapen nails, and seek medical or podiatric attention if signs of ulceration or infection appear. Education is needed to increase awareness of complications of diabetes, such as retinopathy and neuropathy [37]. Patients with diabetes must also receive screening and education regarding PVD [5].

Patient education materials are available from diabetes resource centers and web sites (see Appendix). Nurse educators and podiatrists can help keep patients on track. A multidisciplinary approach is being advocated that would include many physician specialists and allied health care providers.

Community screening events are also in progress. The screenings include questionnaires, ABI examinations, and nurse and physician consultations. Patients and their caregivers are being reached with such programs.

Prevention by treatment is another major category. There are several medications available for treatment of intermittent claudication. Diabetes management and antihypertensive therapy have been shown to decrease morbidity and mortality in patients with PVD. Exercise, especially walking and leg exercises, can increase the pain-free walking distance if pursued for at least 3 months. Dietary modifications are needed, especially lowering fat and cholesterol. Other treatment methods include interventional radiology and surgical techniques to restore circulation. These are usually performed on an inpatient basis.

One area that requires special mention is the problem of heel ulcers. The prevalence of such wounds in the outpatient or inpatient population is not known. Heel ulcers in a dysvascular or diabetic person can lead to amputation. Preventive measures must be taken in the less mobile patients. These methods include providing heel pads, assistance with repositioning, assistance with getting out of bed, and daily inspection of the feet. Early intervention when a wound develops is crucial.

A coordinated, multi-stage program that includes education, screening, provision of off-loading devices, wound care, and progressive ambulation will reduce hospitalization time and costs and amputation-related admissions [79].

Outcomes

Several scales that purport to assess quality of life after amputation [80] or predict ability to function after surgery [64,65,81] have been proposed. Large-scale studies are needed for validation.

There is little written about the economic impact of a comprehensive amputee rehabilitation program. Three studies showed a reduction in length of stay, an improvement in healing time, and a higher percentage of successful ambulators [82]. The differences between the programs for younger amputees and older amputees are the need to accommodate for the older person's decreased physical and (occasionally) mental capacity, the consideration of increased risk to the ischemic remaining leg, the need to control the comorbidities, and the recognition of the greater socioeconomic issues [82,83].

Resumption of employment and high-level activities has been thought of as an appropriate goal for young people. For elderly amputees, improvement in self-care and walking skills, decreased reliance on caregivers, and increased comfort are appropriate goals. Important factors are age, physical condition, psychologic condition/mental status, and social resources [83]. Goals may be modified and the tempo may be slowed to accommodate the patient [84]. According to some authors, older patients are more likely to go to a nursing home after the acute hospital stay, are less likely to use a prosthesis, and are thought to require longer hospital stays and longer periods of rehabilitation [81].

Long-term survival of older persons after amputation has been studied [40]. Some authors claim that people with transtibial amputations have less severe systemic atherosclerosis, so their mortality rate is lower than that of transfemoral amputees [40].

Functioning after provision of a prosthesis has been studied. Based upon review of articles published in 1967 and 1972, one group stated that older people tend to set aside their prostheses shortly after training is concluded [7]. In 1967, it was felt that over one half of amputees discarded their limbs within 6 months after training [13]. A study of people who had undergone amputation between 1987 and 1992 revealed that decreased use of a prosthesis was correlated with advanced age, female gender, possession of a wheelchair, cognitive impairment, level of disability, and patient dissatisfaction with the prosthesis [85]. Retrospective assessment of one clinic's activity revealed that people who were denied prostheses were more likely to have advanced age, decreased cognition, cerebrovascular disease, and need for reamputation. Successful fitting with a prosthesis has been associated with younger age, fewer comorbidities, more distal level of amputation, marriage, and ability to be discharged home [86]. The functional level of the transfemoral amputee declines more rapidly with advancing age than does the functional level of the transtibial amputee [82].

As survival improves and the likelihood of bilateral surgery increases, there needs to be more discussion of levels and of prosthetic components [87]. In addition, more resources need to be allocated to elderly, bilateral amputees to make them more independent in the community [80,88].

Aging with an amputation

The young amputee who ages needs regular follow-up as the manifestations of aging become evident (eg, poor nutrition, fragile skin, restricted joint motion, and more frequent falls). Lighter-weight materials and simpler feet may be useful. Modification of the prosthetic suspension for easier donning and doffing and more stable knee joints may also be required for the aging patient [14,54].

Future areas of inquiry and research

There is little information on how the young amputee ages or how the physiologic changes that accompany aging affect the residual limb. For example, muscle atrophy occurs with aging. Some of the muscles in a residual limb are denervated as a result of surgery. Do those muscles atrophy more quickly? Does preserving the nerve supply where possible have an effect upon the rate of muscle atrophy? One can observe in patients of all ages that some muscles in the residual limb (regardless of level) are under voluntary control. Would instructing patients in regular residual limb muscle "twitching" exercises have an effect upon the rate of muscle atrophy? How would this affect socket fit? Would it decrease the number and type of adjustments needed? This issue has implications for the surgeon, the physiatrist, the physical therapist, the prosthetist, and the patient.

Research with statistically significant numbers of subjects is needed on the effects of different prosthetic components (especially feet and knees) on the gait of older amputees. Another area that needs further exploration is prospective follow-up of young amputees as they age to watch for changes in general function and in the fit and use of a prosthesis [89]. Further, research into socket designs and specific changes made over time as people age is needed.

Summary

There are special aspects of aging with an amputation and with being elderly at the time of an amputation. Older adults who have undergone amputation have many issues to contend with, including comorbidities that affect postoperative care and rehabilitation, general deconditioning and loss of mobility (especially if the onset of rehabilitation is delayed), and lack of social support upon returning to the community. These problems are compounded by a lack of knowledge about caring for the residual limb and prosthesis, maintenance of general health, and management of comorbid conditions.

People who have sustained an amputation at an early age and who are ambulatory may find increasing difficulties as they age. Acquired chronic disease occurs more frequently as people age. These conditions can adversely affect function after amputation. Prosthetic designs may need modification because certain components may become more difficult to use.

The prevention of a (second) amputation results in saving a limb and preserving self-image and independent function. Considering the emotional and economic cost of amputation and lifelong management of a prosthesis, it is worth the time and effort to practice preventive measures. Should amputation become necessary, careful patient assessment, compassionate management, and communication among the team members results in a more favorable outcome. Including the physiatrist early in the clinical course makes this process easier.

Appendix

Useful web sites for education, screening programs, and preventing amputation

American Diabetes Association: www.diabetes.org
WebMD Health: www.diabetes.com
Legs for Life (screening program): www.legsforlife.org
National Diabetes Education Program: www.ndep.nih.gov

References

[1] Wells JL, Seabrook JA, Stolee P, Borrie MJ, Knoefel F. State of the art in geriatric rehabilitation. Part I: review of frailty and comprehensive geriatric assessment. Arch Phys Med Rehabil 2003;84:890–7.
[2] Wells JL, Seabrook JA, Stolee P, Borrie MJ, Knoefel F. State of the art in geriatric rehabilitation. Part II: clinical challenges. Arch Phys Med Rehabil 2003;84:898–903.
[3] Newman AB. Peripheral arterial disease: insights from population studies of older adults. J Am Geriatr Soc 2000;48:1157–62.
[4] Roth EJ, Park KL, Sullivan WJ. Cardiovascular disease in patients with dysvascular amputation. Arch Phys Med Rehabil 1998;79:205–15.
[5] Vinicor F. Diabetes: preventing lower-extremity amputations. inMotion 2001;11:15–6.
[6] Moore TJ, Barron J, Hutchinson F III, Golden C, Ellis C, Humphries D. Prosthetic usage following major extremity amputation. Clin Orthop 1989;238:219–24.
[7] Cutson TM, Bongiorni DR. Rehabilitation of the older lower limb amputee: a brief review. J Am Geriatr Soc 1996;44:1388–93.
[8] Warren R. Early rehabilitation of the elderly lower extremity amputee. Surg Clin North Am 1968;48:807–16.
[9] Anderson AD, Cummings V, Levine SL, Kraus A. The use of lower extremity prosthetic limbs by elderly patients. Arch Phys Med Rehabil 1967;48:533–8.
[10] Inter-Society Commission for Heart Disease Resources. Hospital resources for a quality amputation program. Circulation 1972;46:A293–304.
[11] Fletcher DD, Andrews KL, Hallett JW Jr, Butters MA, Rowland CM, Jacobsen SJ. Trends in rehabilitation after amputation for geriatric patients with vascular disease: implications for future health resource allocation. Arch Phys Med Rehabil 2002;83:1389–93.
[12] Dillingham TR, Pezzin LE, MacKenzie EJ. Limb amputation and limb deficiency: epidemiology and recent trends in the United States. South Med J 2002;95:875–83.
[13] Mazet R Jr. The geriatric amputee. Artif Limbs 1967;11:33–41.

[14] Leonard JA Jr. The elderly amputee. In: Felsenthal G, Garrison SJ, Steinberg FU, editors. Rehabilitation of the aging and elderly patient. Baltimore: Williams & Wilkins; 1994. p. 397–406.

[15] Cutson TM, Bongiorni D, Michael JW, Kochersberger G. Early management of elderly dysvascular below-knee amputees. J Prosthet Orthot 1994;6:62–6.

[16] Feinglass J, Brown JL, LoSasso A, Sohn MW, Manheim LM, Shah SJ, et al. Rates of lower-extremity amputation and arterial reconstruction in the United States, 1979 to 1996. Am J Public Health 1999;89:1222–7.

[17] Van Niekerk LJA, Stewart CPU, Jain ASA. Major lower limb amputation following failed infrainguinal vascular bypass surgery: a prospective study on amputation levels and stump complications. Prosthet Orthot Int 2001;25:29–33.

[18] Pomposelli FB Jr, Arora S, Gibbons GW, Frykberg R, Smakowski P, Campbell DR, et al. Lower extremity arterial reconstruction in the very elderly: successful outcome preserves not only the limb but also residential status and ambulatory function. J Vasc Surg 1998;28: 215–25.

[19] Kistner RL. Management of severe leg ischemia in the elderly patient. Geriatrics 1968;23: 93–6.

[20] Skversky N, Zislis JM. Peripheral-vascular disorders and the aged amputee. Geriatrics 1970; 25:142–9.

[21] Callow AD, Mackey WC. Costs and benefits of prosthetic vascular surgery. Int Surg 1988; 73:237–40.

[22] Robinson KP. Long posterior flap amputation in geriatric patients with ischaemic disease. Ann R Coll Surg Engl 1976;58:440–51.

[23] O'Brien TS, Lamont PM, Crow A, Gray DR, Collin J, Morris PJ. Lower limb ischaemia in the octogenarian: is limb salvage surgery worthwhile? Ann R Coll Surg Engl 1993;75:445–7.

[24] Persson B. Lower limb amputation part 1: amputation methods—a 10 year literature review. Prosthet Orthot Int 2001;25:7–13.

[25] Weiss GN, Gorton A, Read RC, Neal LA. Outcomes of lower extremity amputations. J Am Geriatr Soc 1990;38:877–83.

[26] Margolis IB, Hayes DF. Managing peripheral vascular disease secondary to atherosclerosis. Geriatrics 1977;32:79–82.

[27] Reyes RL, Leahey EB, Leahey EB Jr. Elderly patients with lower extremity amputations: three-year study in a rehabilitation setting. Arch Phys Med Rehabil 1977;58:116–22.

[28] Burgess EM. Knee disarticulation and above-knee amputation. In: Moore WS, Malone JM, editors. Lower extremity amputation. Philadelphia: WB Saunders; 1989. p. 132–46.

[29] Campbell WB, St-Johnston JA, Kernick VFM, Rutter EA. Lower limb amputation: striking the balance. Ann R Coll Surg Engl 1994;76:205–9.

[30] Committee on Prosthetic-Orthotic Education. The geriatric amputee: principles of management. Washington, DC: National Academy of Sciences-National Research Council; 1971.

[31] Clark GS, Blue B, Bearer JB. Rehabilitation of the elderly amputee. J Am Geriatr Soc 1983; 31:439–48.

[32] Wilson AB. Limb prosthetics today. Artif Limbs 1963;7:1–42.

[33] Steinberg FU, Sunwoo IS, Roettger RF. Prosthetic rehabilitation of geriatric amputee patients: a follow-up study. Arch Phys Med Rehabil 1985;66:742–5.

[34] Pohjolainen T, Alaranta H. Ten-year survival of Finnish lower limb amputees. Prosthet Orthot Int 1998;22:10–6.

[35] Marquardt E, Correll J. Amputations and prostheses for the lower limb. Int Orthop 1984;8: 139–46.

[36] Dickstein R, Halevy E, Meir H, Bigon R. Use of the early walking aid as a "geriatric prosthesis" in the community. J Prosthet Orthot 1989;1:110–5.

[37] Dacher JE. Rehabilitation and the geriatric patient. Nurs Clin North Am 1989;24: 225–37.

[38] Bradley RL, Bradley EJ. Amputation in the elderly: analysis of 85 patients. Geriatrics 1966; 21:189–92.

[39] Hoenig H, Nusbaum N, Brummel-Smith K. Geriatric rehabilitation: state of the art. J Am Geriatr Soc 1997;45:1371–81.

[40] Harris PL, Read F, Eardley A, Charlesworth D, Wakefield J, Sellwood RA. The fate of elderly amputees. Br J Surg 1974;61:665–8.

[41] Nicholas JJ, Rybarczyk B, Meyer PM, Lacey RF, Haut A, Kemp PJ. Rehabilitation staff perceptions of characteristics of geriatric rehabilitation patients. Arch Phys Med Rehabil 1998;79:1277–84.

[42] Michael JW. Prosthetic feet: options for the older client. Top Geriatr Rehabil 1992;8:30–8.

[43] Francis R. Geriatric patients: are they getting the best prosthetic choices? O&P Edge 2003;2: 38–40.

[44] Katrak PH, Baggott JB. Rehabilitation of elderly lower-extremity amputees. Med J Aust 1980;1:651–3.

[45] Oh SH. Rehabilitating the geriatric amputee: what the primary MD should know. Geriatrics 1982;37:91–4.

[46] Esquenazi A. Geriatric amputee rehabilitation. Clin Geriatr Med 1993;9:731–43.

[47] Russek AS. Management of lower extremity amputees. Arch Phys Med Rehabil 1961;42: 687–703.

[48] Miller WC, Speechley M, Deathe B. The prevalence and risk factors of falling and fear of falling among lower extremity amputees. Arch Phys Med Rehabil 2001;82:1042–7.

[49] Miller WC, Deathe B, Speechley M, Kovac J. The influence of falling, fear of falling, and balance confidence on prosthetic mobility and social activity among individuals with a lower extremity amputation. Arch Phys Med Rehabil 2001;82:1238–44.

[50] Kosasih JB, Silver-Thorn MB. Sensory changes in adults with unilateral transtibial amputation. J Rehabil Res Dev 1998;35:85–90.

[51] Cochrane H, Orsi K, Reilly P. Lower limb amputation part 3: prosthetics—a 10 year literature review. Prosthet Orthot Int 2001;25:21–8.

[52] Czerniecki JM, Harrington RM, Wyss CR, Sangeorzan BJ, Matsen FA III. The effects of age and peripheral vascular disease on the circulatory and mechanical response of skin to loading. Am J Phys Med Rehabil 1990;69:302–6.

[53] Dunlop DD, Manheim LM, Sohn M-W, Liu X, Chang RW. Incidence of functional limitation in older adults: the impact of gender, race, and chronic conditions. Arch Phys Med Rehabil 2002;83:964–71.

[54] Andrews KL. Rehabilitation in limb deficiency. 3: the geriatric amputee. Arch Phys Med Rehabil 1996;77:S14–7.

[55] Hong C-Z, Tobis JS. Physiatric rehabilitation and maintenance of the geriatric patient. In: Kottke FJ, Lehmann JF, editors. Krusen's handbook of physical medicine and rehabilitation. 4th edition. Philadelphia: WB Saunders; 1990. p. 1209–16.

[56] Kerrigan DC, Todd MK, Della Croce U, Lipsitz LA, Collins JJ. Biomechanical gait alterations independent of speed in the healthy elderly: evidence for specific limiting impairments. Arch Phys Med Rehabil 1998;79:317–22.

[57] Sadeghi H, Prince F, Zabjek KF, Labelle H. Simultaneous, bilateral, and three-point dimensional gait analysis of elderly people without impairments. Am J Phys Med Rehabil 2004;83:112–23.

[58] Lemaire ED, Fisher FR, Robertson DGE. Gait patterns of elderly men with trans-tibial amputation. Prosthet Orthot Int 1993;17:27–37.

[59] Hubbard WA, McElroy GK. Benchmark data for elderly, vascular trans-tibial amputees after rehabilitation. Prosthet Orthot Int 1994;18:142–9.

[60] Squires JW, Johnson WC, Widrich WC, Nabseth DC. Cause of wound complications in elderly patients with above-knee amputation. Am J Surg 1982;143:523–7.

[61] Russek AS. Management of amputees in the older age group. Int J Phys Med 1960;4: 51–6.

[62] Rusk HA. Geriatric rehabilitation. In: Rehabilitation medicine. 3rd edition. St. Louis: Mosby; 1971. p. 663–4.

[63] Anderson AD, Levine SA, Colmer M. The temporary walking device for the mobilization of the elderly amputee. Geriatrics 1966;21:186–8.

[64] Gailey RS, Roach KE, Applegate EB, Cho B, Cunniffe B, Licht S, et al. The amputee mobility predictor: an instrument to assess determinants of the lower-limb amputee's ability to ambulate. Arch Phys Med Rehabil 2002;83:613–27.

[65] Geertzen JHB, Martina JD, Rietman HS. Lower limb amputation part 2: rehabilitation—a 10 year literature review. Prosthet Orthot Int 2001;25:14–20.

[66] Schoppen T, Boonstra A, Groothoff JW, deVries J, Goecken LN, Eisma WH. Physical, mental, and social predictors of functional outcome in unilateral lower-limb amputees. Arch Phys Med Rehabil 2003;84:803–11.

[67] Beekman CE, Axtell LA. Prosthetic use in elderly patients with dysvascular above-knee and through-knee amputations. Phys Ther 1987;67:1510–6.

[68] Gauthier-Gagnon C, Grise M-C, Potvin D. Enabling factors related to prosthetic use by people with transtibial and transfemoral amputation. Arch Phys Med Rehabil 1999;80: 706–13.

[69] Burger H, Marincek C. Functional testing of elderly subjects after lower limb amputation. Prosthet Orthot Int 2001;25:102–7.

[70] Mueller MJ, DeLitto A. Selective criteria for successful long-term prosthetic use. Phys Ther 1985;65:1037–40.

[71] Harris KA, van Schie L, Carroll SE, Deathe A, Maryniak O, Meads GE, et al. Rehabilitation potential of elderly patients with major amputations. J Cardiovasc Surg 1991; 32:463–7.

[72] Chiu C-C, Chen C-E, Wang T-G, Lin M-C, Lien I-N. Influencing factors and ambulation outcome in patients with dual disabilities of hemiplegia and amputation. Arch Phys Med Rehabil 2000;81:14–7.

[73] O'Connell PG, Gantz S. Hemiplegia and amputation: rehabilitation in dual disability. Arch Phys Med Rehabil 1989;70:451–4.

[74] Sioson ER, Kerfoot S, Ziat LM. Rehabilitation outcome of older patients with end-stage renal disease and lower extremity amputation. J Am Geriatr Soc 1993;41:667–8.

[75] Rommers GM, Vos LDW, Klein L, Groothoff JW, Eisma WH. A study of technical changes to lower limb prosthesis after initial fitting. Prosthet Orthot Int 2000;24:28–38.

[76] Williams LS, Lowenthal DT. Clinical problem-solving in geriatric medicine: obstacles to rehabilitation. J Am Geriatr Soc 1995;43:179–83.

[77] Evans SL, Nixon BP, Lee I, Yee D, Mooradian AD. The prevalence and nature of podiatric problems in elderly diabetic patients. J Am Geriatr Soc 1991;39:241–5.

[78] Plummer ES, Albert SG. Focused assessment of foot care in older adults. J Am Geriatr Soc 1996;44:310–3.

[79] Horswell RL, Birke JA, Patout CA Jr. A staged management diabetes foot program versus standard care: a 1-year cost and utilization comparison in a state public hospital system. Arch Phys Med Rehabil 2003;84:1743–6.

[80] Nissen SJ, Newman WP. Factors influencing reintegration to normal living after amputation. Arch Phys Med Rehabil 1992;73:548–51.

[81] Kerstein MD, Zimmer H, Dugdale FE, Lerner E. What influence does age have on rehabilitation of amputees? Geriatrics 1975;30:67–71.

[82] Goldberg RT. New trends in the rehabilitation of lower extremity amputees. Orthot Prosthet 1985;39:29–40.

[83] Hamilton EA, Nichols PJR. Rehabilitation of the elderly lower-limb amputee. BMJ 1972;2: 95–9.

[84] Hutchins PM. The outcome of severe tibial injury. Injury 1981;13:216–9.

[85] Bilodeau S, Hebert R, Desrosiers J. Lower limb prosthesis utilization by elderly amputees. Prosthet Orthot Int 2000;24:126–32.

[86] Fletcher DD, Andrews KL, Butters MA, Jacobsen SJ, Rowland CM, Hallett JW Jr. Rehabilitation of the geriatric vascular amputee patient: a population-based study. Arch Phys Med Rehabil 2001;28:776–9.

[87] Pinzur MS, Smith D, Tornow D, Meade K, Patwardan A. Gait analysis of dysvascular below-knee and contralateral through-knee bilateral amputees: a preliminary report. Orthopedics 1993;16:875–9.

[88] Brodza WK, Thornhill HL, Zarapkar SE, Malloy JA, Weiss L. Long-term function of persons with atherosclerotic bilateral below-knee amputation living in the inner city. Arch Phys Med Rehabil 1990;71:895–900.

[89] Dillingham TR, Pezzin LE, MacKenzie EJ, Burgess AR. Use and satisfaction with prosthetic devices among persons with trauma-related amputations: a long-term outcome study. Am J Phys Med Rehabil 2001;80:563–71.

ELSEVIER
SAUNDERS

Phys Med Rehabil Clin N Am
16 (2005) 197–218

PHYSICAL MEDICINE
AND REHABILITATION
CLINICS OF
NORTH AMERICA

Aging in polio

Matthew N. Bartels, MD, MPH*, Akiko Omura, MD

*Department of Rehabilitation Medicine, Columbia College of Physicians and Surgeons,
Columbia University, Unit #38, 630 West 168th Street, New York, NY 10032*

Although the number of cases of acute poliomyelitis worldwide has dramatically decreased in recent years due largely in part to the success of vaccination programs, late effects of poliomyelitis continue to be a source of widespread disability in the United States and around the world. Although the major epidemics of poliomyelitis occurred in the late 1940s to 1950s, many thousands of polio survivors did not start to experience new neurologic changes and decline in function related to their polio until the late 1970s and early 1980s [1]. The first description of the late effects of polio was noted the French literature in 1875 [1–4]. The term "postpolio syndrome" (PPS) was coined around the time of the First International Post Polio Conference at Warm Springs, Georgia in 1984 [1,5].

PPS is a disorder defined by a collection of neurologic and non-neurologic symptoms, occurring decades after a patient has recovered from the initial infection with the poliovirus. The hallmarks of PPS are new muscle weakness, fatigue, pain, bulbar dysfunction, and decline in exercise capacity and overall function.

Estimates of the incidence and prevalence of PPS vary widely in the literature because accurate numbers of Americans who had paralytic poliomyelitis are not available. The best estimate of the number of polio survivors is based on data from the National Center for Health Statistics. The National Health Interview Survey in 1987 contained specific questions for persons given the diagnosis of poliomyelitis with or without paralysis. Based on the results of this survey, an estimate of 1.63 million polio survivors with 641,000 persons having had paralytic poliomyelitis was derived [1,6]. No recent surveys have been conducted; however, it has been estimated that 5% to 10% of the polio population has died since 1987 [1]. A consensus statement by the Post Polio Task force noted, "Retrospective studies using objective

This work was supported by the VIDDA Foundation.
* Corresponding author.
E-mail address: mnb4@columbia.edu (M.N. Bartels).

criteria have estimated that PPS will develop in 20-40% of acute paralytic polio survivors" [1,7]. Based on this information, approximately 200,000 to 400,000 individuals are likely to be experiencing symptoms of PPS.

Epidemiology

On average, the onset of PPS occurs approximately 35 years after the initial polio infection; the delay can range between 8 to 71 years [8]. Studies have shown that those who experienced severe paralytic poliomyelitis and whose original losses were largely regained during the period of recovery were most likely to develop PPS. However, it is not unusual to see individuals with PPS who had mild paralytic disease or even nonparalytic poliomyelitis. Other risk factors include greater length of time since original polio infection, older age at time of initial diagnosis, presence of permanent impairment after recovery, recent weight gain, and female sex [1,8–10]. There have been no good estimates of the costs of PPS and treatments. Because many individuals are retired, the losses due to unemployment are limited, but the ongoing costs of treatment are likely considerable.

Pathophysiology of poliomyelitis in aging

Role of central and peripheral structures

Fatigue and weakness are the most common sequelae of polio with aging. The fatigue described by PPS patients is separated into two forms: (1) a physical tiredness and weakness associated with the new muscle weakness, and (2) a "central fatigue" that is associated with decreased attention and cognition. In view that these separate symptom components, the pathology and physiology of the two different types of fatigue is explored after a review of the effects of acute infection with poliomyelitis. A brief review of the course of acute poliomyelitis is presented as a background for the understanding of the physiologic changes seen with aging. The basic research into PPS pathophysiology is good but limited in that most studies can be done only in postmortem studies. Even though good animal models are limited because the disease takes a long time to present, many things have been learned about PPS.

History of the acute pathology and treatment of polio

Poliomyelitis is an acute generalized viral illness. In the past it was the most common form of viral illness, but due to vaccination it is now rare. The clinical syndrome is characterized by a flaccid paralysis during a febrile illness [11]. Paralysis is relatively rare, occurring in 1/100 infected persons, and many with patients paralysis had minimal or transient weakness [12]. Diagnosis was usually confirmed with a spinal tap and evaluation of the CSF. Mortality was usually due to bulbar and respiratory involvement, which are areas of special concern in individuals with aging in polio. Among the notable signs during an acute infection were marked tenderness of the affected muscles, Babinski reflexes, and increased deep tendon reflexes. Paralysis was more prominent in the legs than in the arms and happened in a random distribution with areas of sparing, but electromyographic examination usually revealed far more widely distributed effects. There were rare reports of cerebellar signs, mental status changes, sensory changes, and pain syndromes. The recovery period usually lasted from months to years. The random and widespread nature of the syndrome is pertinent to the understanding of PPS, particularly the chronic fatigue, pain, and progression of disability.

Some of the treatments that were used may have some effect in the subsequent issues that present in patients aging with polio. The early standard of care often involved whole-body splinting with subsequent disuse atrophy. It was only in 1940 that more active treatment regimens were advocated [13,14]. Irradiation of affected muscles was done with possible deleterious side effects [15]. Residual deficits were usually treated with bracing, and often orthopedic surgical procedures would be done to fixate joints, adjust limb length, alter circulation, and transfer tendons. Ventilatory management with the iron lung was introduced in the 1930s and allowed for the survival of individuals with respiratory and bulbar disease, allowing for some of the late effects in those areas to manifest themselves [11].

Acute motor neuron injury in poliomyelitis

In even mild cases of acute polio, there is a diffuse effect upon the motor neurons. Studies by Bodian [16,17] from the 1940s to the 1980s described the generalized effect of the disease and belied the clinical observation of a spotty distribution of the disease. After the acute infection with polio, there are five groups of neurons that remain: (1) normal unaffected neurons away from the areas of lost neurons, (2) normal unaffected neurons near the areas of lost neurons, (3) neurons originally affected but now appearing to be fully recovered, (4) moderately affected neurons that survive but with decreased size, and (5) severely affected neurons that fail to fully recover. The neurons in groups 1 and 2 are morphologically normal but have larger than normal motor units. Their lifespan may be mildly decreased or normal. Group 3 neurons have less resistance to metabolic stress and shorter life spans than normal motor units. Group 4 cells have a decreased capacity to maintain normal synapses and motor units and have decreased life expectancy. The Group 5 neurons have abnormal function and life expectancy. In addition to the neuronal changes, the terminal axons in postpolio survivors have up to five times the number of muscle fibers per motor unit.

Electrophysiologic findings

The documentation of the electrophysiology of PPS is complete in the literature. Usual EMG observations have shown that postpolio patients demonstrate motor units of increased amplitude and duration in all muscles, even those that are not clinically affected [18]. The fiber clusters can be as large as 200 fibers, and single-fiber EMG demonstrates an increase in jitter and block in stable and newly weakening muscles. This represents a variation in the time of the action potential propagating into two or more branches of an axon at the axonal branching point [19]. The histologic correlate of abnormal jitter is the presence of the neural cell adhesion molecule (N-CAM) [20,21]. This factor is expressed by a muscle fiber within 2 days of loss of innervation and is a sign of recent denervation [22]. The muscle fibers that do not achieve effective re-innervation lose the expression of N-CAM and become atrophic.

The EMG findings in the muscle cannot explain the universal and early finding of fatigue in the muscles of individuals with PPS. The actual mechanism is not clear and is not defined by findings on pathology. The possible mechanism of the fatigue may be impaired neuromuscular transmission, which is present in PPS and can be improved with treatment with anticholinesterases [23]. Individuals with fatigue show a decrease in oxidative capacity with a decrease in the ability to carry out oxidative phosphorylation, and this is associated with decreased phosphocreatinine in steady-state exercise [24].

Motor unit degeneration in the distal motor unit in aging with polio

Although the causes of the loss of distal axonal regeneration in PPS that lead to new weakness are unclear, there are several theories of how this may progress (Box 1). Attrition is a favored theory and is consistent with the classic clinical appearance of PPS about 30 years after the onset of the disease [25]. Attrition probably accounts for the majority of the decline in muscle strength over time. The instability of motor neurons results from excessive distal sprouting resulting in the inability to form truly effective synapses with all of the motor fibers. This yields an ongoing innervation and denervation that after many years leaves the surviving neurons with a decreased reserve and an inability to metabolically maintain all of the sprouts. This leads to the creation of muscle fiber patches that can no longer be re-innervated, with an associated gradual progression of weakness and atrophy.

Box 1. Causes of new motor degeneration and weakness in PPS

- Attrition of motor neurons
- Normal aging and loss of motor neurons
- Immune dysregulation causing active destruction of motor neurons
- Response to persistent poliovirus RNA and possible mutants causing persistent infection

---

Even though aging is a process that is normally associated with the loss of motor neurons, postpolio motor neurons may have a shortened life span, which leads to an acceleration of the normal process of axonal dropout. Generally, the loss of motor neurons is a process seen only in individuals after the age of 60, but it may occur earlier in individuals with PPS due to the abnormalities of the recovered neurons [26]. The onset of PPS is more closely linked to the duration of survival postpoliomyelitis, not the chronologic age of the individual. This supports the length of time from injury as a factor in the accelerated dropout of neurons [27]. Thus, earlier injury and heavier metabolic loads are likely contributing factors to the atrophy and weakness seen in PPS.

Immune dysregulation has been hypothesized to play a role in the establishment of PPS weakness. Individuals who have died years after polio of unrelated causes have ongoing inflammatory processes in the spinal cord. The inflammation is in the perivascular area of the gray matter and is associated with gliosis out of proportion to the neuronal loss. There are also abnormal surviving neurons and accumulation of lipofuscin [28–30]. Endomysial inflammation is also seen in muscle biopsies in PPS, with CD4+ and CD8+ cells around healthy muscle fibers with MHC1 on their surfaces [31]. The distribution of the inflammation is in a pattern consistent with that seen in some inflammatory myopathies. The MHC-1 expression is also similar to the expression that can be seen in acute polio infection [32]. Additionally, there are some peripheral lymphocyte abnormalities and increased IgM antiganglioside antibodies in individuals with PPS and acute polio [33]. The significance of all these subtle varied abnormalities in immune function is unclear but hints at a smoldering inflammatory process.

Possible role of persistent poliovirus

Poliomyelitis is a monophasic disease without a clear reactivation syndrome, and because the virus is highly lytic in culture, the possibility of a persistent infection has been felt to be unlikely. There are models of persistent infection in animals and in immunocompromised human hosts [34,35]. Although unlikely, a model could be created of a dormant, possibly mutated version of the RNA that activates years later in the CNS and leads to a low-grade immune response similar to that already described. There is no clear evidence of this, and further research remains to be done.

In summary, the findings in PPS demonstrate that the process of deterioration is an active and continuing process of the spinal motor neurons and results in ongoing denervation and remodeling of the terminal axons. Eventually, the need for reinnervation outstrips the capacity of the remaining motor neurons to adequately reinnervate the myocytes, leading to a syndrome of atrophy and progressive weakness. This is an area of research that is in evolution, and definitive work has not been done.

Central fatigue in postpolio syndrome

Fatigue is the most commonly reported symptom in PPS. In surveys, 91% of individuals with PPS report new or increased fatigue, 41% report fatigue significant enough to interfere with the performance or the completion of work, and 25% report fatigue interfering with the performance of activities of daily living (ADLs) [36,37]. Fatigue was often triggered by overexertion (91%) or emotional stress (62%). The exact mechanism of fatigue is not clear. Several hypotheses exist to look for mechanisms in the central nervous system to explain this fatigue.

The acute infection of poliomyelitis was associated with central changes in the majority of cases. The changes included damage to neurons in the hypothalamus, thalamus, caudate, putamen, globus pallidus, locus ceruleus, substantia nigra, and cerebellum [38]. The components of the reticular activating system, including the reticular formation, the thalamus, the hypothalamus, and the locus ceruleus are often severely involved, corresponding to reports in acute polio infection of drowsiness, lethargy, somnolence, and even coma [39,40]. It may be a progression of the damage in these areas combined with aging that causes a significant part of the central fatigue experienced in PPS. Recent studies comparing PPS with chronic fatigue syndrome have shown an overlap in the defects in attention and memory that may be correlated with an impact upon the reticular activating system [38].

The new fatigue seen in PPS 20 to 30 years after the acute infection needs further exploration. The onset of the late central fatigue may be due to age-related attrition of neurons in the setting of abnormal and injured neurons after acute poliomyelitis. This could correlate to the known rate of loss of neurons in the substantia nigra of 33% by 50 years of age, which contributes to the onset of Parkinson disease [41,42]. The age-related loss of neurons and dendritic connections in the already depleted reticular activating system could lead to the crossing of a threshold where reticular activation is impaired, leading to fatigue and the mild neurocognitive impairments seen in PPS. There may be a role for treatment with dopaminergic agents for fatigue in PPS as has been done in chronic fatigue syndrome [38,43,44]. The success of the treatments in chronic fatigue may be an indicator of treatments for PPS fatigue because there may be an overlap in the pathology of these syndromes.

Evaluation for postpolio syndrome

Criteria for postpolio syndrome

Establishing a diagnosis of PPS can be challenging because symptoms vary from patient to patient and are often nonspecific. Furthermore, the lack of diagnostic tests to confirm the diagnosis of PPS makes the evaluation more difficult.

Criteria for diagnosing PPS have been proposed by the Post Polio Task Force and include (1) a prior episode of poliomyelitis with residual motor neuron loss (confirmed though patient history, neurologic examination, or electromyography); (2) neurologic recovery followed by a period (usually ≥15 years) of neurologic and functional stability; (3) a gradual or sometimes abrupt onset of new weakness or abnormal muscle fatigue, muscle atrophy, pain, or generalized fatigue; and (4) exclusion of other medical, orthopedic, or neurologic conditions that may cause similar symptoms [1,7,8].

New weakness is the hallmark of PPS, and the diagnosis cannot be made without a clear history of new muscle weakness [1]. Symptoms of PPS such as pain and fatigue are nonspecific, and it is not practical to rule out all possible causes for a patient's symptomatology. The clinician must develop a list of reasonable alternative explanations for each symptom and perform diagnostic tests to exclude or confirm these diagnoses.

Medical history

The first step in evaluating individuals with possible PPS is to confirm the original diagnosis of poliomyelitis, the extent and severity of deficits at the time of the acute infection, and the extent of recovery [45]. It is imperative to obtain a quantitative history of a patient's function over a number of years to determine the extent of current deficits. The hallmark of PPS is new muscle weakness, which manifests as a decrease in muscle endurance. Questions should focus on activities that require repetitive or sustained muscle contractions such as standing, walking, stair climbing, dressing, and lifting.

Generalized fatigue is the most common manifestation of PPS and is present in over 80% of patients [1,8]. Joint and muscle pain caused by muscle weakness and overuse leading to subsequent joint instability and degeneration are also common. New muscle weakness, the cardinal symptom of PPS, can be see in previously affected and clinically unaffected muscles. The weakness is usually slowly progressive and asymmetric and can affect the proximal or distal musculature. Patients may report abnormal muscle fatigue with increased weakness after overuse followed by a prolonged recovery period. New weakness can also lead to respiratory and bulbar dysfunction. Cold intolerance is also a common manifestation and is present in 29% to 56% of PPS patients surveyed [8].

Physical examination

It is important to perform a thorough physical examination with a focus on the neurologic evaluation and any musculoskeletal abnormalities. Motor strength should be documented to assess distribution and severity of involvement. Although previously affected muscles are more likely to become weak in PPS, clinically unaffected muscles should be carefully examined because they may have sustained damage from subclinical poliomyelitis and therefore may have become affected in PPS [1]. Muscles should be examined for evidence of atrophy and fasciculations. Sensation is normal except in a severely paralyzed limb where it may be increased. Deep tendon reflexes are often diminished in weak, atrophied muscles.

PPS patients report myalgias and often have muscles that are tender on palpation. Joints should be evaluated for range of motion and alignment because contractures and degenerative joint disease are common. Patients with significant spinal curvature may have respiratory compromise and require further examination. Gait abnormalities may be caused by leg length discrepancy, muscle weakness, or pain.

Diagnostic studies

Based on findings from the medical history and physical examination, a reasonable differential diagnosis is developed for each of the major symptoms of PPS. Confirmation of a history of previous poliomyelitis is the first step in the evaluation for PPS. Although electrodiagnostic findings are not specific for poliomyelitis, studies are recommended to document signs of previous motor neuron loss, especially if the medical history and physical examination is not suggestive of a history of poliomyelitis. Evaluation of muscles thought to be spared by the original infection may reveal that these areas were affected by subclinical poliomyelitis. Such findings are helpful when formulating appropriate exercise programs for PPS patients.

Laboratory tests are normal in PPS except for serum creatine kinase (CK) concentrations, which can be mildly elevated after exercise. High elevations in serum CK should raise concern for a myopathy [11]. Laboratory tests are helpful in excluding other diagnoses that can present with similar symptoms as PPS, such as anemia, thyroid dysfunction, and rheumatologic disorders. Imaging studies, such as CT scans and MRI, can be used to evaluate for nerve root entrapment, spinal stenosis, or spinal cord abnormality. Plain radiographs should be ordered for individuals with significant scoliosis or evidence of degenerative joint disease. Pulmonary function tests with arterial blood gases should be performed on patients with a history of respiratory involvement at the time of acute infection. Patients with current pulmonary disease or scoliosis and smokers should be evaluated. Evaluation by a speech pathologist is beneficial if bulbar symptoms are present.

The diagnosis of PPS is complicated by the lack of specific diagnostic tests. Because it is not practical to rule out all possible causes for a patient's symptoms, a careful differential diagnosis is formulated based upon information obtained from the medical history and physical examination, and tests are selected to rule out or confirm the most likely diagnoses. PPS is a diagnosis of exclusion (see Box 1).

Respiratory issues in aging with polio

Although acute respiratory failure in polio is no longer an issue in the United States, individuals with PPS may have respiratory compromise.

Ventilatory limitation in PPS is widespread but often underappreciated. A recent study of respiratory capacity in ambulatory individuals with PPS demonstrated that ventilatory limitations exist in the majority of people studied [46]. The need for ventilator management and the types of treatment available have increased in recent years. There may be a late respiratory decompensation in PPS with or without a history of ventilator dependence during the acute episode of polio [47–49]. Up to 42% of individuals with PPS report new breathing problems, and the need for ventilatory support among survivors of poliomyelitis is increasing because a number of previously ventilator-dependent survivors need ventilatory support [50]. The clinical cutoff for screening for the development of respiratory failure in individuals with PPS is a vital capacity of 50% or less [51]. Individuals in this range may benefit from screening and treatment as needed. The objective numbers from pulmonary function tests are helpful, especially in individuals who are sedentary because their lack of metabolic demand may prevent the recognition of significant respiratory limitation until they present with an acute episode of respiratory failure. The use of the cutoff is useful in individuals who are ambulatory with declining function, even though they are far more likely to demonstrate symptoms earlier and receive attention and treatment.

The largest group of patients who come to need ventilator support are the survivors of respiratory failure with their initial episode, although there is also a group of individuals who have never had respiratory compromise who are also becoming late-onset PPS, ventilator-assisted individuals [52]. The causes of the respiratory failure are mostly related to a decrease in respiratory muscle strength and mass and fatigue of the ventilatory muscles. The mechanisms of the decline are the same as for peripheral muscle weakness. The clinical manifestations of the weakness include decreased pulmonary volumes, decreased maximal inspiratory and expiratory pressures, and decreased peak airflows. There is controversy over whether individuals with PPS lose ventilatory capacity at greater rates with age than normal individuals, but overall capacities are usually lower than for age-matched control subjects [53]. The chronic decrease in vital capacity leads to microatelectasis and decreased pulmonary compliance and increased chest wall stiffness [54]. This, in combination with inspiratory muscle weakness, leads to chronic alveolar hypoventilation and the potential for possible acute respiratory failure. Scoliosis, which is commonly seen in PPS, exacerbates the situation.

Cough flows are often compromised due to the mechanisms described, and this can impair the ability to manage airway secretions. Any decrease of the inspiratory capacity below 2.5 L places an individual at risk for issues of decreased secretion/airway clearance and, in combination with the possibility of impaired bulbar function, may be a setup for respiratory compromise [55]. The addition of smoking, COPD, reactive airways disease, or other underlying pulmonary condition compounds the issues in the PPS patient with respiratory compromise. The most effective means to maintain adequate secretion clearance is by maintaining a peak cough flow of more than 3.0 L/s, and in individuals with compromise, manual and assisted cough techniques may have to be considered [56]. The pulmonary function cutoffs for the use of ventilatory support are shown in Box 2.

The management of respiratory insufficiency in PPS is divided into noninvasive and invasive ventilatory support. The possibilities for ventilatory support are shown in Table 1. The noninvasive forms of ventilatory support are better tolerated and have a good record of efficacy. The glossopharyngeal breathing has limitations but can be a good alternative for an individual who has bulbar function to be able to achieve a period of ventilator-free existence. The equipment for noninvasive intermittent positive pressure ventilation has also improved, and portable units may allow for community mobility and continued employment. The use of tracheostomy with ventilator management is less common because it has many negative side effects and because in PPS patients equivalent ventilatory support can be achieved noninvasively [52].

Due to advances in pulmonary medicine, quality of life can be maintained with the appropriate use of noninvasive ventilatory support and early detection of individuals at risk. The use of ventilatory support with management of alveolar hypoventilation and improving airway clearance in a preventive fashion can prevent episodes of acute respiratory failure and the subsequent morbidity. The goals of good pulmonary management in

---

Box 2. Cutoff points for evaluation for ventilatory support in PPS respiratory failure

Evaluation
- Vital capacity (VC): <50%
- Peak expiratory cough flow: <3.0 L/s
- Inspiratory capacity: <2.5 liters
- Symptomatic decrease in respiratory function
- Elevation of Pco_2 on arterial blood gas: Pco_2 > 45 or $etco_2$ > 50
- Evidence of chronic alveolar hypoventilation: VC < 50% and Sao_2 < 95%

Treatment
- Maximum insufflation capacity: <2.5 L
- VC: < 50%
- Forced expiratory volume in 1 second: <1000 mL
- Peak expiratory cough flow: <3.0 L
- Capnometry or Pco_2: Pco_2 > 45 or $etco_2$ > 50
- Hemoglobin oxygen saturation or Po_2: Sao_2 < 95% or Po_2 < 65

Table 1
Modalities for ventilatory support in PPS respiratory failure

Modality	Advantages	Disadvantages	Delivery alternatives
Noninvasive			
Glossopharyngeal	Inexpensive	Must train patient	
Breathing	Patient controlled	Only when awake	
Intermittent positive	More reliable	Expensive	Mouthpiece,
pressure ventilation	Well tolerated	Noisy	nosepiece
	Noninvasive	Non cosmetic	
Negative pressure	More physiologic	Only in supine	
ventilation/cuirass	Reliable	Less well tolerated	
Invasive			
Tracheostomy with	Reliable	Invasive	
ventilator	Good airway access	Lose speech	
		Less well tolerated	

Data from Halstead LS. Diagnosing postpolio syndrome: inclusion and exclusion criteria. In: Silver JK, Gawne AC, editors. Postpolio syndrome. 1st edition. Philadelphia: Harley and Belfus; 2004. p. 1–20.

PPS are to avoid hospitalization, tracheal intubation, bronchoscopy, and pulmonary infections. Timely use of intermittent noninvasive ventilation and education of patients in self-monitoring can prolong the quality and duration of life for individuals with ventilatory failure and PPS.

Psychologic issues in aging with polio

Aging is a psychologically stressful situation, and aging with a disability is especially so. Because individuals with a history of paralytic poliomyelitis may develop new disability and fatigue in PPS, the psychologic issues also have to be addressed. Mild fatigue and weakness may effect up to 90% of polio survivors, and depression and anxiety are common, especially among individuals with new limitations [57,58]. The incidence of depression was found to range from 16% to 23% in several studies, using several different indices to study depression. These studies did not have matched controls, so the ability to draw meaningful conclusions is limited [59,60]. One study with controls did not find any difference in the rates of depression in PPS versus normal control subjects [58].

Neuropsychologic evaluation of patients with PPS indicates that there are some subtle changes in the cognitive and psychologic function after polio and that there may be some contributions from the symptoms of pain and fatigue and the physiology of the infection with the poliovirus. Coping mechanisms in PPS patients are intact, and the general level of depression is not elevated above the normal population. Yet, the onset of the new disability from their disease places them at risk, and close individual follow-up is needed for individuals who are distraught over new symptoms or the loss of independence and function.

The neuropsychologic status of individuals with PPS has been studied to a limited degree. Several studies have shown that the evaluations of cognitive function have been on the low end of the normal range for nonverbal recall and inhibition of automatic processes, with slightly better than normal associative encoding and speed of information of processing [61]. None of these findings were out of the normal range. In a study by Bruno et al [62], a significant number of PPS patients self-reported problems with concentration, memory, attention, and thinking clearly. None of these patients was depressed, and evaluation of individuals demonstrated decreased functioning in many neuropsychologic scales. The most fatigued PPS patients did the worst, and the authors suspected a possible attention deficit disorder in the PPS patients. In looking to see if there might be a central component to the mild abnormalities seen on the neuropsychologic tests, Bruno et al have undertaken PET, MRI, and other studies without clear evidence of true neurocognitive dysfunction in the brain. Most of the attention-deficit findings are likely to be explicable on the basis of fatigue, and further studies are being done in this area.

Musculoskeletal issues in aging with polio

Due to the weakness and the deformity caused by differential growth of effected limbs with polio, aging with polio can manifest with many musculoskeletal complaints. For weakness and limb length discrepancies, bracing and lifts can accommodate the majority of deformities. Despite these interventions, many patients with a history of polio develop musculoskeletal complications that require attention. The number one complaint of musculoskeletal origin in PPS is pain in the muscles or in the bones and joints of surrounding muscles [63]. Pain occurs in 38% to 86% of PPS patients, and joint pain occurs in 42% to 80% of PPS patients [64]. The pain is severe enough in about 25% of patients that it governs the day and seriously affects daily activities [65]. Muscle pain is caused by muscle cramps, fasciculations, and overuse. The pain in joints is caused by the presence of overuse in certain joints and the uneven forces of unbalanced muscle strength. These problems can be compounded by improper bracing or overuse, which occur frequently in PPS patients [66]. In a multivariate analysis of joint pain in PPS patients, female gender, longer duration of symptoms, younger age, lower isometric strength, and lower SF-36 score were associated with higher risk of joint pain [63]. Even with this understanding, the mechanisms seem to be the usual degenerative conditions seen in overused joints and muscles. Treatment of these issues is limited to avoidance of overuse and supporting affected joints with bracing, accommodation, and, in the case of severe joint damage, joint replacement as needed.

Another musculoskeletal issue seen in postpolio survivors with aging is an increase in fractures and a rise in osteopenia in the affected limbs. As in other neurologic conditions, paresis of an affected limb leads to bone loss and an increase in the risk of fracture. Care recommendations include screening for osteopenia and osteoporosis in patients aging with polio [67]. An evaluation of fracture incidence in patients with PPS done by the Mayo Clinic demonstrated that in nonaffected limbs the rates of fracture were the same as in an age- and gender-matched control group, but the incidence of fracture in affected limbs was about 50% greater than in the control limbs. There was no association of fracture with use of assistive devices or bracing. The findings of increased fracture in affected limbs agree with other studies where 21% of aging polio survivors had a fracture [68]. The reasons for the increased fractures in affected limbs may be caused by disuse atrophy and, in individuals with childhood polio, by abnormal development and failure to achieve peak bone mass in the affected limbs. Treatments for the increased risk of fracture are the same as for any individual with decreased bone mineralization: safety; fall prevention; calcium replacement; hormone replacement if needed; bone-forming agents; and gentle, progressive weight-bearing exercises.

Dysphagia in aging with polio

The onset or worsening of bulbar symptoms of dysphagia can cause profound difficulties [69–71]. The presence of previous bulbar polio increases the incidence of progressive symptoms in later years, and the degree of impairment can range form mild to severe. The patient with mild dysfunction may be unaware of their limitations and may have compensated adequately for many years. It is with the onset of aging and the progression to PPS that individuals can have severe symptoms that can cause aspiration, malnutrition, or other severe manifestations of dysphagia. Because the findings can be subtle, it has been suggested that individuals at risk (eg, patients with a past history of bulbar polio) may benefit form the monitoring of swallowing function [72]. Any evidence of aspiration in a postpolio patient may indicate that the swallowing disorder may be related to the antecedent polio, and investigation and management can take that into account.

The prevalence of dysphagia in PPS has never been fully studied, but from several investigations, the rates can be estimated as 10% to 15% in individuals with acute polio and between 18% and 22% of new swallowing disorders in postpolio survivors [73–75]. Although there is a significant degree of dysphagia that can be detected with complete studies, the incidence of symptomatic dysphagia is low. The majority of the abnormalities discovered did not cause life-threatening events, and most patients were able to continue to eat with minor interventions, such as swallowing techniques and education. These patients should be followed closely because the few longitudinal studies have demonstrated a progression of the symptoms if present [71].

Treatments in poliomyelitis with aging

Pharmacologic treatment

Large-scale studies have not shown benefits of pharmacologic intervention for the treatment of PPS [8,76–79]. Some agents investigated include pyridostigmine, insulin-like growth factor-I (IGF-I), amantadine, bromocriptine, and prednisone.

Many patients with history of paralytic poliomyelitis have neuromuscular junction transmission defects, and this is thought to be a possible cause for muscle weakness and fatigue [76]. It was hypothesized that pyridostigmine may reduce muscular fatigue by improving neuromuscular transmission and by increasing IGF-I concentrations. IGF-I is necessary for the regeneration of peripheral nerves and axonal sprouting [77]. Initial studies conducted on a small group of PPS patients found significant improvement of subjective fatigue with the use of pyridostigmine [80–82]. However, a large multicenter, randomized, double-blind, placebo-controlled study of 126 patients by Trojan et al [77] showed no significant difference with regard to perceived quality of life and generalized fatigue between the pyridostigmine- and placebo-treated patients at 6 months [77]. There was a trend toward improved strength in the very weak muscles with pyridostigmine use. Circulating IGF-I levels were increased in compliant patients, but the difference was not significant. Similar results were observed in a single-center, randomized, placebo-controlled, double blind trial of 67 PPS patients [83].

Amantadine is an antiviral agent used for the treatment of fatigue resulting from neurologic disorders such as multiple sclerosis. A randomized, placebo-controlled trial in 25 PPS patients treated for 6 weeks showed no significant difference in subjective fatigue [84].

Prednisone has been proposed as a treatment because of the immunologic abnormalities seen in PPS. No significant improvement in muscle strength or subjective fatigue has been noted with high-dose treatment [85].

One component of the generalized fatigue seen in PPS may be due to central mechanisms. It has been hypothesized that damage to the reticular activating system of the brain by the poliovirus may be responsible for CNS dysfunction and fatigue, referred to as "brain fatigue" by PPS patients. Reduced secretion of dopamine has been thought to play a role in the decreased attention, concentration, and memory seen in some individuals with PPS [86]. Bruno et al [87] studied the dopamine-2 receptor agonist bromocriptine in a placebo-controlled trial involving five PPS patients. Three patients reported marked symptom improvement on bromocriptine [87]. A larger, randomized, double blind, placebo-controlled study is needed to confirm the efficacy of bromocriptine in the treatment of PPS-related cognitive dysfunction.

Even though small trials have yielded promising results for the use of some pharmacologic agents in the treatment of PPS-related weakness and fatigue, larger studies have failed to demonstrate any efficacy. Further research using larger sample sizes, longer duration, and defined outcome measures is necessary to determine the efficacy of these medications.

Energy conservation

Generalized fatigue is one of the most commonly reported manifestations of PPS and is present in >80% of PPS patients [1,8]. Management consists of energy conservation measures and pacing of daily activities with frequent rest periods. Examples of energy conservation techniques include eliminating unnecessary energy-consuming activities, making ergonomic modifications at home and at the workstation, using handicap license plates, decreasing standing time when feasible, and using a motorized wheelchair or scooter to travel longer distances. Lifestyle changes, such as changing jobs, working from home, or working part-time, may be necessary. Weight loss and the avoidance of weight gain are important measures in decreasing mechanical load and energy expenditure, thereby reducing fatigue.

Quality of sleep should be improved to minimize daytime somnolence and fatigue. Relaxation techniques and medications can be introduced to meet this goal. If sleep apnea or nocturnal hypoventilation is suspected as reasons for nonrestorative sleep, a sleep study should be performed so appropriate treatment can be initiated early.

The judicious use of assistive devices such as lower-extremity orthoses, canes, walkers, and wheelchairs are important measures of energy conservation. Studies have shown that energy expenditure during ambulation can be reduced by as much as two thirds with the use of proper lower-extremity orthoses [88,89]. In a study of 104 PPS patients, Waring et al [90] found that 18% of the patients were using an orthosis at the time of presentation to the postpolio clinic even though most of these individuals had used an orthosis in the past. After evaluation, recommendations were made to each patient, including new lower extremity orthoses for 37 patients (36%), of which 32 responded to a questionnaire at a later time. Nineteen patients reported using the orthosis daily, and 13 patients reported used them sporadically. With daily use of the orthosis, patients reported improved fatigue, weakness, and ability to walk. Pain symptoms were also reduced. These studies demonstrate the reluctance that often exists in patients with PPS to use bracing. Although there is no research to support this, clinical experience often shows a hesitance on the part of patients to use new bracing technologies that may function better. This reluctance can sometimes be overcome, but usually accommodation is the best technique.

Patients should be educated about the harmful effects of overexertion and should be taught to attend to their perception of fatigue throughout the day. For example, the Borg Rating Scale of Perceived Exertion can be used, recommending patients to end their activity when the score reaches 14 ("hard") [76]. In this way, patients are better able to pace their activities and take rest periods and naps as needed.

With lifestyle modifications, energy conservation measures, and the use of proper assistive devices, patients can conserve energy and reduce fatigue.

Exercise

Many studies document the benefit of exercise in selected postpolio individuals [88,91,92]. Physical therapy has been shown to reduce muscle fatigability by optimizing muscle function. Isotonic and isokinetic strengthening can be used on muscles that are ≥3 on the Medical Research Council scale, and isometric exercises can be used over painful joints. Aerobic exercise should involve an activity that the patient enjoys. Cross training can be of benefit in avoiding the overuse of a particular muscle group. Stretching can be useful to maintain or improve range of motion; however, caution should be used because certain contractures may be compensatory for a patient and should not be stretched [76]. Initially, the patient should be monitored closely to ensure that exercises are being performed correctly and that muscles are not being overused. Overuse of muscles in PPS patients has been reported to produce muscle weakness that can be permanent [93]. Exercise should be performed for short intervals with adequate rest between sessions to promote recovery.

There has been controversy regarding the type and intensity of exercises appropriate for patients with PPS. In a study by Agre et al [94], 12 PPS patients participated in a low-intensity, alternate-day, 12-week quadriceps muscle-strengthening program. Muscle strength and endurance improved without adverse effects on EMG or serum CK concentrations. Einarsson [95] studied the effects of high-intensity isokinetic and isometric exercises in PPS patients and found significant improvements in strength. There is evidence that low- and high-intensity exercise programs, when coupled with adequate rest, can be effective in reducing muscle fatigue.

Many postpolio patients are severely deconditioned due to their sedentary lifestyles. Studies have shown that the use of upper and lower extremity ergometers leads to improved strength and oxygen use without deleterious effects on muscle. Patients report improvement in fatigue with increased conditioning [88,96–98].

Beneficial effects of aquatic exercise in PPS patients were discovered in Warm Springs, Georgia during the polio epidemics in the 1940s and 1950s, and more recent studies have confirmed the efficacy of this type of rehabilitation [88,99]. Exercises in these studies included swimming, strengthening, stretching, balancing, and relaxation. Increases in strength in some muscle groups were noted, as were increases in range of motion of some joints. In the study by Willen et al [99], a reduction in heart rate at exercise was observed. Patients reported less pain and an increased sense of well-being. Programs were well tolerated, and no adverse effects were reported. Unique properties of water make it a comfortable and beneficial environment in which PPS patients can exercise to improve their land mobility and ADL skills.

Other conditions

Management of the postpolio patient should include the identification and treatment of conditions that occur more frequently in this population. A retrospective chart review of 88 postpolio patients by Gawne et al [100] showed that PPS patients have a high prevalence of two or more coronary heart disease risk factors, with the prevalence of dyslipidemia being higher than United States population estimates. These findings are possibly due to the sedentary lifestyle of many PPS patients, deconditioning, and obesity [101]. Evaluation of the PPS patient should include screening for hyperlipidemia and education regarding the elimination of modifiable cardiac risk factors. Behavioral modifications, such as dyslipidemia treatment, weigh loss, diet, and exercise, should be implemented as part of the rehabilitation plan. In view of possible respiratory compromise, administration of the pneumococcal and influenza vaccines is recommended. In view of cardiac and pulmonary limitations, smoking cessation should be encouraged [76].

The prevalence of osteoporosis in PPS patients is not known; however, Delahunt [102] found that the weakest PPS patients are at the greatest risk for developing osteoporosis. A bone mineral density test is recommended to identify those who are affected or at risk. Prophylaxis and treatment of osteoporosis does not differ from the general population and includes weight-bearing exercises, adequate calcium and vitamin D intake, and possible use of bisphosphonates.

Focal entrapment neuropathies occur frequently in PPS patients. Gawne et al [103] evaluated electrodiagnostic findings of 108 PPS patients and found that 32% of patients had evidence of carpal tunnel syndrome. Reduction of repetitive motion and avoidance of pressure on the nerve coupled with the use of splints can help alleviate symptoms and halt progression.

Postpolio patients are not immune to the other medical conditions found in the older adult population, and such disorders can account for some or even all of their new symptoms. Any new symptoms must be investigated fully before they are attributed to progression of PPS. To assist in their management, it is imperative that PPS patients keep their routine medical care up to date.

Summary

For a disease that was "conquered" some 40 years ago with the onset of effective vaccination, the issues of long-term survivors of paralytic polio as they age continue to present challenges to rehabilitation specialists. Aging with polio is a definition of PPS. There are over a million patients with PPS in the United States. Management has to include the appropriate use of exercises, appropriate bracing and support, and, in the case of bulbar and respiratory symptoms, the appropriate use of speech therapy services and ventilatory support. There are no prospective randomized trials studying the treatment of weakness and fatigue in PPS. Pharmacologic interventions are limited at this time but include anticholinergics for muscle weakness and dopaminergic agents or amantadine to control central fatigue. The pathophysiology of aging with polio is consistent with neuronal loss and denervation lying at the heart of the developing disorder, whereas the central nervous system components of the fatigue syndrome may be related to central changes with neuronal loss in the basal ganglia and reticular-activating system.

Many of the survivors of the polio epidemics are in their later retirement years, and their needs will increase as they have other disabilities due to natural aging. Sensitivity to some of the special issues in PPS may help to avoid complications. Polio is an active infection in the third world. Although great strides have been made, the disease is endemic in eight nations and is threatening to spread. The lessons learned in treating PPS now will be useful in years to come as these individuals age and manifest PPS in the future.

References

[1] Halstead LS. Diagnosing postpolio syndrome: inclusion and exclusion criteria. In: Silver JK, Gawne AC, editors. Postpolio syndrome. 1st edition. Philadelphia: Hanley and Belfus; 2004. p. 1–20.

[2] Carriere M. Des amytrophies spinales secondaire: contribution a l'etude de la diffusion des lesion irritaves du systeme nerveu. These de Montpeliere, France, 1875.

[3] Cornil V, Lepine R. Sur un cas de paralysie generale spinale anterieure subaigue, suivi d'autopsie. Gaz Med (Paris) 1875;4:127–9.

[4] Raymond M, Charcot JM. Paralysie essentiele de l'enfance: Strophie musculaire consecutive. Gaz Med (Paris) 1875.

[5] Cashman NR, Raymond CA. Decades after polio epidemics, survivors report new symptoms. JAMA 1986;255:1397–404.

[6] Parsons PE. National Center for Health Statistics. Letter to the editor. N Engl J Med 1991; 325:1108.

[7] Post-Polio Task Force. Post-polio syndrome. New York: BioScience Communications; 1999.

[8] Jubelt B, Agre JC. Characteristics and management of postpolio syndrome. JAMA 2000; 284:412–4.

[9] Klingman J, Chui H, Corgiat M, Perry J. Functional recovery: a major risk factor for the development of postpoliomyelitis muscular atrophy. Arch Neurol 1988;45:645–7.

[10] Shefner JM, Jubelt B. Post-polio syndrome. Available at:www.utdol.com. Accessed January 10, 2004.

[11] Mulder DW. Clinical observations in acute poliomyelitis. Ann N Y Acad Sci 1995;753: 1–10.

[12] Paul JR. A history of poliomyelitis. New Haven (CT): Yale University Press; 1971.

[13] McSweeney CJ. A visit to poliomyelitis centers in the USA. Ir J Med Sci 1951;120:65–73.

[14] Cohn V. Sister Kenny: the woman who challenged the doctors. Mineapolis (MN): University of Minnesota Press; 1976.

[15] Weinstein L. Diagnosis and treatment of poliomyelitis. In: Poliomyelitis: papers and discussions. Proceedings of the First International Poliomyelitis Conference. Philadelphia: J.B. Lippincott; 1948. p. 1377–402.

[16] Bodian D. Hisopathologic basis of clinical findings in poliomyelitis. Am J Med 1949;6: 563–78.

[17] Bodian D. Poliomyelitis: pathologic anatomy. In: Poliomyelitis: papers and discussions. Proceedings of the First International Poliomyelitis Conference. Philadelphia: J.B. Lippincott; 1962. p. 66–73.

[18] Lange DJ. Post polio muscular atrophy: an electrophysiological study of motor unit architecture. Ann N Y Acad Sci 1995;753:151–7.

[19] Stalberg E. Electrophysiological studies of reinnervation in amyotrophic lateral sclerosis. In: Rowland LP, editor. Motor neuron diseases. New York: Raven Press; 1982. p. 47–59.

[20] Cashman NR, Maselli SD, Wollman RL, et al. Late denervation in patients with antecedent paralytic poliomyelitis. N Engl J Med 1987;317:7–12.

[21] Trojan DA, Gendron D, Cashman NR. Stimulation frequency dependent neuromuscular transmission defects in patients with prior poliomyelitis. J Neurol Sci 1993;118:150–7.

[22] Maselli RA, Cashman NR, Wallman EF, et al. Neuromuscular transmission as a function of motor unit size in patients with prior poliomyelitis. Muscle Nerve 1992;15:648–55.

[23] Trojan D, Cashman NR. Anticholinesterases in post poliomyelitis syndrome. Ann N Y Acad Sci 1995;753:285–95.

[24] Sivakumar KR, Sinnwell T, Yildiz E, et al. Study of fatigue in muscles of patients with post polio syndrome by in vivo 31P magnetic resonance spectroscopy: a metabolic cause for fatigue. Ann N Y Acad Sci 1995;753:397–401.

[25] Dalakas MC. The post polio syndrome as an evolved clinical entity. Ann N Y Acad Sci 1995;753:68–79.

[26] Tomlinson BE, Irving D. The numbers of limb motor neurons in the human lumbosacral cord throughout life. J Neurol Sci 1977;34:213–9.

[27] Halstead LS, Weichers DO. Research and clinical aspects of the late effects of poliomyelitis. White Plains (NY): March of Dimes; 1987.

[28] Pezeshkpour GH, Dalakas MC. Long term changes in the spinal cord of patients with old poliomyelitis: signs of continuous disease activity. Arch Neurol 1988;45:505–8.

[29] Miller DC. Post polio syndrome spinal cord pathology. Case report with immunopathology. Ann N Y Acad Sci 1995;753:186–93.

[30] Kaminski HJ, Tresser N, Hogan RE, et al. Pathologic analysis of the spinal cords form survivors of poliomyelitis. Ann N Y Acad Sci 1995;753:390–3.

[31] Dalakas MC. Polymyositis, dermatomyositis, and inclusion body myositis. N Engl J Med 1991;325:1487–98.

[32] Dalakas MC. Pathogenic mechanisms of post polio syndrome: morphological, electrophysiological, virological, and immunological correlations. Ann N Y Acad Sci 1995;753: 167–85.

[33] Ginsberg AH, Gale MJ, Rose LM, et al. T-cell alteration in late post poliomyelitis. Arch Neurol 1989;46:497–501.

[34] Miller JR. Prolonged intracerebral infection with polio virus in asymptomatic mice. Ann Neurol 1981;9:590–6.

[35] Colbere-Garapin F, Christodoulou C, Craniac R, et al. Persistent poliovirus infection of human neuroblastoma cells. Proc Natl Acad Sci USA 1989;86:4354–9.

[36] Parsons PE. Data on polio survivors from the National Health review Survey. National Center for Health Statistics. Washington, DC: US Government Printing Office; 1989.

[37] Bruno RL, Frick NM. Stress and type A behavior as precipitants of post polio sequelae. In: Halstead LS, Weichers DO, editors. Research and clinical aspects of the late effects of poliomyelitis. White Plains (NY): March of Dimes; 1987. p. 145–56.

[38] Bruno RL, Sapolsky R, Zimmerman JR, Frick NM. Pathophysiology of a central cause of post-polio fatigue. Ann N Y Acad Sci 1995;753:257–75.

[39] Baker AB. Neurologic signs of bulbar poliomyelitis. In: Poliomyelitis. Proceedings of the First International Poliomyelitis Conference. Philadelphia: Lippincott; 1949. p. 241–4.

[40] Holmgren BE. Electroencephalography in poliomyelitis. In: Poliomyelitis. Proceedings of the First International Poliomyelitis Conference. Philadelphia: Lippincott; 1949. p. 448–52.

[41] Mann DM, Yates PO, Hawkes J. The pathology of the human Locus Ceruleus. Clin Neuropathol 1983;2:1–7.

[42] Vincent FM, Myers WG. Poliomyelitis and parkinsonism. N Engl J Med 1978;298:688–9.

[43] Alexander GE, Crutcher MD, DeLong MR. Basal ganglia-thalamo-cortical circuits. Brain Res 1990;85:119–46.

[44] Bruno RL, Frick NM. The psychology of polio as prelude to post polio sequellae. Orthopedics 1991;14:1185–93.

[45] Trojan DA, Finch L, Da Costa D, Cashman NR. Evaluating and treating symptomatic postpolio patients. In: Silver JK, Gawne AC, editors. Postpolio syndrome. 1st edition. Philadelphia: Hanley and Belfus; 2004. p. 21–35.

[46] Weinberg J, Morg J, Bevegard SA, Sinderby C. Respiratory response to exercise in post polio patients with severe inspiratory muscle dysfunction. Arch Phys Med Rehabil 1999;80: 1095–100.

[47] Hamilton EA, Nichols PJR, Tait GBW. Late onset of respiratory insufficiency after poliomyelitis: a preliminary communication. Ann Phys Med 1970;10:223–9.

[48] Fischer D. Poliomyelitis: late respiratory complications and management. Orthopedics 1985;8:891–4.

[49] Dolmage TE, Avendano MA, Goldstein RS. Respiratory function during wakefulness and sleep among survivors of respiratory and non respiratory poliomyelitis. Eur Respir J 1992; 5:864–70.

[50] Bach JR, Alba AS. Pulmonary dysfunction and sleep disordered breathing as post polio sequelae. Orthopedics 1991;14:1329–37.

[51] Braun NMT, Arora NS, Rochester DF. Respiratory muscle and pulmonary function in poliomyelitis and other proximal myopathies. Thorax 1983;38:616–23.

[52] Bach JR. Management of post polio respiratory sequelae. Ann N Y Acad Sci 1995;753: 96–101.

[53] Midgren B. Lung function and clinical outcome in postpolio patients: a prospective cohort study during 11 years. Eur Respir J 1997;10:146–9.

[54] Estenne M, DeTroyer A. The effects of tetraplegia on chest wall statics. Am Rev Respir Dis 1986;134:121–4.

[55] Leith DE. Lung biology in health and disease: respiratory defense mechanisms, part 2. In: Brian JD, Proctor D, Reid L, editors. Cough. New York: Marcel Dekker; 1977. p. 545–92.

[56] Bach JR. Mechanical Insufflation-exsufflation: comparison of peak expiratory flows with manually assisted and unassisted coughing techniques. Chest 1993;104:1553–62.

[57] Parsons RE. Data on polio survivors from the national health intensive survey. Washington, DC: US Government Printing Office; 1989.

[58] Kemp BJ, Adams BM, Campbell ML. Depression and life satisfaction in aging polio survivors versus age matched controls: relation to post polio syndrome, family functioning, and attitude toward disability. Arch Phys Med Rehabil 1997;78:187–92.

[59] Tate DG, Forchheimer M, Kirsch N, et al. Prevalence and associated features of depression and psychological distress in polio survivors. Arch Phys Med Rehabil 1993;74: 1056–60.

[60] Conrady LJ, Wish JR, Agre JC, et al. Psychologic characteristics of polio survivors: a preliminary report. Arch Phys Med Rehabil 1989;72:115–8.

[61] Freidenberg DL, Freeman D, Huber SJ, et al. Postpoliomyelitis syndrome: assessment of behavioral features. Neuropsychiatr Neuropsychol Behav Neurol 1989;40:272–81.

[62] Bruno RL, Galski T, DeLuca J. The neuropsychology of post polio fatigue. Arch Phys Med Rehabil 1993;74:1061–5.

[63] Vasiliades HM, Collet JP, Shapiro S, Venturini Am Trojan DA. Predictive factors and correlates for pain in postpoliomyelitis syndrome patients. Arch Phys Med Rehabil 2002; 83:1109–15.

[64] Gawne AC, Halstead LS. Post polio syndrome: pathophysiology and clinical management. Crit Rev Phys Rehabil Med 1995;7:S47–99.

[65] Ahlstrom G, Karlsson U. Disability and quality of life in individuals with post polio syndrome. Disabil Rehabil 2000;22:416–22.

[66] Trojan DA, Cashman NR. Current trends in post-poliomyelitis syndrome. New York: Milestone Medical Communications; 1996. p. 1–51.

[67] Silver JK, Aiello DD. What internists need to know about post polio syndrome. Cleve Clin J Med 2002;69:704–706, 709–12.

[68] Cosgrove JL, Alewxander MA, Kitts EL, Swan BE, Klein MJ, Bauer RE. Late effects of poliomyelitis. Arch Phys Med Rehabil 1987;68:4–7.

[69] Buchholz DW. Postpolio dysphagia. Dysphagia 1994;9:99–100.

[70] Sonies BC, Dalakes MC. Dysphagia in patients with the post polio syndrome. N Engl J Med 1991;324:1162–7.

[71] Sonies BC, Dalakas MC. Progression of oral motor and swallowing symptoms in the post-polio syndrome. Ann N Y Acad Sci 1995;753:87–95.

[72] Silbergleit AK, Warring WP, Sullivan MJ, et al. Evaluation, treatment, and follow up results of post polio patients with dysphagia. Otolaryngol Head Neck Surg 1991;104:333–8.

[73] Baker AB, Matzke HA, Brown JR. Bulbar poliomyelitis: a study of medullary function. Arch Neurol Psychiatry 1950;63:257–61.

[74] Halstead LS, Weichers DO, Rossi CD. Results of a survey of 201 polio survivors. Southern Medical Journal 1985;78(11):1281–7.

[75] Coehlo CA, Ferranti R. Incidence and nature of dysphagia in polio survivors. Arch Phys Med Rehabil 1991;72:1071–5.

[76] Trojan DA, Finch L, Da Costa D, Cashman NR. Evaluating and treating symptomatic postpolio patients. In: Silver JK, Gawne AC, editors. Postpolio syndrome. 1st edition. Philadelphia: Hanley and Belfus; 2004. p. 21–35.

[77] Trojan SA, Collet JP, Shapiro S, Jubelt B, Miller RG, Agre JC, et al. A multicenter, randomized, double-blinded trial of pyridostigmine in postpolio syndrome. Neurology 1999;53:1223–33.

[78] Nollet F, Horemans H, Beeleb A. A multicenter, randomized, double-blinded trial of pyridostigmine in postpolio syndrome. Neurology 2000;55:899–900.

[79] Dalakas MC. Why drugs fail in postpolio syndrome: lessons from another clinical trial. Neurology 1999;53:1166–7.

[80] Trojan DA, Cashman NR. Anticholinesterases in post-poliomyelitis syndrome. Ann N Y Acad Sci 1995;753:285–95.

[81] Trojan DA, Cashman NR. An open trial of pyridostigmine in a post-poliomyelitis clinic. Can J Neurol Sci 1995;22:223–7.

[82] Trojan DA, Gendron D, Cashman NR. Anticholinesterase-responsive neuro-muscular junction transmission defects in post-poliomyelitis fatigue. J Neurol Sci 1993; 114:170–7.

[83] Nollet F, Horemans HLD, Beelen A. Pyridostigmine in postpolio syndrome: a randomized double-blinded trial [abstract]. Neurology 2002;58(Suppl 2):199–200.

[84] Stein DP, Dambrosia JM, Dalakas MC. A double-blind, placebo-controlled trial of amantadine for the treatment of fatigue in patients with post-polio syndrome. Ann N Y Acad Sci 1995;753:296–302.

[85] Dinsmore S, Dambrosia J, Dalakas MC. A double-blind, placebo-controlled trial of high dose prednisone for the treatment of post-poliomyelitis syndrome. Ann N Y Acad Sci 1995; 753:303–13.

[86] Borg K. Postpolio fatigue. In: Silver JK, Gawne AC, editors. Postpolio syndrome. 1st edition. Philadelphia: Hanley and Belfus; 2004. p. 77–85.

[87] Bruno RL, Zimmerman JR, Creange SJ, Lewis T, Molzen T, Frick NM. Bromocriptine in the treatment of post-polio fatigue: a pilot study with implications for the pathophysiology of fatigue. Am J Phys Med Rehabil 1996;75:340–7.

[88] Agre JC. Exercise in the treatment of postpolio syndrome. In: Silver JK, Gawne AC, editors. Postpolio syndrome. 1st edition. Philadelphia: Hanley and Belfus; 2004. p. 117–43.

[89] Luna-Reyes OB, Reyes TM, So FY. Energy cost of ambulation in healthy and disabled Filipino children. Arch Phys Med Rehabil 1998;69:946–9.

[90] Waring WP, Maynard F, Grady W, Grady R, Boyles C. Influence of appropriate lower extremity orthotic management on ambulation, pain, and fatigue in a post-polio population. Arch Phys Med Rehabil 1989;70:371–5.

[91] Fillyaw MJ, Badger GJ, Goodwin GD. The effects of long-term non-fatiguing resistance exercises in subjects with post-polio syndrome. Orthopedics 1995;14:1553–6.

[92] Gross MT, Schuch CP. Exercise programs for patients with post-polio syndrome: a case report. Phys Ther 1989;69:72–6.

[93] Trojan DA, Finch L. Management of post-polio syndrome. Nuerol Rehabil 1997;8:93–105.

[94] Agre JC, Rodriguez AA, Franke TM, Swiggum ER, Harmon RL, Curt JT. Low-intensity, alternate-day exercise improves muscle performance without apparent adverse affect in postpolio patients. Am J Phys Med Rehabil 1996;75:50–8.

[95] Einarsson G. Muscle conditioning in late poliomyelitis. Arch Phys Med Rehabil 1991;72: 11–4.

[96] Jones DR, Speier J, Canine K. Cardiorespiratory responses to aerobic training by patients with post-poliomyelitis sequelae. JAMA 1989;261:3255–8.

[97] Kriz JL, Jones DR, Speier JL. Cardiorespiratory responses to upper extremity aerobic training by post-polio subjects. Arch Phys Med Rehabil 1992;73:49–54.

[98] Ernstoff B, Wetterqvist H, Kvist H, Grimby G. Endurance training effect on individuals with postpoliomyelitis. Arch Phys Med Rehabil 1996;77:843–8.

[99] Willen C, Sunnerhagen KS, Grimby G. Dynamic water exercises in individuals with later poliomyelitis. Arch Phys Med Rehabil 2001;82:66–72.

[100] Gawne AC, Wells KR, Wilson KS. Cardiac risk factors in polio survivors. Arch Phys Med Rehabil 2003;84:694–6.

[101] Agre JC, Rodrigues AA, Sperling KB. Plasma lipid and lipid concentrations in symptomatic post-polio patients. Arch Phys Med Rehabil 1990;71:393–4.

[102] Delahunt JW, Falkner ME, Krebs J. Correlations between bone mineral content, bone area, and lean tissue in individual limbs of subjects with limb weakness after acute poliomyelitis in the past [abstract]. Proc Endocr Soc Australia 1999;10:18.

[103] Gawne AC, Pham BT, Halstead LS. Electrodiagnostic findings in 108 consecutive patients referred to a post-polio clinic: the value of routine electrodiagnostic studies. Ann N Y Acad Sci 1995;753:383–5.

ELSEVIER
SAUNDERS

Phys Med Rehabil Clin N Am
16 (2005) 219–234

PHYSICAL MEDICINE
AND REHABILITATION
CLINICS OF
NORTH AMERICA

Aging with multiple sclerosis

Michelle Stern, MD

Department of Physical Medicine and Rehabilitation, Columbia University,
College of Physicians and Surgeons, New York Presbyterian Hospital,
180 Fort Washington Ave HP1-180, New York, NY 10032, USA

Multiple sclerosis (MS) is the most common cause of acquired neurologic disability in young adults. Symptoms emerge between 20 and 40 years of age in 70% of individuals with the disease. The current understanding of MS is that it is an autoimmune disease with lesions that are disseminated by time and space. The hallmark of MS is central nervous system (CNS) inflammation, demyelination, and gliosis that cause a wide array of brain and spinal cord syndromes. The etiology of the disease may be due to a genetically predetermined susceptibility to MS that is triggered by an environmental factor. MS is an unpredictable and chronic disease. Aging is associated with its own physiologic changes; aging combined with a diagnosis of MS presents unique challenges for the clinician and the patient [1–3].

The major symptoms of MS are cognitive impairment, depression, spasticity, weakness, ataxia, heat intolerance, visual disturbances, fatigue, pain, and bowel and genitourinary dysfunction. The symptoms that occur with MS have many similarities with the aging process. The physiologic changes that occur with aging can lead to diminished muscle strength, balance difficulties, changes in vision, reduced sensation, cognitive impairment, and alteration of bowel and bladder. Weakness and fatigue from MS is compounded by age-related changes such as muscle atrophy, reduced cardiopulmonary reserve, impaired temperature regulation, and depression. The aging population is sensitive to the side effects of many medications. This is due to the physiologic changes that involve liver and kidney function and the absorption and body distribution of medications. The risk-to-benefit ratio of medications used for aging MS patients needs to be considered thoroughly. There are many issues the clinician must address for the older MS patient to help minimize the disability and morbidity caused by aging with this chronic and progressive disease [4–6].

E-mail address: ms1127@columbia.edu

Epidemiology

The disease has a prevalence of less than 1 per 100,000 in equatorial areas; 6 to 14 per 100,000 in the southern United States and southern Europe; and 30 to 80 per 100,000 in Canada, northern Europe, and the northern United States. Incidence in the United States is 250,000 to 350,000, with 10,000 persons diagnosed with the disease every year. It is twice as likely to affect women, with the highest incidence in the early fourth decade and the highest prevalence in the fifth decade. Monozygotic twins have 20% to 40% concordance rates, whereas the risk of a child developing MS when one parent has the disease is 3% to 5% [1–3,7].

A diagnosis of MS is generally not a death sentence. The effect of MS on life expectancy varies in different studies. One study suggested a reduced life expectancy by 14 years, whereas other studies have shown life expectancy to be reduced by 6 to 7 years. Fifty percent of patients survive 30 years or more after disease onset [8].

MS patients need to be educated about their disease process. They must be aware of the impact of their condition and how it will alter their lifestyle. Approximately 50% of patients with MS can expect the following over time: They will be unable to carry out household and employment responsibilities after 10 years, they will require an assistive device to walk after 15 years, and they will be unable to walk after 25 years [9,10].

Indicators of a poor prognosis at onset are progressive course, age >40 years, cerebellar involvement, multiple system involvement, and male sex. Indicators of a favorable prognosis include minimal disability 5 years after onset, complete and rapid remission of initial symptoms, age ≤35 years at onset, only one symptom in the first year, and onset with sensory symptoms or mild optic neuritis [2,11].

Classification of multiple sclerosis

Eighty-five percent of patients have an abrupt onset of the disease. After the initial presentation, the disease can follow different courses. There can be acute episodes of worsening (exacerbations or relapses) or a gradual progression of the disease. There are four major subtypes of MS that can be characterized by their disease course: relapsing remitting (RRMS), secondary progressive (SPMS), progressive relapsing (PRMS), and primary progressive (PPMS) [2,3,12,13].

RRMS is diagnosed in 85% of patients on initial diagnosis; 55% have this subtype. The relapses occur with or without complete recovery, and the patient is clinically stable between episodes. The longer a patient has MS, the greater the chance that the relapses will be associated with residual deficits and increasing disability. Predictors of an unfavorable course include more than five relapses in the first 2 years; increasing relapses after 5 years; short duration between relapses; multiple neural systems involved; incomplete relapse recovery; and motor, cerebellar, and bowel/bladder involvement. Most patients recover from relapses within 4 weeks. There is a subtype of RRMS called benign MS. Benign MS occurs in 10% to 20% of patients. This group has relatively few attacks and excellent recovery between attacks. There is usually minimal disability 20 years after onset, but a majority of patients develop significant disability after 25 years. RRMS patients usually transition to secondary progressive disease [3,12,13].

SPMS occurs in 30% of patients and is characterized by a gradual progression of disability with or without superimposed relapses. If RRMS is left untreated, 50% of patients develop SPMS in 10 years and 90% in 25 years. It is speculated that the disease progression is secondary to ongoing axonal loss despite a lower rate of inflammatory lesions as compared with RRMS [3,12,13].

PPMS is defined by the gradual progression of disability from onset without superimposed relapses. This form occurs in 10% of patients and is most likely to have later onset (40–60 years of age). There are minimal cognitive changes because the spinal cord region is primarily affected. It occurs equally in men and women [3,12,13].

PRMS is characterized by the gradual accumulation of neurologic deficits from initial disease onset with additional intermittent exacerbation. This type affects 5% of patients [3,12,13].

Studies used in the diagnosis of multiple sclerosis

MRI with gadolinium is commonly used to aide in the diagnosis by demonstrating disseminated white matter lesions in the CNS with a characteristic demyelination pattern. Gadolinium enhancement can demonstrate the breakdown in the blood-brain barrier that occurs during active MS. T1 gadolinium–enhancing lesions indicate acute disease activity (<6 weeks). T2 hyperintense lesions demonstrate the extent of MS lesions. Demyelination on MRI is not a unique finding for MS. MRI studies have revealed that aging is associated with increased prevalence of subcortical hyperintense foci in T2 weighted images. These hyperintense lesions develop mainly in periventricular deep white matter. Subcortical white matter hyperintensities in the brain increase by 5% to 9% per year in older adults. Lesions in MS are commonly found extending outward from the ventricular surface, within the brainstem, corpus callosum, cerebellum, and spinal cord. Lesions of the anterior corpus callosum are useful diagnostically because this site is usually spared in cerebrovascular disease. Older patients may present a challenge in differentiating between a new MS lesion and a stroke, but changes in MRI due to an ischemic stroke typically follow a vascular territory [3,14].

Examination of the cerebrospinal fluid (CSF) and evoked potentials (visual, brainstem auditory, and somatosensory) are also used in diagnosing MS. The presence of oligoclonal bands in the CSF is not exclusive to MS. Evoked potentials reveal an increase in latency that is indicative of a demyelinating process. With late-onset MS, there is a higher frequency of oligoclonal banding in the CSF and asymptomatic evoked potential abnormalities compared with a younger age-matched MS population [15,16].

Scales used in multiple sclerosis

There are many different scales used in the literature, but there has been paucity of data investigating their validity and reliability in older individuals. There are three common scales. The Kurtzke Expanded Disability Status Scale (EDSS) is a method of quantifying disability in MS. A patient is evaluated on the EDSS according to the signs and symptoms seen on a neurologic examination. Grading is from 0 (normal) to 10 (death from MS) and increases in 0.5 increments across eight neurologic systems. The eight functional systems that are used in the grading are pyramidal, cerebellar, brainstem, sensory, bowel and bladder, visual, cerebral, and other. The limitations of the EDSS include the overemphasis on lower extremity function and being insensitive to changes in quality of life issues. The Multiple Sclerosis Functional Composite consists of three parts: timed 25-foot walk, nine-hole peg test, and the paced auditory serial addition test. The MS Quality of Life Inventory (MSQLI) consists of 10 individual scales providing a quality of life measure that is generic and MS specific. Studies have shown that MSQLI is a reliable and valid instrument for use in older individuals, but more research is warranted [17–21].

Symptoms of multiple sclerosis

Sensory disturbance and pain

Sensory disturbance seen in MS includes paresthesia, dysthesias, and proprioception loss. Sensory symptoms are a common initial symptom and are present during some point in a majority of patients. Chronic and acute pain syndromes are experienced by more than half of MS patients. The etiology of the pain syndromes can be due to the direct effect of the disease or secondary to the disability created by the disease process. Pain can be characterized into four categories: neuropathic pain, acute pain due to the inflammatory process, pain caused by increased muscle tone, and musculoskeletal pain from poor body posture or improper positioning. Pain is associated with longer disease duration and with pronounced spinal cord involvement. The older population often reports pain as the most distressing symptom. Aging is associated with musculoskeletal degeneration, which can further aggravate painful conditions. Studies have shown that MS patients are often undertreated for pain, which can result in increased morbidity [22–24].

Medication useful for treating pain in this population includes opioid analgesics, nonsteroidal anti-inflammatory drugs (NSAIDs), anti-seizure medication, antidepressants, and anti-spasticity agents. An intrathecal pump may be beneficial for intractable pain and spasms.

Reduced doses of opioids may be required to limit adverse reactions in elderly MS patients. Typical side effects are constipation, respiratory depression, and confusion. Carbamazepine and other anticonvulsants may increase confusion and ataxia in elderly patients. Tricyclic antidepressants (TCAs) may lead to urinary retention, confusion, cardiac symptoms, and autonomic instability. NSAIDs should be used with caution in elderly patients due to the increase risk of hypertension, gastrointestinal bleeding, and impaired renal function [25].

Even though many different pain syndromes can be solely due to MS, pain complaints in an aging population should be evaluated for other possible etiologies. Cervical spondylosis may occur in conjunction with MS. Clues to help identify cases of cervical spondylosis in addition to MS include neck pain, radicular pain in the upper extremity, muscle atrophy in a segmental distribution in the upper extremity, and the loss of deep tendon reflexes in the upper extremity. Surgery is useful for some MS patients [26].

Fatigue

Fatigue is present in two thirds of patients, with one half describing fatigue as the most disabling symptom. Common features of MS fatigue include reduced energy, malaise, motor weakness during sustained activity, and difficulty maintaining concentration. An aging MS patient who complains of fatigue should have a thorough evaluation. Secondary causes, such as infection, cancer, anemia, hypothyroidism, rheumatologic disorders, and diseases of the cardiovascular, pulmonary, renal, or hepatic system, should be ruled out. Medications that can contribute to fatigue include TCAs, benzodiazepines, anticonvulsants, beta-blockers, interferons, and the anti-spasticity medications. Other factors that can lead to fatigue include depression, pain, physical deconditioning, and exposure to a heated environment. Once other causes have been ruled out, treatment of fatigue includes energy conservation, an exercise program, and medication. Medications include amantadine, pemoline, modafinil, and methylphenidate. Stimulants in the aging population should be used with caution due to the increased risk of cardiac side effects. Amantadine has been associated with an increase risk of confusion and edema in elderly patients [27,28]. Aerobic exercises have been shown to be beneficial in reducing fatigue [29].

Depression

Mood changes can be caused by neuroanatomic and neurochemical changes from MS or can result from having to adapt to living with the disease. Depression is the most common mood disorder, affecting more than half of patients. Incidence of depression in MS is three times higher than the general population and more common even when compared with other chronic disease states. Depression may be overlooked because there are symptoms common to depression and MS, such as fatigue, reduced activity, and poor concentration. MS is associated with a 7.5 times higher suicide rate than in the general population, which cannot be explained fully by a reactive depression. In general, suicide rates increase with age, and completed suicide is more common in men. Risk factors for suicide include major depression, living alone, and alcohol abuse. Duration of MS, severity of physical disability, and cognitive impairment do not affect the risk of suicide. Drugs that can cause depressive symptoms include anxiolytics, beta-blockers, methyldopa, clonidine, reserpine, and steroids. Depression rating scales may have limited utility in the MS population. The widely used Beck Depression Inventory evaluates depression based on responses to 21 questions, but the questions may overlap with the symptoms of MS, such as fatigue. The same is true for the Geriatric Depression Scale. How the common depression scales should be modified to better evaluate the MS patient is unclear [22,30–32].

Cognitive dysfunction

Fifty percent of patients with MS suffer from cognitive dysfunction. Changes in cognitive ability can significantly impair relationships and the ability to work and to live independently. Even though mild cognitive dysfunction occurs frequently, only 5% to 10% of patients develop severe cognitive dysfunction [22]. Cognitive deficits involve loss of short-term memory, reasoning, verbal fluency, visuospatial functions, abstract reasoning, and speed of information processing. Intellectual functions and language skills are generally unaffected. Decreased short-term memory is the most common finding. Patients demonstrate slowed retrieval of formed memories and often require cueing. Aging causes a slowing in the frontal lobe, which can lead to a slower learning rate. Thus, the aging MS patient may be at a greater risk for significant cognitive disturbance. Patients should be encouraged to use lists, daily journals, and appointment books for activities. The mini-mental examination may be useful in tracking changes in cognition, but it may not detect subtle cognitive changes occurring in most MS patients. The patient medication list should be assessed for possible impact on cognitive function. Medications that can contribute to cognitive slowing, especially in the aging population, include anticholinergics, antispasmodics, opioids, benzodiazepines, and TCAs. Consideration should be given to changing to the long-acting anticholinergic preparations and to the use of intrathecal medications or botulinum toxin injections to reduce high doses of oral antispasticity agents. The clinician should monitor for signs of depression, anxiety, or fatigue, which may exacerbate these difficulties [33–39].

Ophthalmologic symptoms

Disturbances of the visual system are among the most common manifestations of MS, affecting up to 80% of patients at some time during the disease course. These abnormalities can result in significant disability, culminating in an inability to work and compromising the patient's activities of daily living. The most common visual manifestations of MS are optic neuritis, internuclear ophthalmoplegia, and nystagmus. Symptoms may include blurred vision, scotoma, impaired color vision, and diminished contrast sensitivity. Visual changes are also common in the aging population and include the development of cataracts, presbyopia, macular degeneration, and glaucoma, which can lead to further social isolation and difficulty in self-care. Useful recommendations may include the outlining of doorways, steps, and wall switches with tape or markers; the use of magnifiers; and glare reduction. Eyeglasses with prisms or patching one eye can help minimize diplopia [22,40].

Cerebellar symptoms

Cerebellar lesions are seen in one third of patients with MS. The tremors in MS can be one of the more disabling symptoms of the disease and can affect any muscle group. Tremors can increase fatigue by causing an increase in energy consumption. Although there is no effective treatment, medications used have included Inderal, Klonopin, Mysoline, and isoniazid (the risk of hepatitis increases with age >35 years). Stereotactic surgery is not recommended. Aging is also associated with a decline in balance. Fall precautions should be reviewed [22].

Motor loss and spasticity

Corticospinal tract involvement is present in 62% of patients with progressive disease. Spasticity and weakness usually have a greater impact on the lower extremities. The weakness associated with aging is caused by lower motor neuron denervation and muscle atrophy [22].

The energy requirement for an activity is increased with the presence of spasticity. The aging patient with increased spasticity needs to be evaluated to rule out secondary causes such as infections, skin breakdown, spinal stenosis with myelopathy, or other disease processes. The use of oral medications for spasticity may be less tolerated in the older population and should be monitored closely. Baclofen use in an elderly patient requires an initial lower dose and a slower titration to decrease the risk of sedation and confusion. Tizanidine should also be used with caution in elderly patients because clearance of the drug is decreased fourfold. Monitoring for hypotension and sedation is essential. The benzodiazepines are traditionally poorly tolerated in the older population and are associated with an increased half-life and a higher association of paradoxic reactions, agitation, and disequilibrium [5,22].

Bladder disturbance

Ninety-six percent of patients with MS for over 10 years will have some form of urologic symptoms, with detrusor hyper-reflexia being the most common. The use of oxybutynin and tolterodine in the treatment of detrusor hyperreflexia in clinical studies did not reveal overall differences in safety between the older and younger patients. Anatomic and physiologic changes due to aging can cause urinary frequency, hesitancy, retention, and nocturia. Incontinence may also be due to delirium, atrophic vaginitis, enlarged prostrate, constipation, and endocrine disorders. Women should be evaluated for estrogen replacement, and men should have routine prostate evaluation. Elderly patients are especially sensitive to the urologic side effects of other medications used to treat MS. The alpha-blocking agents that are used to treat sphincter dysergia may have a higher incidence of orthostasis in elderly patients, and blood pressure should be monitored. Urinary tract dysfunction can lead to the formation of bladder stones, renal stones, and frequent urinary tract infection. Frequent urinary tract infections and antibiotic use can lead to the development of resistant organisms. Treatment of urologic symptoms should take into account the patients level of disability, degree of reversibility of symptom, ability to function independently, manual dexterity, other medical problems, and social support networks. Before placing a patient on a program of clean intermittent catheterization, a careful assessment of the patient's coordination, vision, cognitive function, and manual dexterity needs to be completed. If intermittent catheterization is impractical, an indwelling catheter can be used. Choices include a suprapubic or a urethral catheter. Chronic indwelling catheters can lead to colonization of the urinary tract, which should be kept in mind when obtaining a urine culture. Other disadvantages include bladder calculi and the development of squamous cell carcinoma. In patients with poor mobility, poor dexterity, or significant lower extremity spasticity, an augmentation cystoplasty with a catherizable abdominal stoma may be considered to ease catheterization [22,41].

Bowel disturbance

Constipation is the most common bowel dysfunction. Constipation can result from pelvic floor spasticity, decreased gastro-colic reflex, inadequate hydration, medication, immobility, and weak abdominal muscles. Elderly persons are at risk for constipation due to slowed motility of the gastrointestinal tract. Many medications can exacerbate constipation, especially in elderly patients. The anticholinergics, TCAs, anti-hypertensives (especially the calcium-channel blockers), iron, calcium, and opioid agents are common offenders. Fecal incontinence can result from sphincter dysfunction, constipation with rectal overflow, and diminished rectal sensation. A regular bowel program may be necessary. Any aging patient, including MS patients, should undergo routine colonoscopy. Changes in bowel habits need to be investigated to exclude colon cancer and diverticular disease, and patients should be screened for thyroid disease and other medical causes [22,42].

Sexual disturbance

A majority of MS patients and their partners suffer from some form of sexual dysfunction. Primary sexual dysfunction is due to lesions in the CNS that cause loss of libido, decreased genital sensation, decreased orgasmic response, difficulty achieving an erection in men, and decreased vaginal lubrication in women. Secondary sexual dysfunction occurs due to other symptoms of MS, such as bowel and bladder problems, spasticity, etc. Tertiary sexual dysfunction is related to psychosocial and cultural issues. Sexual changes that occur commonly in the elderly population include impotence in men and orgasmic dysfunction and dyspareunia in women. A sexual history should be taken routinely, and treatment options should be discussed with the patient and their partner. The phosphodiesterase 5 inhibitors should be used with caution in elderly patients due to a reduced clearance of these medications and possible cardiac side effects [41,43].

Heat intolerance

MS is associated with an increase in severity of symptoms with heat. Weather, over-exercising, or fever can produce symptoms. Elderly patients are vulnerable to hyperthermia due to loss of homeostatic temperature-regulating control, a decline in function of the autonomic nervous system, decrease in sweat gland function, and regional loss of subcutaneous fat. To help manage heat intolerance, outside activities should be timed for early morning, energy conservation techniques should be used, and air conditioning should be used in homes and cars. Cooling vests and light-colored clothes may be useful, and saunas and hot tubs should be avoided. Pool temperature should be 85°F [6,22].

Swallowing

Swallowing disorders have been estimated to affect 3% to 20% of MS patients. Oral intake and nutritional status should be closely monitored in these patients. Appropriate swallowing studies may be needed for evaluation, and patients with severe dysphagia may require enterostomal feedings. Elderly patients can develop deficits that can exacerbate the dysphagia associated with MS, such as ineffective pharyngeal peristalsis and reduced motility of the esophagus leading to reflux, achalasia, and hiatal hernia [22].

Other related conditions

Falls

Leg weakness, impaired balance, and older age lead to an increased risk of falling. There are limited data on the effects of exercise on reducing fall risk in the MS population. A recent study suggested that gait speed is a predictor for fall risk in MS and that the introduction of a home exercise program may lead to a fall reduction. Fall prevention in the elderly MS patient can include a home safety evaluation, proper footwear, and orthotic use. Medications that can contribute to fall risk include benzodiazepines, antihypertensives, TCAs, and tizanidine. Home modifications include nonslip floors, low carpet, absence of area rugs, and a bedside commode [44].

Osteoporosis

The effects of aging, limited ambulation ability, and the use of corticosteroids are common causes of bone loss. The aging MS patient with impaired balance and ambulation is at increased risk for fractures. MS patients of both genders usually have decreased bone density in the spine and femoral neck. Patients need to be screened regularly for osteoporosis. Studies have shown that hip fractures can be reduced with the use of a hip protector in elderly patients, but this study did not look at MS patients [45,46].

Cardiac

Cardiac disease risk increases in the aging population. Some patients with MS have lower participation in physical activity and may be at an increased risk for coronary artery disease as they age. A low- or high-intensity exercise program was associated with reducing the coronary artery disease risk in women with MS. Patients with lower physical activity had higher abdominal fat, and an increase in exercise led to lower glucose and triglyceride levels. Patients with MS should be encouraged to participate in low- to moderate-intensity activity to reduce the risk of coronary disease. Patients with MS benefit from physical activity, but the current research has mainly been conducted on patients younger 65 years of age, and its effect on the elderly MS patient is unknown [47].

Vaccination

There has been reluctance in the medical community to administer routine vaccinations to MS patients due to concern that it may lead to an exacerbation of MS symptoms. Multiple clinical studies have not linked vaccinations as a cause of MS exacerbations. Patients with MS should be advised against routine casual vaccination, especially if previous exacerbations have been preceded by vaccination, but medically indicated vaccines should be given [48,49].

Medication used to treat multiple sclerosis

There is no cure for MS, but there are disease-modifying agents, each with its own side-effect profile and efficacy. Exacerbations are usually treated with a short course of intravenous corticosteroids with or without a prednisone taper. Side effects of high-dose steroid use include mood changes, hypertension, glucose abnormalities, and fluid retention. Repetitive use of steroids can predispose to the development of osteoporosis and cataracts [22,50].

Once a patient is diagnosed with RRMS, there are a number of agents that can be used to decrease the frequency of relapses and reduce the degree of disability. These agents are the interferons and glatiramer acetate. There are three interferons on the market: Betaseron, Avonex, and Rebif. Side effects include flu-like symptoms, local reaction at the injection site, elevated liver function test, and an abnormal CBC. The usefulness of these medications may be limited over time by the development of neutralizing antibodies [50].

Glatiramer acetate (Copaxone) is a collection of random peptides of four amino acids designed to mimic myelin basic protein. Side effects include injection site reaction and a short-lived, post-injection reaction characterized by chest tightness, palpitations, flushing, and anxiety [50].

Most studies that evaluated these disease-modifying agents used patients with a mean age of 34 to 47 years. Therefore, the effects of these medications on an aging population are not fully understood. Studies are needed to confirm that these agents are effective and well tolerated with long-term use.

Immunosuppressants are mainly used for progressive MS, but their risk-to-benefit ratio may outweigh their usefulness in the older population [50]. Mitoxantrone is an anthracycline analog that shows promise for the MS population, although the optimal use of this drug is not known. The major side effect of this drug is the development of a cardiomyopathy, which limits use to 2 years. The long-term effect of this drug on an aging MS population is unknown, but patients should be monitored closely for cardiac dysfunction [51].

The use of azathioprine as a treatment for MS remains controversial because of mixed research results. Side effects can include nausea, anemia or leukopenia, liver damage, and a long-term increased risk of developing cancers such as leukemia or lymphoma. This medication is less likely to be tolerated in an older population and if used requires monitoring for cancers as the patient ages. Cyclophosphamide has shown only a modest benefit. It seems to be most effective in patients younger than 40 years of age, especially in those who have been in the progressive phase for <1 year. The duration of treatment is limited by the risk of bladder cancer, which seems to rise with time and may depend upon the total accumulated drug dose [50,52].

There is debate in the MS community as to the best allocation of money in caring for patients with progressive MS. Is it better to spend money on current treatment, which has limited results at best, or to put the money into financing the complex home care that these patients will likely require, especially as they age?

Assistive devices

Reports have shown that gait disturbance is caused by the following four symptoms (in order of importance): muscle weakness, ataxia, sensory loss, and spasticity [22]. There are many devices to help aide the MS patient in mobilization, including canes, crutches, walkers, scooters, and manual or motorized wheelchairs. Lofstrand crutches, although useful in the younger MS population, have limited utility in the older patients. Older patients generally benefit from canes or walkers. A rolling walker helps to conserve energy, and the addition of hand brakes, a seat, and a basket can be beneficial. Patients with ataxia may require the use of weighted equipment. Orthotics such as an ankle foot orthosis (AFO) may be helpful in improving toe clearance. AFOs can add knee stability without much additional weight. Orthotics with high-energy demands such as the hip-knee-ankle-foot orthosis should be avoided, especially in the elderly MS patient. Wrist-hand orthoses are useful in the treatment of upper extremity paresis and spasticity. Other equipment that may be required for safety or for energy conservation includes bathtub benches, shower chairs, grab bars, Hoyer lifts, and stair lifts [53].

The use of self-propulsion wheelchairs, even lightweight manual wheel-chairs, may be difficult for this patient population, especially as they age, and a motorized wheelchair should be considered. Before being prescribed a motorized wheelchair, the patient should be evaluated for deficits in cognition, vision, and manual dexterity, which can effect a patient's ability to safely operate this device. The safety of these devices needs to be assessed periodically as the disease progresses. Patients may prefer a scooter to a motorized wheelchair because there is less perception of a disability with a scooter. The disadvantage of a scooter is that it is not designed for prolonged seating. A wheelchair is more useful for patients who rely solely on motorized devices for locomotion. Patients with MS who have risk factors for a progressive course should be advised to consider wheelchair/handicap accessible housing as early as possible [53].

Vocational issues

Seventy-five percent of patients with MS are employed at the time of diagnosis, but only 30% to 40% of people with MS remain in the work force 10 years after diagnosis. Not all jobs can be recommended for MS patients. Patients should be counseled regarding training for a less physically or intellectually demanding job and should be advised to apply for disability benefits [22,54].

Driving with multiple sclerosis

MS patients have a higher number of traffic accidents and offenses compared with healthy adults. Assessment for driving ability needs to be done periodically, especially as MS patients age, to ensure sufficient cognitive and physical for safe automobile operation. A formal driving evaluation may be necessary. Referral for a handicap parking plaque should be done as early as possible. This helps conserve energy in the early phase of the disease and can be useful as ambulation becomes impaired. Car adaptation may be needed as the disability progresses. The clinician should prepare the MS patient for the future if it seems likely they will no longer be able to drive. Alternative transportation options should be discussed [55,56].

Family

Family dynamics may change after a diagnosis of MS. Compromises from family members is necessary to successfully adapt to the deficits brought on by the disease. There should be open communication of how care will be managed at home as the patient progresses and as the caregiver ages. Appropriate referrals to home care agencies and social workers should be arranged. Support groups or counseling can help the patient and family deal with difficult decisions and help with coping strategies. Long-term placement may need to be explored for patients with severe disability [22].

Summary

The chronic and progressive nature of MS may be overwhelming to the patient and the family. It is vital for the clinician to develop a system of periodic evaluations and interventions that monitor the disease and address the effects on the patient's physical, psychologic, social, and vocational functioning. MS patients are susceptible to other diseases of aging, such as stroke, cancer, heart disease, and diabetes, and need to be evaluated and treated for these conditions. Obtaining appropriate routine medical care may become difficult in less mobile patients because many clinicians' offices are unable to accommodate handicapped patients. Careful coordination and referral to handicap-accessible centers may be required to ensure adequate treatment.

Nearly half of MS patients die from complications of their disease. Other major causes of mortality are malignancy (16%), suicide (15%), and myocardial infarction (11%). Age-appropriate cancer screenings and cardiac evaluation are necessary. Depression is an important factor in geriatric MS patients despite the fact that most MS patients have an easier time adjusting to the aging process than the general population [57]. There are many unanswered questions for the older MS population due to the paucity of research, but future studies may rectify this situation. Although there is no cure for MS, the clinician can play a key role in helping the patient and family adapt to the illness and improve their quality of life. Resources are available for the clinician, the patient, and family members (Box 1).

Box 1. Resources for dealing with MS

- Multiple Sclerosis Association of America (MSAA)—800-532-7667; www.msaa.com
- National Multiple Sclerosis Society (NMSS)—800-FIGHT-MS (800-344-4867); www.nmss.org
- American Nystagmus Network—www.nystagmus.org
- The Lighthouse—800-829-0500; www.lighthouse.org
- Low Vision Information Center—301-951-4444; www.lowvisioninfo.org

---

References

[1] Williams R, Rigby AS, Airey M, Robinson M, Ford H. Multiple sclerosis: its epidemiological, genetic, and health care impact. J Epidemiol Community Health 1995;49: 563–9.

[2] Frohman E. Multiple sclerosis. Med Clin N Am 2003;87:867–97.

[3] Hauser S, Goodkin D. Multiple sclerosis and other demyelinating diseases. In: Braunwald E, Fauci A, Isselbacher K, et al, editors. Harrison's principles of internal medicine. 15th edition. Columbus (OH): McGraw-Hill; 2001. p. 1096–33.

[4] Joy J, Johnston R. Characteristics and management of major symptoms in multiple sclerosis current status and strategies for the future. Washington, DC: National Academy Press; 2001. p. 115–76.

[5] Paty D. Initial symptoms. In: Burks J, Johnson K, editors. Multiple sclerosis: diagnosis, medical management, and rehabilitation. New York: Demos; 2000. p. 75–9.

[6] Hazelwood M, Fielstein E. Physiological aspects of aging. In: Maloney F, Means K, editors. Physical med and rehab: state of the art review. Rehabilitation and the aging population. Philadelphia: Hanley and Belfus; 1990. p. 19–28.

[7] Kurtzke J, Wallin M. Epidemiology. In: Burks J, Johnson K, editors. Multiple sclerosis: diagnosis, medical management, and rehabilitation. New York: Demos; 2000. p. 75–9.

[8] O'Connor P. Canadian Multiple Sclerosis Working Group. Key issues in the diagnosis and treatment of multiple sclerosis: an overview. Neurology 2002;59:S1–33.

[9] Weinshenker BG. Natural history of multiple sclerosis. Ann Neurol 1994;36(Suppl): S6–11.

[10] Weinshenker BG. The natural history of MS. Neurol Clin 1995;13:119–46.

[11] Amato MP, et al. A prospective study on the natural history of multiple sclerosis: clues to the conduct and interpretation of clinical trials. J Neurol Sci 1999;168:96–106.

[12] Lublin FD, et al. Defining the clinical course of multiple sclerosis: results of an international survey. Neurology 1996;46:907–11.

[13] Joy J, Johnston R. Clinical and biological features in multiple sclerosis current status and strategies for the future. Washington, DC: National Academy Press; 2001. p. 29–114.

[14] Miller D. Magnetic resonance imaging in multiple sclerosis. In: Cohen J, Rudick R, editors. Multiple sclerosis therapeutics. New York: Martin Dunitz; 2003. p. 81–97.

[15] Polliak M, Barak Y, et al. Late-onset multiple sclerosis. J Am Geriatr Soc 2001;49:168–71.

[16] Noseworthy J, Paty D, Wonnacott T, et al. Multiple sclerosis after age 50. Neurology 1983; 33:1537–44.

[17] Hoogervorst EL, van Winsen LM, Eikelenboom MJ, et al. Comparisons of patient self-report, neurologic examination, and functional impairment in MS. Neurology 2001; 56:934–7.

[18] Kurtzke JF. Rating neurological impairment in multiple sclerosis: an expanded disability status scale EDSS. Neurology 1983;33:1444–52.

[19] Cohen JA, Cutter GR, Fischer JS, et al. Use of the multiple sclerosis functional composite as an outcome measure in a phase 3 clinical trial. Arch Neurol 2001;58:961–7.

[20] Fischer JS, Rudick RA, Cutter GR, et al. The Multiple Sclerosis functional composite measure (MSFC): an integrated approach to MS clinical outcome assessment. National MS Society Clinical Outcomes Assessment Task Force. Mult Scler 1999;5:244–50.

[21] Dilorenzo T, Halper J, Picone MA. Reliability and validity of the multiple sclerosis quality of life inventory in older individuals. Disabil Rehabil 2003;25:891–7.

[22] Cobble N, Miller E, Grigsby J, et al. Aging with multiple sclerosis. In: Felsenthal G, Garrison S, Steinberg F, editors. Rehabilitation of the aging and elderly patient. Philadelphia: Williams and Wilkins; 1994. p. 427–39.

[23] Ehde DM, Jensen MP, Engel JM, Turner JA, Hoffman AJ, Cardenas DD. Chronic pain secondary to disability: a review. Clin J Pain 2003;19:3–17.

[24] Jeffrey D. Pain and dysthesia. In: Burks J, Johnson K, editors. Multiple sclerosis: diagnosis, medical management, and rehabilitation. New York: Demos; 2000. p. 425–31.

[25] Boop W. Pain management in the geriatric patient. In: Maloney F, Means K, editors. Physical med and rehab: state of the art review. Rehabilitation and the aging population. Philadelphia: Hanley and Belfus; 1990. p. 83–92.

[26] Bashir K, Hadley MN, Whitaker JN. Surgery for spinal cord compression in multiple sclerosis. Curr Opin Neurol 2001;14:765–9.

[27] Krupp L. Fatigue in multiple sclerosis. In: Cohen J, Rudick R, editors. Multiple sclerosis therapeutics. New York: Martin Dunitz; 2003. p. 599–608.

[28] Van den Noort S, Fisk JD, Pontefract A, Ritvo PG, et al. The impact of fatigue on patients with MS. Can J Neurol Sci 1994;21:9–14.

[29] Mostert S, Kesselring J. Effects of a short-term exercise training program on aerobic fitness, fatigue, health perception and activity level of subjects with multiple sclerosis. Mult Scler 2002;8:161–8.

[30] Minden S, Frumin M, Erb J. Treatment of disorders of mood and affect in multiple sclerosis. In: Cohen J, Rudick R, editors. Multiple sclerosis therapeutics. New York: Martin Dunitz; 2003. p. 651–89.

[31] Sadovnick AD, Eisen K, Ebers GC, Paty DW. Cause of death in patients attending multiple sclerosis clinics. Neurology 1991;41:1193–6.

[32] Feinstein A. An examination of suicidal intent in patients with multiple sclerosis. Neurology 2002;59:674–8.

[33] Rao SM. Neuropsychology of MS. Curr Opin Neurol 1995;8:216–20.

[34] Bolbholz JA, Rao S, et al. Cognitive decline in MS: an eight year longitudinal study. J Int Neuropsych Soc 1998;16:435–40.

[35] Rao SM, Hammeke T, et al. Memory disturbance in chronic progressive MS. Arch Neurol 1984;41:625–31.

[36] Rao S, Leo G, et al. Cognitive dysfunction in MS: I. frequency, patterns and prediction. Neurology 1991;41:685–91.

[37] Amato MP, Ponzianni G, et al. Cognitive impairments in early-onset MS: pattern predictors and impact on every day life in a 4-year follow-up. Arch Neurol 1995;52:168–72.

[38] Amato MP, Ponzianni G, et al. Cognitive impairments in early-onset MS: a reappraisal after 10 years. Arch Neurol 2001;58:602–6.

[39] Schwid S. Management of cognitive impairments in MS. In: Cohen J, Rudick R, editors. Multiple sclerosis therapeutics. New York: Martin Dunitz; 2003. p. 715–25.

[40] Frohman E, Zimmerman C, et al. Neuro-opthalmic signs and symptoms. In: Burks J, Johnson K, editors. Multiple sclerosis: diagnosis, medical management, and rehabilitation. New York: Demos; p. 341–77.

[41] DasGupta R, Fowler CJ. Sexual and urological dysfunction in multiple sclerosis: better understanding and improved therapies. Curr Opin Neurol 2002;15:271–8.

[42] Wiesel PH, Norton C, Glickman S, Kamm MA. Pathophysiology and management of bowel dysfunction in multiple sclerosis. Eur J Gastroenterol Hepatol 2001;13:441–8.

[43] Zorzon M, Zivadinov R, et al. Sexual dysfunction in MS: a 2-year follow-up study. J Neurol Sci 2001;187:1–5.

[44] DeBolt L, McCubbin J. The effects of home-based resistance exercise on balance, power and mobility in adults with multiple sclerosis. Arch Phys Med Rehabil 2004;85:290–7.

[45] Cosman F, Nieves J, et al. Fracture history and bone loss in patients with MS. Neurology 1998;51:1161–5.

[46] Kanus P, Parkkari J, et al. Prevention of hip fracture in elderly people with the use of a hip protector. NEJM 2000;343:1506–13.

[47] Slawta JN, McCubbin JA, Wilcox AR, Fox SD, Nalle DJ, Anderson G. Coronary heart disease risk between active and inactive women with multiple sclerosis. Med Sci Sports Exerc 2002;34:905–12.

[48] Confavreux C, Suissa S, Saddier P, et al. Vaccinations and the risk of relapse in multiple sclerosis. New Engl J Med 2001;344:319–26.

[49] Miller A, Morgante L, Buchwald L. A multicenter, randomized, double-blind, placebo-controlled trial of influenza immunization in multiple sclerosis. Neurology 1997;48:312–4.

[50] Noseworthy JH. Management of multiple sclerosis: current trials and future options. Curr Opin Neurol 2003;16:289–97.

[51] Ghalie RG, Edan G, Laurent M, et al. Cardiac adverse effects associated with mitoxantrone (Novantrone) therapy in patients with MS. Neurology 2002;59:909–13.

[52] Galetta SL, Markowitz C, Lee AG. Immunomodulatory agents for the treatment of relapsing multiple sclerosis: a systematic review. Arch Intern Med 2002;162:2161–9.

[53] Strobel W. Issues in assistive technology. In: Rumrill D Jr, Hennessey M. Multiple sclerosis: a guide for rehabilitation and health care professionals. Springfield (IL): Charles C Thomas; 2002. p. 179–208.

[54] Rumrill P. Impact on employment and career development. In: Rumrill D Jr, Hennessey M. Multiple sclerosis: a guide for rehabilitation and health care professionals. Springfield (IL): Charles C Thomas; 2002. p. 137–78.

[55] Bobholz J, Rao S. Cognitive dysfunction in MS: a review of recent developments. Curr Opin Neurol 2003;16:283–8.

[56] Schultheis M, Garay E, et al. The influence of cognitive impairment on driving performance in MS. Neurology 2001;56:1089–94.

[57] Sadounick A, Eisen K, et al. Cause of death in patients attending MS clinic. Neurology 1991; 41:1193–6.

ELSEVIER
SAUNDERS

Phys Med Rehabil Clin N Am
16 (2005) 235–249

PHYSICAL MEDICINE
AND REHABILITATION
CLINICS OF
NORTH AMERICA

Aging with cerebral palsy

Celeste D. Zaffuto-Sforza, DO[a,b,*]

[a]*Department of Rehabilitation Medicine, Mount Sinai School of Medicine,
One Gustave L. Levy Place, New York, NY 10029, USA*
[b]*Elmhurst Hospital Center, 79-01 Broadway, Elmhurst, NY 11373, USA*

Cerebral palsy (CP) has been defined as the result of an injury or nonprogressive lesion to the immature, developing brain, causing a disorder of movement and posture [1,2]. The diagnostic sign is classically that of a motor deficit, but other symptom complexes of cerebral dysfunction may be associated with CP. CP has a spectrum of clinical syndromes, all of which are characterized by abnormalities in muscle tone, deep tendon reflexes, primitive reflexes, and postural reactions [3,4]. It is classified by the type of neurologic dysfunction (spastic, hypotonic, athetotic, dystonic, or a combination of these) and by the extremities involved (monoplegia, hemiplegia, diplegia, triplegia, and quadriplegia) [5]. There is a paucity of information in the literature regarding adults with CP, and most primary care physicians and specialists in the adult health care system have not received special training dealing with adults with developmental disabilities. This article calls attention to the needs that are unique to this population and aids the health care provider's basic approach to these patients.

Epidemiology

CP has been reported to be the leading cause of childhood disability, with estimates that 8000 babies are diagnosed with the condition each year. However, it is no longer a disorder affecting newborns and adolescents. Although the number of adults with CP is unknown, it is estimated to be 400,000 [6]. Approximately 764,000 children and adults manifest at least one symptom of CP [7]. The number of adults with CP is increasing, likely due to the increased survival of low-birth-weight infants and increased longevity of the adult population in general. Ninety percent of children with CP survive

---

* Department of Rehabilitation Medicine, Mount Sinai School of Medicine, One Gustave L. Levy Place, New York, NY 10029.

1047-9651/05/$ - see front matter © 2004 Elsevier Inc. All rights reserved.
doi:10.1016/j.pmr.2004.06.014   pmr.theclinics.com

to age 20 [8]. Ninety-five percent of children with diplegia and 75% of children with quadriplegia survive to 30 years of age [9]. By contrast, 65% of severely mentally retarded and 90% of mildly mentally retarded children survive to 38 years of age [9]. This means that although CP is second to mental retardation as the most frequent developmental disability in children [10], it is becoming more prevalent in the adult population. Because there is a growing trend to transfer adults with CP to the community from long-term care facilities [11], health care providers must become more educated in the problems that this portion of the population faces.

Secondary conditions

Secondary conditions are defined as injuries, impairments, functional limitations, or disabilities that occur as a result of a primary condition or pathology [12]. The primary condition in patients with CP is the brain insult with ensuing effects on musculoskeletal growth and motor control. Because many body systems are affected during a child's development, a child is at a high risk for secondary conditions as an adult.

Pain

Pain has been identified by individuals with CP as one of the most common secondary conditions. Turk et al [13] found that 84% of women surveyed reported pain. This is significantly higher than the 25% reported for the general American adult population [14]. Causes of pain can include musculoskeletal deformities, overuse syndromes, and arthritis. The pain may be acute or chronic. The most common areas are the hip, knee, ankle, lumbar spine, and cervical spine [6,12]. The majority of subjects in a study by Turk et al [12] reported that they experienced pain daily, and one third reported that the pain was constant. Patients with the spastic type of CP had an increased number of sites and worse pain than those with other types of CP. Exceptions were those with joint subluxations, dislocations, or degenerative joint disease [12].

Hip pain is a significant issue for adults who are nonambulatory. Forty-seven percent of adult individuals with CP have hip pain [15]. In a cross-sectional, multicenter study, Hodgkinson et al [15] found that pain provoked by mobilization, palpation, and lower extremity weight bearing was the most frequent. They also found that positional pain was reported in 19% of their subjects. These patients reported pain with prolonged maintenance of one position or when changing position.

Chronic pain is also a serious problem for many adults with CP. Tenuta et al [16] reported that 41% of 27 adults with CP who underwent triple arthrodesis as children complained of pain as adults. Schwartz et al [17] found that 67% of their subjects reported pain of 3 or 4 months duration in one or more sites.

An important question to be addressed is whether the pain of these patients is being managed adequately. For patients with CP, pain may be unrecognized or mismanaged by health care providers [18]. Communicative and cognitive impairments in some patients can make the assessment and management of pain difficult [19]. For this reason, it is often useful to have the patient's caregiver present for the history and physical examination, in order to uncover nuances in the patient's nonoral communication.

CP-related pain is known to be undertreated in the adult population. Less than half of patients with moderate to severe pain make visits to their physicians or nurse practitioners specifically for pain [20]. Although the frequency of pain in adults with CP is high, there is little research regarding the efficacy of treatments for pain. Engel et al [20] found that adult patients with CP are more likely to use passive interventions for pain, such as medications. Few patients used active interventions like biofeedback, counseling, or exercise to manage their pain, even though the patients rated these interventions to be at least somewhat to moderately helpful.

Musculoskeletal deformities and arthritis

Among the musculoskeletal deformities associated with CP are hip dislocation and subluxations, foot abnormalities, patella alta, pelvic obliquity, scoliosis, degenerative changes in the spine, and contractures [12,13,21]. Although these conditions may not produce pain during childhood, they can become painful with daily activities in adulthood. It has been suggested that some musculoskeletal deformities be corrected in childhood in order to prevent progression into adulthood and limited mobility [21].

Hips that are dislocated are far more likely to cause pain than those that are stable. Often, surgical intervention is needed. Procedures include tendon releases, tendon transfers, open reduction, and femoral or pelvic osteotomies. However, hip arthritis can develop if the joint does not maintain its stability, leading to a total hip replacement [22].

Various foot and knee abnormalities are common in children with CP and can cause pain and loss of function in the adolescent and adult. Cavus foot deformities can cause metatarsal pain. Patella alta is common due to walking with knee flexion. The long-term effect can be chondromalacia and pain [23], which can result in functional losses such as difficulty getting out of a chair or climbing stairs.

Scoliosis is a common secondary condition of CP. Because it is usually of neuromuscular origin, it will likely progress even after skeletal maturity. Curves over 50° progress at a rate of about 1° per year [21]. The rate of progression is more rapid in individuals with C-shaped curves than in those with S-shaped curves [24]. Nonambulatory individuals with CP are more likely to develop scoliosis than ambulatory individuals. Patients with CP should be monitored for scoliosis and its progression throughout their lives.

The abnormal relationship of joint surfaces and excessive joint compression can lead to osteoarthritis and pain. Murphy et al [6] suggested that early development of degenerative arthritis in 40-year-old individuals with CP could explain their pain in weight-bearing joints. Cathels and Reddihough [25] reported clinical evidence of arthritis in 27% of subjects between 15 and 25 years of age. It was more prevalent in people who were ambulatory than in those who were not. This is likely due to the effects of ambulation on weight-bearing joints.

Nerve entrapments and overuse syndromes

Persons with CP have limited strength and patterns of movement. This places them at risk for overuse syndromes, nerve entrapments, fatigue, radiculopathies, and myelopathies [6]. Individuals with athetotic and spastic types of CP are at risk for cervical myelopathies, although they are less common in those with spastic CP [26,27]. Compressive and shearing forces associated with the repetitive and involuntary motions of rotation, flexion, and extension can lead to cervical instability, disc herniation, spondylosis, osteophytes, and cervical spinal stenosis [28].

Individuals with dyskinesis are more likely to have signs and symptoms of overuse than patients with spasticity. Nerve compression is a result of the repetitive movements that the individual uses for their daily activities. For example, carpal tunnel and cubital tunnel have been described in patients with CP [6,29].

Fractures

It has been well documented that persons with CP have a higher incidence of fractures throughout their lifespan than their able-bodied counterparts. Most fractures occur in the lower extremities and are nontraumatic. This is due to the combination of contractures, osteoporosis, and long lever arms. Brunner and Doderlein [30] found that the most common site of pathologic fractures was the supracondylar region of the distal femur. Predisposing factors were hip dislocations or contractures of major joints. Postsurgical fractures accounted for 41% of the fractures identified and occurred most frequently during physical therapy sessions, likely as a result of osteoporosis that developed from prolonged immobility. Other fractures were associated with daily care or nursing activities. Ambulatory individuals are at risk for fractures due to falling as well as stress fractures. In this group, adults with dyskinetic CP were more likely to suffer fractures than adults with spastic CP [6]. Brunner and Doderlein [30] described two ambulatory individuals with spastic diplegia who suffered bilateral patellar stress fractures. The overactivation of the quadriceps muscle seen with crouched gait was thought to be the cause.

Individuals with CP are unable to protect their joints and soft tissues during movement because they do not have the normal neurologic control of their uninvolved peers. Daily life affects their musculoskeletal systems in a far harsher manner than it does people without disabilities.

Loss of function

Twenty percent of adults with CP are ambulatory, 40% ambulate with assistance, and 40% are nonambulatory [31]. Functional deterioration has been described in 35% of adults with CP, with a higher percentage among older patients and individuals with decreased independence in activities of daily living (ADLs) [32]. Ando and Ueda [32] studied the relationship between the functional deterioration in adult patients with CP who work at community workshops in Japan and the type of paresis, finding a low incidence in spastic hemiplegics. Through interviews and physical examinations, the study also revealed a higher incidence of functional deterioration in patients with exaggerated involuntary movements of the head and neck, increased neck tone during transfers, and in those who reported an inadequate work environment.

Cathels and Reddihough [25] reported that young adults with CP had ongoing impairment and disability. They suggest that the lack of contact with health services after they left school may be responsible for the decrease in health status. Individuals who receive regular physical training in adulthood have reported increased walking ability [33]. Turk et al [13] found that 80% of participants in their study were active in at least one physical activity (swimming, walking, using exercise equipment, and weightlifting), but improvements in function after these activities were not reported. Further study is necessary to evaluate the effects of physical training on adults with CP.

Fatigue

Fatigue is defined as a decreased ability to sustain force or power output; reduced capacity to perform multiple tasks over time; and the experience of feeling tired, weak, exhausted or lacking energy [34]. Although fatigue is frequently reported as it relates to such other neurologic diseases as poliomyelitis and multiple sclerosis [35], little has been reported on fatigue in adults with CP. Jahnsen et al [36] studied fatigue in 406 individuals with CP in Norway. The results of their questionnaire revealed that adults with CP have significantly more physical—but not more mental—fatigue than the general population. Associations were found with increasing age, low physical function, no physical activity, general health problems, and low life satisfaction. Fatigue in individuals with CP may have a physical etiology. Duffy et al [37] reported that individuals with CP consume three to five times more energy (O_2 rate and O_2 cost) during ambulation than individuals without CP.

Lifetime care issues and the general effects of aging

The life expectancy of the population is constantly improving, with the average adult living to an average of 78 years. Although CP affects primarily the neuromuscular system, other body systems are also involved due to the general effects of aging or due to the disease itself. A small change in the body can cause a large loss in function, particularly in the adult with CP who already has borderline functioning abilities. Conversely, a small change to the body can translate into a large gain in function. Adult health care for individuals with CP deals with the gradual decline in function. Therefore, a review of body systems is particularly important in the evaluation and management of this population, and the caregiver or family member should be available to aid in the history.

Cardiovascular system

It is estimated that 10% of patients with CP have hypertension and coronary artery disease. Increased mortality from ischemic heart disease has been documented in adults with CP [38]. Agitation and poor skin color may be subtle clues for ischemic heart disease and are usually given by caretakers. Lower extremity swelling, discoloration, or temperature change may be noted. Proper skin and toenail care as well as suitable shoes and compression stockings are essential to prevent such problems as mycotic and hypertrophic toenails, pressure ulcerations, cellulitis, and phlebitis.

Pulmonary system

Aspiration is a complication seen in patients with quadriparesis [31] and may be the result of swallowing dysfunction or delayed gastric emptying. Indications of aspiration may include nasal regurgitation, lethargy, fever, and slowly progressive dyspnea. The health care provider should ask about coughing during or immediately after a meal. Swallowing dysfunction can be identified by a speech pathologist with a clinical swallowing evaluation or video fluoroscopic examination. Interventions include proper positioning during and after meals, teaching airway protection techniques, and changing the consistency of the diet to prevent aspiration.

Gastrointestinal system

Vomiting and constipation are the primary gastrointestinal complaints of adults with CP. Vomiting is often the result of delayed gastric emptying, predisposing the patient to esophagitis and gastroesophageal reflux. An association has been found between constipation and abnormal autonomic control of gastrointestinal motility [39], immobilization, inadequate oral intake, and prolonged colonic transit [40]. Because the individual with CP is at risk for all the above, a query into nutrition and bowel habits should be made, with appropriate dietary changes and laxative implementation if necessary.

Musculoskeletal system

Scoliosis has been noted to be common in institutionalized individuals with CP. Uncorrected scoliosis may cause impairment of ambulation and decubiti [24] and should be followed regularly by an orthopedic surgeon.

Abnormalities of the foot, ankle, and hip are also common and should be monitored regularly. Proper footwear and orthotics are essential to allow for maintenance of alignment, to prevent progressive deformity, and to allow for maximal function in transfers and ambulation. Referral to an orthopedist should be made when suitable.

Osteopenia and low bone density have been reported in nonambulatory individuals with CP and can worsen with age. Adults with CP have been noted to have a lower dietary intake of calcium [41]. In addition, decreased exposure to sunlight, immobility, spasticity, and use of anticonvulsant medications may predispose the patient to fractures. Patients who would benefit from an osteoporosis work-up include those with a positive family history, postmenopausal state, and fracture. If osteoporosis is detected, an appropriate exercise regimen should be prescribed, and referral to an endocrinologist should be considered.

Urinary system

Bladder dysfunction can lead to infection and incontinence in adults with CP. Neurogenic bladder can be seen in up to 15% of the population and is more common in those with bilateral involvement. Mainstays of treatment include anticholinergics and intermittent catheterization, and Botox and surgical options are being explored. Brodak et al [42] have reported that structural abnormalities leading to recurrent infection are rare. Rather, poor learning capacity results in an inability to train the bladder and leads to incontinence. In addition, difficulty with toileting accessibility, transfers, and positioning can result in issues with continence because of volitional retention of urine. Dysuria as a sign of infection may be difficult to assess if the patient is cognitively impaired; the caregiver may describe the patient grimacing or in distress upon urination. Another diagnostic sign may be a change in the frequency of urination. If any of these are present, cultures should be taken and the infection treated as appropriate.

Neurologic system

Thirty percent of patients with CP have seizures [43]; patients with diplegia and athetosis least commonly experience them [44]. The type, frequency, and duration of seizures should be noted at each visit. If patients have been seizure-free for 2 or more years, a referral to a neurologist is advisable to determine the necessity of continuing anticonvulsant medications.

Any neurologic change may indicate a progressive condition. Symptoms such as a change in seizure frequency or balance or a change in functional status must be investigated.

Reproductive system

Young adults with CP have been documented to have abnormalities in sexual maturation such as precocious puberty or delayed puberty. Poor nutrition has been cited as a cause for delayed and prolonged puberty [45]. Disabled patients have the same or more diseases as found in the general population but are less likely to get routine care and screening.

For many women with CP, there is a lack of routine gynecologic follow-up. Equipment (eg, mammogram devices and tables) is not accessible for persons with disabilities. Women with CP may need alternative positioning for pelvic examination, and examination under anesthesia may be necessary due to spasticity or behavioral issues. After the initial examination, a pelvic ultrasound may be substituted for the following 2 years before the next pelvic examination provided no pathology is found [46]. Self-breast examination may be difficult or impossible, so the caregiver or spouse should be trained to perform it. Turk et al [13] found that during menstruation, 35% of women with CP reported increased spasticity, and 24% reported increased urinary incontinence.

Men with CP have a higher incidence of cryptorchidism (53%) at the age of 21 years compared with the general population [47]. If the testes are not palpated or visualized when the patient is examined in the standing position, referral to a urologist for further evaluation is necessary.

Dental issues

Many factors contribute to the oral health of persons with CP. It is important to consider the functional abilities of the patient. Many patients lack adequate hand control and attendant care, which can affect the ability of the patient to allow regular dental treatment and to perform regular oral hygiene. Caries and periodontal disease may be caused by the combination of mouth breathing, poor hygiene, and enamel dysplasia. Bruxism, abnormal dental development, and poor control of the oral musculature contribute to problems with overall oral health. Many patients lack routine dental care; possible explanations include difficulty finding dental care due to reimbursement and positioning issues.

The routine use of certain medications can also affect oral health. Turk et al [13] found an association between poor dental hygiene and seizure history. The belief is that the harmful effect of anticonvulsant medications on the teeth and gums (gingival hyperplasia) is responsible. In addition, decreased saliva due to medication side effects can affect oral health.

Nutrition and diet

It has been well documented that many children with CP do not consume enough food to meet their nutritional requirements, with the result being a decrease in fat-free mass. Low caloric intake in adolescents can result in poor growth and decreased muscle mass at maturity [48]. In addition, patients with the athetoid type of CP have higher caloric requirements. The adult with low fat-free mass and malnutrition is additionally compromised by decreased appetite and weight. A sedentary lifestyle and diet low in fruits and vegetables also lead to nutritional problems.

Speech and swallowing problems

Cognitive impairments or oral motor incoordination lead to speech and communication difficulties in many patients. The incoordination is manifested by retraction or thrusting of the tongue, poor lip closure, and decreased tongue movements [2]. The individual will demonstrate difficulty managing oral secretions, dysphagia, and mild to severe dysarthria.

The adult with CP may require more time for feeding than an unaffected individual. If this time is not allowed by the caregiver, the result is poor caloric intake and weight loss.

Hearing and vision

Twenty-five percent to 39% of adults with CP have visual defects [31,49]. Although a review of the literature failed to identify the etiology in adults, it is known that the causes in children include cataracts, retinitis, and optic atrophy [50]. A history of difficulty handling small objects may indicate the need for further evaluation by an ophthalmologist.

Eight percent to 18% of adults with CP have hearing problems [31,49]. The usual hearing loss is a sensorineural impairment caused by congenital nervous system infections [51]. The individual's reaction or response to noise gives a gross idea of auditory function, but formal audiologic evaluation is necessary to diagnose and treat hearing loss.

Exercise

Researchers have observed the benefits of regular exercise in patients with CP. These individuals must maintain higher levels of physical fitness than the general population to counteract declining function from the natural aging process (eg, decreased endurance and strength) and from changes related to their underlying condition (eg, decreased mobility, spasticity, pain, contractures) [52]. Rimmer [53] reported that regular exercise can improve functional status and decrease the level of assistance required by people with disabilities to perform ADLs. Exercise increases muscular endurance and strength, flexibility, balance, and respiratory and cardiovascular efficiency. In addition, exercise can decrease the incidence of secondary conditions in persons with disabilities, thus enhancing or at least maintaining their quality of life [54]. Turk et al [13] found that more than half of the women surveyed in their study reported that they did not engage in stretching or range-of-motion exercises. Unfortunately, fitness centers and fitness equipment are often not accessible to persons with CP, and most exercise instructors have minimal, if any, training in working with people with CP. Rimmer et al [55] found that women with one or more physical disabilities were interested in increasing their activity level, but barriers prevented them from participating in regular exercise activities. The barriers were identified as the cost of the exercise program, transportation, and lack of information regarding exercise facilities. Much remains to be studied regarding the specific effect of regular exercise on individuals with CP. In addition, the various barriers to exercise for individuals with CP must be investigated.

Social issues

Recent studies show that more adults with CP, even those with moderate to severe disability, are attaining independent living and competitive employment (defined as holding a job in an able-bodied market earning wages appropriate for their education and skills). Murphy et al [56] studied 101 adults with CP between the ages of 27 and 74 years living independently in the community. A detailed history and physical examination, functional rating, and questionnaire were performed on all participants. The study found that 67% of adults live independently, and 34% of them with a home attendant. Van der Dussen et al [57] studied the functional levels of 80 young adults in the Netherlands through a structured questionnaire. Almost half of the respondents live in an unadapted house. Ten subjects were married or lived with their partner. Approximately one third of adults with CP live with their parents [31]. Many parents of adults with CP are aging or elderly and are physically unable to care for their children. In these cases, contingency plans for future care should be made.

Fifty-three percent were competitively employed, with the most important factor in achieving this being education beyond high school [56]. Of those, 22% earned an income high enough that an increase would cause termination of disability benefits. The type of CP also seems to be important in achieving employment. Individuals with hemiparesis have been found to have the highest employment rate [58].

Murphy et al [56] found that about one quarter of their subjects had been married at some point in their lives. In most cases the spouses also had CP. Four of the couples produced developmentally normal children.

Adaptive equipment

In addition to the patient's health care needs, the presence and appropriateness of adaptive equipment can have a vital impact on the quality of life. The equipment owned by many adults with CP is often inappropriate, outgrown, or broken [6]. Murphy et al [6] found that few ambulatory adults had appropriate lower extremity orthoses and ambulatory aids. In addition to those who used wheelchairs, only 3 of 67 had solid seats or adaptive postural supports. The rest had sling seats and wheelchairs that were of improper size. Many of these patients complained of back pain that subsided when proper adaptations were made.

For employed individuals, new and different equipment may be necessary to assist them in maintaining current jobs or learning new work skills. Murphy et al [56] found that half of those who were competitively employed worked in jobs that relied almost exclusively on the use of computers. Eighty-six percent of the nonambulatory individuals who were competitively employed used a power wheelchair. Half of them were independent in manual wheelchair propulsion but preferred to use the power wheelchair to save energy for the physical demands of their job.

A common consequence of aging for many individuals with CP is the loss of function, especially mobility. Many individuals require the use of a wheelchair or adaptive equipment to maintain independence in daily care. However, obtaining and maintaining these may be difficult [59]. Unfortunately, private and governmental insurance plans excessively restrict the approval of equipment for adults with developmental disabilities, making it difficult to obtain equipment that is more accessible to children.

Life expectancy

Long-term survival is expected for the majority of individuals with CP, including those who are severely disabled. Those involved in the health care of adults with CP need information about life expectancy to better counsel the caregivers and best treat these patients. However, at this point, little is known about the life expectancy of these adults. Recent studies agree that the most important factors influencing survival are immobility, severe mental retardation, and epilepsy [60–62]. Gender seems to play no role in survival time for persons with CP [62].

CP is most often recorded as the underlying cause of death in afflicted adults. Approximately 60% of individuals died from respiratory problems in a study in Australia [63]. A recent study has documented excess mortality in adults with CP from stroke, cancer, and ischemic heart disease [38]. A possible explanation is the lack of early detection and routine health care.

Areas for future investigation

CP was once considered to be a disease of childhood, but we are becoming aware of the implications for adolescents and adults. Adult health care deals with the gradual decline in function and multisystem organ failure. We are beginning to learn about conditions seen in adults aging with CP, and we know little about the prevention of many of these conditions. Although the amount of attention given to CP in the literature has been increasing, much remains to be investigated. Studies are needed regarding causes of age-related hearing and vision loss in adults with CP. There is limited information regarding the impact of use of anti-spasticity drugs and pregnancy. Only anecdotal evidence exists for causes, effects, and treatments for lower extremity edema. More studies are needed to address the current methods of management of neurogenic bladder in adults with CP. The studies available for review are mostly surveys and consist of small study populations. In general, adults with CP do not receive the physical therapy and adaptive equipment that they need. Perhaps a prospective study comparing individuals who receive proper physical therapy and adaptive equipment with those who do not might be valuable to see if the proper services increase functional independence and quality of life in these individuals.

Summary

Before the mid-twentieth century, few people with CP survived to adulthood. Now, 65% to 90% of children with CP survive. Because of improvements in intensive care techniques leading to the increased survival of very low-birth-weight infants and the increased longevity of the general population, there are a large number of disabled adults requiring medical care.

Adults with CP have medical and social issues that are unique to them. Although there is an increasing awareness of the rights of people with disabilities, there is more work to be done particularly as relates to the cost and availability of adaptive equipment and exercise. In recent years, more attention has been given to studying the needs of this growing part of the population. However, much remains to be investigated to improve the quality of life for these patients.

Resources for clinicians

Table manners: a guide to the pelvic examination for disabled women and health care providers. Planned Parenthood Golden Gate. 815 Eddy St., Suite 300, San Francisco, CA 94109.

United Cerebral Palsy web site (www.ucp.org)

New York State Commission on Quality of Care web site (www.cqc.state.ny.us)

American Association of Mental Retardation web site (www.aamr.org)

The Arc web site (www.thearc.org)

National Institute of Neurological Disorders and Stroke web site (www.ninds.nih.gov)

References

[1] Bax MCO. Terminology and classification of cerebral palsy. Dev Med Child Neurol 1964;11: 295–7.

[2] Molnar GE. Cerebral palsy. In: Molnar GE, editor. Pediatric rehabilitation. 3rd edition. Baltimore: Williams & Wilkins; 1999. p. 193–217.

[3] Blasco PA. Primitive reflexes: their contribution to the early detection of cerebral palsy. Clin Pediatr 1994;33:388–97.

[4] Harris SR. Early neuromotor predictors of cerebral palsy in low birth weight infants. Dev Med Child Neurol 1987;29:508–19.

[5] Carter S, Low NL. Cerebral palsy and mental retardation. In: Merritt's textbook of neurology. 8th edition. Philadelphia: Lea and Febiger; 1989.

[6] Murphy KP, Molnar GE, Lankasky K. Medical and functional status of adults with cerebral palsy. Dev Med Child Neurol 1995;37:1075–84.

[7] United Cerebral Palsy website. Available at: www.ucp.org/ucp_generaldoc.cfm/1/9/37/ 37-37/447. Accessed February 21, 2004.

[8] Evans PM, Evans SJW, Alberman E. Cerebral palsy: why we must plan for survival. Arch Dis Child 1990;65:1325–33.

[9] Crighton J, MacKinney M, Light CP. The life expectancy of persons with cerebral palsy. Dev Med Child Neurol 1995;37:567–76.

[10] Prevalence rate of developmental disabilities among children aged 3–10 years by type of developmental disability. MMWR 1993;45:130–1.

[11] McDonald EP. Medical needs of severely developmentally disabled persons residing in the community. Am J Ment Defic 1985;90:171–6.

[12] Turk MA, Geremski CA, Rosenbaum PF. Secondary conditions of adults with cerebral palsy: final report. Syracuse (NY): State University of New York; 1997.

[13] Turk MA, Geremski CA, Rosenbaum PF, Weber RJ. The health status of women with cerebral palsy. Arch Phys Med Rehabil 1997;78(Suppl 5):S-10–7.

[14] Ortho McNeil. Pain management survey. Available at: www.orthomcneil.com/healthinfo/ painmanagement/related/survey.html. Accessed February 21, 2004.

[15] Hodgkinson I, Jindrich ML, Duhaut P, Vadot JP, Metton G, Berard C. Hip pain in 234 non-ambulatory adolescents and young adults with cerebral palsy: a cross-sectional multicentre study. Dev Med Child Neurol 2001;43:806–8.

[16] Tenuta J, Shelton YA, Miller F. Long-term follow-up of triple arthrodesis in patients with cerebral palsy. J Pediatr Orthop 1993;13:713–6.

[17] Schwartz L, Engel JM, Jensen MP. Pain in persons with cerebral palsy. Arch Phys Med Rehabil 1999;80:1243–6.

[18] Murphy KP. Medical problems in adults with cerebral palsy: case examples. Asst Technol 1999;11:97–104.

[19] Oberlander TF, O'Donnell ME, Montgomery CJ. Pain in children with significant neurological impairment. J Dev Behav Pediatr 1999;20:235–43.

[20] Engel JM, Kartin D, Jensen MP. Pain treatment in persons with cerebral palsy: frequency and helpfulness. Am J Phys Med Rehabil 2002;81:291–6.

[21] Bleck EE. Where have all the CP children gone? The needs of adults. Dev Med Child Neurol 1984;26:674–6.

[22] Buly RL, Huo M, Root L, Binzer T, Wilson PD. Total hip arthroplasty in cerebral palsy: long-term follow-up results. Clin Orth Rel Res 1993;296:148–53.

[23] Villani C, Pappalardo S, Meloni C, Amorese V, Romanini L. Patellofemoral dysplasia in infantile cerebral palsy. Ital J Orthop Traumatol 1988;14:201–10.

[24] Majd ME, Muldowny DS, Holt RT. Natural history of scoliosis in the institutionalized adult cerebral palsy population. Spine 1997;22:1461–6.

[25] Cathels BA, Reddihough DS. The health care of young adults with cerebral palsy. Med J Aust 1993;159:444–6.

[26] Fuji T, Yonenobu K, Fujiwara K, Yamashita K, Ebara S, Ono K, et al. Cervical radiculopathy or myelopathy secondary to athetoid cerebral palsy. J Bone Joint Surg 1987; 69-A:815–21.

[27] Reese M, Msall M, Owen S, Pictor S, Paroske M. Acquired cervical spine impairment in young adults with cerebral palsy. Dev Med Child Neurol 1991;33:153–66.

[28] Harada T, Ebara S, Anwar MM, Okawa A, Kajiura I, Hiroshima K, et al. The cervical spine in athetoid cerebral palsy: a radiological study of 180 patients. J Bone Joint Surg 1996;78-B:613–9.

[29] Alvarez N, Larkin C, Roxborough J. Carpal tunnel syndrome in athetoid-dystonic cerebral palsy. Arch Neurol 1982;39:311–2.

[30] Brunner R, Doderlein L. Pathological fractures in patients with cerebral palsy. J Pediatr Orthop 1996;5:232–8.

[31] Brown MC, Bontempo A, Turk MA. Secondary consequences of cerebral palsy: adults with cerebral palsy in New York State. Albany (NY): Developmental Disabilities Planning Council; 1992.

[32] Ando N, Ueda S. Functional deterioration in adults with cerebral palsy. Clin Rehabil 2000; 14:300–6.

[33] Andersson C, Mattsson E. Adults with cerebral palsy: a survey describing problems, needs, and resources, with special emphasis on locomotion. Dev Med Child Neurol 2001;43:76–82.

[34] Kaasa S, Loge JH, Knobel H, Jordhay MS, Brenne E. Fatigue: measures and relation to pain. Acta Anesthesiol Scand 1999;43:939–47.

[35] Packer TL, Sauriol A, Brouwer B. Fatigue secondary to chronic illness: post-polio syndrome, chronic fatigue syndrome and multiple sclerosis. Arch Phys Med Rehabil 1994; 75:1122–6.

[36] Jahnsen R, Villien L, Stanghelle JK, Holm I. Fatigue in adults with cerebral palsy in Norway compared with the general population. Dev Med Child Neurol 2003;45:296–303.

[37] Duffy CM, Hill AE, Cosgrove AP, Corry IS, Graham HK. Energy consumption in children with spina bifida and cerebral palsy: a comparative study. Dev Med Child Neurol 1996;38: 238–43.

[38] Strauss D, Cable W, Shavelle R. Causes of excess mortality in cerebral palsy. Dev Med Child Neurol 1999;41:580–5.

[39] Goyal R, Hirano I. The enteric nervous system. N Engl J Med 1996;334:1106–15.

[40] Giudice ED. Cerebral palsy and gut functions. J Pediatr Gastroenterol Nutr 1997;24:522–3.

[41] Ferring TM, Johnson RK, Ferarra MS. Dietary and anthropometric assessment of adults with cerebral palsy. J Am Diet Assoc 1992;92:1083–6.

[42] Brodak PP, Scherz HC, Packer MG, Kaplan GW. Is urinary tract screening necessary for patients with cerebral palsy? J Urol 1994;152:1586–7.

[43] Alesu F. Nature and prognosis of seizures in patients with cerebral palsy. Dev Med Child Neurol 1990;32:661–8.

[44] Krageloh-Mann I, Hagberg G, Meisner C, Schelp B, Haas G, Eeg-Olofsson KE, et al. Bilateral spastic cerebral palsy: a comparative study between south-west Germany and western Sweden. I: Clinical patterns and disabilities. Dev Med Child Neurol 1993;35: 1037–47.

[45] Daniels SM, Cornelius D, Makes E. Sexuality and disability: the need for services. Annu Rev Rehabil 1981;2:83–112.

[46] Bradshaw KD, Elkins TE, Quint EH. The gynecologic exam in the patient with mental retardation: a continuing education monograph. Dallas: University of Texas Medical Center at Dallas; 1996.

[47] Smith JA, Hutson JM, Beasley SW, Reddihough DS. The relationship between cerebral palsy and cryptorchidism. J Pediatr Surg 1989;24:1303–5.

[48] Bandini LG, Schoeller DA, Fukagawa NK, Wykes LJ, Dietz WH. Body composition and energy expenditure in adolescents with cerebral palsy or myelodysplasia. Pediatr Res 1991; 29:70–7.

[49] Granet KM, Balaghi M, Jaeger J. Adults with cerebral palsy. N J Med 1997;94:51–4.

[50] Ingram TS. Pediatric aspects of cerebral palsy. Edinburgh: E & S Livingstone Ltd; 1964.

[51] Robinson RO. The frequency of other handicaps in children with cerebral palsy. Dev Med Child Neurol 1973;15:305–12.

[52] Leibold S. Achieving and maintaining body systems integrity and function: personal care skills. In: Lollar DJ, editor. Preventing secondary conditions associated with spina bifida and cerebral palsy. Washington, DC: Spina Bifida Association of America; 1994.

[53] Rimmer JH. Health promotion for people with disabilities: the emerging paradigm shift from disability prevention to prevention of secondary conditions. Phys Ther 1999;79: 495–502.

[54] Noreau L, Shephard RJ. Spinal cord injury, exercise and quality of life. Sports Med 1995;20: 226–50.

[55] Rimmer JH, Rubin SS, Braddock D. Barriers to exercise in African-American women with physical disabilities. Arch Phys Med Rehabil 2000;81:182–8.

[56] Murphy KP, Molnar GE, Lankasky K. Employment and social issues in adults with cerebral palsy. Arch Phys Med Rehabil 2000;81:807–11.

[57] van der Dussen L, Nieuwstraten W, Roebroeck M, Stam HJ. Functional level of young adults with cerebral palsy. Clin Rehabil 2001;15:84–91.

[58] Nielsen HH. A follow-up of young cerebral palsied patients: some psychological, educational and vocational aspects. Scand J Psychol 1975;16:217–24.

[59] Stevenson CJ, Pharoah PO, Stevenson R. Cerebral palsy: the transition from youth to adulthood. Dev Med Child Neurol 1997;39:336–42.

[60] Evans PM, Evans SJ, Alberman E. Cerebral palsy: why we must plan for survival. Arch Dis Child 1990;65:1329–33.

[61] Maudsley G, Hutton JL, Pharoah PO. Cause of death in cerebral palsy: a descriptive study. Arch Dis Child 1999;81:390–4.

[62] Crichton JU, Mackinnon M, White CP. The life-expectancy of persons with cerebral palsy. Dev Med Child Neurol 1995;37:567–76.

[63] Blair E, Watson L, Badawi N, Stanley FJ. Life expectancy among people with cerebral palsy in Western Australia. Dev Med Child Neurol 2001;43:508–15.

ELSEVIER
SAUNDERS

Phys Med Rehabil Clin N Am
16 (2005) 251–265

PHYSICAL MEDICINE
AND REHABILITATION
CLINICS OF
NORTH AMERICA

Aging with cardiopulmonary disease: the rehab perspective

Isaac J. Kreizman, MD[a,b,*], Douglas Allen, DO[c]

[a]*Department of Rehabilitation Medicine, SUNY-Health Science Center of Brooklyn, 450 Clarkson Avenue, Brooklyn, NY 11220, USA*
[b]*Department of Pain and Rehabilitation Services, 5223 9th Avenue, Brooklyn, NY 11220, USA*
[c]*St. Vincent's Hospital, 350 Park Avenue South, New York, NY 10010, USA*

It is expected that the number of individuals 65 years or older will more than double in the next 50 years. Older patients with coronary artery disease (CAD) have high rates of disability, mobility limitations, and recurrent coronary events. The increased incidence of coronary heart disease (CHD) with advancing age is clear. Disability rates are particularly high in women, persons older than 75 years of age, and patients with angina pectoris or chronic heart failure [1,2]. Cardiopulmonary rehabilitation has been shown to reduce mortality by 20% to 25% [3]. Although older patients after coronary events are substantially less fit than younger patients, they obtain a similar relative improvement with aerobic conditioning programs in corroboration with other aspects of secondary prevention, including resistance training [4–6]. The benefits of cardiopulmonary rehabilitation in the elderly population has been extensively reviewed, but physicians fail to treat this group aggressively. This article emphasizes the pathophysiology of CAD in the elderly population, risk factor assessment and stratification, exercise prescription for specific cardiac patients, geriatric cardiopulmonary rehabilitation program, future trends, and recommendations to improve participation in cardiac rehabilitation programs in the geriatric population.

Pathophysiology

The mechanism of physiologic adaptations to aerobic exercise conditioning in older patients with CAD is different from younger populations [7].

---

* Corresponding author. Department of Rehabilitation Medicine, Maimonides Medical Center, 5223 9th Avenue, Brooklyn, NY 11220.

E-mail address: docijk@aol.com (I.J. Kreizman).

1047-9651/05/$ - see front matter © 2004 Elsevier Inc. All rights reserved.
doi:10.1016/j.pmr.2004.08.001
pmr.theclinics.com

Vascular disease of the myocardium and peripheral vasculature is superimposed by age-related factors, including ventricular and arterial wall thickness and stiffness [8,9]. It is estimated that atherosclerosis progresses at a rate of 1.5% occlusion in arterial diameter per year [10]. Recent arteriographic secondary prevention trials showed that aggressive modification of risk factors may slow the rate of atherosclerosis progression, stabilize vulnerable plaques, and induce partial regression [10]. The Poiseuille equation states that resistance to flow is inversely proportional to the radius raised to the fourth power. Therefore, a minor reduction in stenosis yields dramatic improvement in myocardial perfusion. Improvements in myocardial perfusion with aggressive modification are thought to be related to improved endothelial-mediated coronary artery and arteriolar vasomotor function [11–13]. Recent studies have shown improved endothelial function after exercise training in elderly healthy persons, patients with congestive heart failure, and patients with CAD [14–17].

The aging process affects the oxygen transport system dramatically (Table 1). Physical performance and Vo_{2max} decline with age. This largely is secondary to a decrease in cardiac output [18]. Cardiac output is a product of heart rate and stroke volume. With increasing age, a reduction of sympathetic activity and decreasing viscoelasticity slows heart rate. This results in myocardium wall stiffness. Factors affecting stroke volume include reduction in venous return with subsequent reduction of pre-ejection filling, myocardial wall stiffness, increased arterial pressure, reduction of mitochondrial enzyme activity, infiltration of muscle by collagen fibers, and loss of coordinated contraction. The Vo_{2max} declines approximately 9% per decade. A 50% reduction of this decline can be achieved with regular aerobic exercise [19].

Table 1
Changes in biologic functions in response to aging, inactivity, weightlessness, and exercise

Function	Aging	Inactivity	Weightlessness	Exercise
Vo_{2max}	Decreased	Decreased		Increased
Cardiac output	Decreased	Decreased		Increased (not for older)
Systolic BP	Increased		Increased	Decreased
Orthostatic tolerance	Decreased	Decreased	Decreased	Increased
Body water	Decreased	Decreased	Decreased	
RBC mass	Decreased	Decreased	Decreased	
Thrombosis	Increased	Increased		Decreased
Serum lipids	Increased	Increased		Decreased
HD lipoprotein (>80 yr old)	Increased			Increased
Lean body mass	Decreased	Decreased	Decreased	
Muscle strength	Decreased	Decreased	Decreased	Increased
Calcium	Decreased	Decreased	Decreased	
Glucose tolerance	Decreased	Decreased		Increased
EEG dominant frequency	Decreased	Decreased		Increased

Epidemiology

The Framingham study 30-year follow-up shows an age-related rise in the incidence of nearly all manifestations of heart disease and circulatory disease. It is considered the most significant longitudinal study in cardiovascular research. In men, CHD increases linearly with age. In women, rates increase more steeply at advanced age, approximating an exponential function. Myocardial infarction (MI) is the most common initial manifestation for CHD in older men, whereas angina pectoris is the most common initial complaint in women. The Framingham study outlines the proportion of MI events that go "unrecognized." The infarctions were noted by unequivocal electrocardiographic changes consistent with infarction during routine examination with the examiner and patient unexpecting. Half of all cases were associated with symptoms including, but not limited to, musculoskeletal chest discomfort, upper gastrointestinal upset, or gall bladder disease. The other half was reported as completely "silent" [20].

Risk factors for CAD are listed in Box 1. Table 2 outlines the impact of specific risk factors on CHD in the Framingham Study, 30-year follow-up.

Box 1. Risk factors of coronary artery disease

Irreversible risks
- Male gender
- Family history of premature CAD ≤55 years of age in a parent or sibling
- Past history of CAD
- Past history of occlusive peripheral vascular disease
- Past history of cerebrovascular disease
- Ethnic characteristics

Reversible risks
- Cigarette smoking
- Hypertension
- Low HDL cholesterol (<35 mg/dL)
- Hypercholesterolemia >200 mg/dL
- High lipoprotein A
- Abdominal obesity
- Hypertriglyceridemia >250 mg/dL
- Hyperinsulinemia
- Diabetes mellitus
- Sedentary lifestyle
- Psychosocial factors

Table 2
Impact of risk factors on incidence of coronary heart disease

| | Bivariate standardized regression coefficients (age adjusted) | | | |
| | Ages 35–64 | | Ages 65–94 | |
Risk factors	Men	Women	Men	Women
Systolic pressure	0.338***	0.418***	0.401***	0.285***
Diastolic pressure	0.321***	0.363***	0.296***	0.082
Serum cholesterol	0.322***	0.307***	0.121	0.213***
Cigarettes	0.259***	0.095	−0.017	−0.034
Blood glucose	0.043	0.206***	0.166***	0.209***
Vital capacity	−0.112*	−0.331***	−0.127	0.253***
Relative weight	0.190***	0.254***	0.177**	0.124*

* $P < 0.05$; ** $P < 0.01$; *** $P < 0.001$.

Hypertension

The seventh report of the joint national committee on prevention, detection, evaluation, and treatment of high blood pressure provides a new guideline for hypertension prevention and management. Individuals who are not hypertensive at 55 years of age have a 90% lifetime risk for developing hypertension. The risk of cardiovascular disease, beginning at 115/75 mm Hg, doubles with each increment of 20/10 mm Hg. In elderly persons, systolic blood pressure above 140 mm Hg is a much more important cardiovascular disease risk factor than diastolic BP. Individuals with borderline hypertension (systolic 120–139 mm Hg or diastolic 80–89 mm Hg) should be considered as "prehypertensive" and require health-promoting lifestyle modifications. Thiazide-type diuretics should be used as first-line treatment for most patients with uncomplicated hypertension alone or in combination with drugs from other classes, especially if pressures are more than 20/10 mm Hg above goal. Most patients require more than one class of agent for adequate blood pressure control. Patient compliance with medication and lifestyle modification is required for long-term blood pressure control [22].

Five randomized trials conducted in patients over 60 years of age show the direct effects of antihypertensive treatment on vascular disease in older patients [21]. A 15/6 mm Hg difference in blood pressure between study and control groups was achieved over an average follow-up period of 4.7 years. Stroke incidence was reduced by 34%, and CHD incidence was reduced by 19% among the treated groups. The absolute benefits observed in older patients were more than twice those observed in younger patients. The results suggest that over a 10-year period, treatment would prevent at least one major vascular event among every 10 elderly patients at similar risk to those enrolled in the trials [21].

Lipids

There is solid evidence validating total serum cholesterol being a predictor of CHD events in older men and women [23–26]. According to the Framingham study, the relationship of cholesterol in CHD decreases with age (see Table 1). Women have an overall lower incidence of CHD at corresponding levels of cholesterol in comparison to men.

Aggressive medical treatment for reducing the incidence of recurrent cardiovascular events has been studied [25,26]. Major coronary events after 5 years were reduced 8.4% with administration of pravastatin versus placebo for patients who had MI between 65 and 75 years of age [27]. Pravastatin lowers serum levels of total cholesterol and LDL and, according to outcome trials, reduces coronary events in elderly patients with hypercholesterolemia or normal cholesterol levels [28]. In the Scandinavian Simvastatin Survival Study, a small cohort of patients older than 65 years of age were compared with a younger patient population. The study concluded that simvastatin produced similar reductions in relative risk for major coronary events in women compared with men and in elderly compared with younger patients. The absolute risk reduction in mortality of simvastatin treated subjects was approximately twice as great in the elderly patients [29].

Lipoprotein subfractions, including serum triglyceride levels, are routine laboratory measurements and should be used to assess risk. The Framingham study emphasizes total serum cholesterol/HDL ratio to provide an accurate risk assessment for CHD. The dynamic equilibrium of the lipid transport system is better understood using this ratio. Triglyceride level as an independent predictor remains controversial in both sexes. However, elevated serum triglycerides represent a risk marker for obesity, glucose intolerance, and low HDL levels, which confer risk for CHD [30,31].

Diabetes

CHD is the most common manifestation of atherosclerosis related to diabetes, and the majority of deaths in diabetic patients are attributable to CHD. Glucose intolerance is observed in 30% to 40% of patients over 65 years of age [31]. Insulin resistance is a significant risk factor for CHD but has not proven to be a causal risk factor [32]. Aging is frequently associated with the development of peripheral insulin resistance and deterioration of glucose tolerance [33]. Loss of glycemic control may result in dramatic elevations of triglycerides and low levels of high-density lipoproteins [31]. The structure, composition, and function of lipids and lipoproteins are often altered, accelerating atherosclerotic formation in the diabetic patient. This phenomenon may occur without elevation of lipid and lipoprotein levels. Triglyceride enrichment or glycosylation of lipoproteins may contribute to foam cell formation and stimulate platelet aggregation [34]. Independent of mechanism, diabetics have higher rates of CHD and subsequent complications including atypical presentation of cardiac events [31,32]. This warrants a greater responsibility of the practitioner to monitor these patients during a cardiac rehabilitation exercise regimen.

Regular exercise alone is effective in reducing hyperinsulinemia and improving insulin action in patients 65 years of age or older to levels typical of young people [35]. Results of cardiac rehabilitation in patients with diabetes mellitus have emphasized the importance of comprehensive care during a cardiac rehabilitation program [37]. Diabetics have a greater risk profile, including body mass index, waist circumference, hypertension, triglycerides, peripheral vascular disease, lower fitness levels, and an overall lower program adherence rate [37]. Therefore, weight management, lipid lowering, and glycemic control are needed in combination with the rehabilitation protocol. Identification of the diabetic patient in the rehabilitation setting, in coordination with aggressive risk factor management, optimizes medical benefit [36].

Smoking

In men and women ≥65 years of age, cigarette smoking fails to show strong risk associations for total CHD events in the Framingham study; however, risk associations are discerned between cigarette smoking and death due to CHD [20]. Explanations for this phenomenon may be more closely related to lethal events alone than to outcomes comprised of morbidity and lethal events. Another explanation is that the cross-sectional pooling used in the Framingham study may have classified nonsmokers as those who were long-term smokers and discontinued smoking. This would dilute the strength of the analysis. The most reliable approach for assessing smoking risk is documenting a current smoker, former smoker, and never smoker along with time intervals. This approach yields strong risk association with CHD, stroke, and peripheral arterial disease [30]. In a study looking at risk factors for 5-year mortality in older adults, a >50 pack-year smoker was a strong independent cardiovascular disease risk factor. Smoking cessation should be a priority in a comprehensive cardiac rehabilitation program [36]. The literature shows that patient-specific, tailored interventions during routine medical care can be effective in smoking cessation in midlife and older smokers [35]. Smoking cessation at any age prevents and reduces the impact of acute and chronic illnesses that limit independence [36].

Psychologic factors

Studies have proven that psychosocial factors directly contribute to the pathogenesis of CHD. These factors relate cardiovascular disease with five specific psychosocial domains: depression, anxiety, personality and character traits, social isolation, and chronic life stress [38]. The prevalence of these factors increases with age [38]. There is increasing evidence that mental stress plays a role in endothelial dysfunction and progression of atherogenesis. In a study with healthy subjects, brief episodes of mental stress may cause transient (up to 4 hours) endothelial dysfunction [39]. Depression is a significant predictor of overall cardiac rehabilitation participation, and its prevalence increases with age. The importance of depression alone in older cardiac patients demonstrates that these patients are less likely to follow behavior and lifestyle recommendations after MI [40]. In the year after a hospital admission for heart failure, emotional support is a strong independent predictor of the occurrence of fatal and nonfatal cardiovascular events [41]. Therefore, clinician's assessment and intervention of a patient's psychosocial function is an important aspect of a comprehensive cardiac rehabilitation program.

Metabolic X syndrome

The National Cholesterol Education Program-Adult Treatment Panel (ATP III) has defined metabolic syndrome as consisting of three or more characteristics, as listed in Table 3. The metabolic syndrome is a culmination of risk factors that should be targeted in addition to cholesterol-lowering therapy to reduce the incidence of CHD [42]. The criteria listed are the usual consequences seen with increasing insulin resistance. The management has a twofold objective: (1) to reduce underlying causes and (2) to treat associated nonlipid and lipid risk factors [42]. First-line treatments are weight reduction and increased physical activity. The incorporation of a cardiac rehabilitation program directly addresses the ATP III's recommendation for management of metabolic X syndrome.

Exercise screening and training

A practitioner implementing a cardiac rehabilitation program needs to pay particular attention to patient-specific modification of an exercise protocol.

Table 3
Characteristics used to define metabolic syndrome

Risk factor	Defining level
Abdominal obesity	
Men	Waist circumference >105 cm (40 in)
Women	Waist circumference >88 cm (35 in)
Triglycerides	>150 mg/dL
HDL cholesterol	
Men	<40 mg/dL
Women	<80 mg/dL
Blood pressure	≥130/85 mm Hg
Fasting serum glucose	≥110 mg/dL

Patients at high risk require careful ECG monitoring for early ischemic changes (eg, ST-segment depression, patient complaint of angina symptoms, decrease in oxygen saturation with blood pressure) and heart rate monitoring (Box 2). In many cardiac rehabilitation programs, the initial evaluation involves an exercise stress test. After this test, the Karvonen formula is used to set the appropriate target heart rate based on cardiac risk stratification.

During the initial evaluation, the practitioner can assess limitation parameters and customize an exercise protocol that maximizes workload. Normally, the initial training program is used to determine a target heart rate for exercise training. If the maximum heart rate achieved is limited by a benign endpoint such as fatigue, musculoskeletal pain, or angina preceding ECG changes, a target heart rate as high as 85% of the actual maximum heart rate tested can be used. Heart rate as low as 60% of maximum can result in effective training [43]. Adjustments made with exercise prescription to maintain at least 60% heart rate may include limiting total exercise time, increasing workout frequency to meet exercise time requirements, oxygen supplementation, or limiting resistance training. Aerobic choices include treadmills, a walking course, cycles, air-dynes, and rowers; each is capable of providing a desired work load catering to the individual's limitations. Special consideration in elderly patients includes training regimens adjustment to accommodate comorbidities.

An exercise heart rate range or scales of perceived exertion such as the Borg scale often guide aerobic exercise. The Borg scale is a perceived level of exertion by the participant on a numeric scale 6 to 20, with 6 being very, very light activity and 18 rated as very, very hard. Older coronary patients are less likely to exercise to a physiologic maximum at their baseline as compared with younger patients; therefore, a strict adherence to an exercise heart rate range is often not appropriate [44]. A perceived exertion scale is often a useful guide to exercise intensity in older patients. Duration of the exercise stimulus can begin with brief, intermittent bouts of exercise, gradually increasing to 20 to 25 minutes or longer. Resistance training often begins with the use of elastic tubing and stretching and progresses to include dumbbells and stationary weights. Resistance training protocols are often quantified by the measurement of single-repetition maximal (1-RM) lift for a given exercise, with subjects performing eight repetitions [43]. The presence of osteoarthritis does not contraindicate resistance exercise unless a specific motion is limited by pain. Upper body resistance exercise is often delayed for at least 3 months after coronary artery bypass surgery to allow for sternal healing.

Exercise training studies

In the absence of CHD, physical fitness decreases by approximately 10% per decade after the age of 25 years. With chronic heart disease and other comorbidities, older coronary patients present with extremely low fitness

Box 2. Cardiac rehabilitation participation risk stratification

Characteristics of patients at lowest risk for exercise participation
- Absence of complex ventricular arrhythmias during exercise testing and recovery
- Absence of angina or other significant symptoms
- Presence of normal hemodynamics during exercise testing and recovery
- Functional capacity $\geq$7 METs

Nonexercise testing findings:
- Rest ejection fraction $\geq$50%
- Uncomplicated MI or revascularization procedure
- Absence of complicated ventricular arrhythmias at rest
- Absence of CHF
- Absence of signs or symptoms of post-event or post-procedure ischemia
- Absence of clinical depression

Characteristics of patients at moderate risk for exercise participation
- Presence of angina or other significant symptoms
- Mild to moderate level of silent ischemia
- during exercise testing or recovery
- Functional capacity <5 METs

Nonexercise testing findings:
- Rest ejection fraction 40% to 49%

Characteristics of patients at high risk for exercise participation
- Presence of complex ventricular arrhythmia during exercise testing and recovery
- Presence of angina or other significant symptoms
- High level of silent ischemia during exercise testing or recovery
- Presence of abnormal hemodynamics during exercise testing and recovery

Nonexercise testing findings:
- Rest ejection fraction <40%
- History of cardiac arrest or sudden death
- Complex dysrhythmias at rest
- Complicated MI or revascularization procedure
- Presence of CHF
- Presence of signs or symptoms of post-event or post-procedure ischemia
- Presence of clinical depression

From Williams MA. Exercise testing in cardiac rehabilitation: exercise prescription and beyond. Cardiol Clin 2001;19:415–31; with permission.

levels. This is often compounded by a fear of exercise and physical activity often derived from inappropriate advice of family and physician [45].

The cardiac rehabilitation literature supports the safety and efficacy of exercise-training regimens in older patients, with relative training benefits documented to be similar to younger patients. In the studies of Williams, Ades, and Lavie, increases in peak exercise intensity of 34% to 53% were demonstrated over a 3-month training period in response to an aerobic conditioning protocol with no apparent increase in exercise-related morbidity [44]. Some researchers recommend longer training regimens in elderly patients due to lower absolute training intensities and to the briefer training sessions often performed early in the training program [44].

Resistance training regimens have been less well studied in elderly coronary populations despite the attraction of a training modality that can increase strength and endurance in this population. In a recently published study, older coronary patients (68 ± 3 years of age) improved their strength to a similar degree as did younger coronary patients (48 ± 7 years of age) after 11 weeks of resistance training. The training protocol involved one set of 8 to 10 repetitions of seven separate exercises at an intensity of 50% of 1-RM, with 1-RMs updated monthly [44]. In a study of healthy deconditioned elderly subjects (mean age 70 ± 4 years), resistance training resulted in an increase in strength and muscle mass of the trained limb and in improved walking endurance [44]. This makes a compelling case to incorporate resistance training to treat or prevent disability in older patients with CHD.

Cardiac rehabilitation participation

Older patients are less likely to participate in cardiac rehabilitation programs [45]. Physician's recommendation for participation is the most powerful predictor of cardiac rehabilitation participation [45,46].

In a systematic review of the literature, predictor variables were identified and categorized as socio-demographic, medical, and psychologic [47]. Non-attenders were more likely to be older, to have lower income/greater deprivation, and to deny the severity of their illness. Job status, gender, and health concerns play an indirect role in attendance behavior [47]. For cardiac rehabilitation programs to attract a greater percentage of older patients for participation, programs have to become more attractive and accessible to individuals in this age group. Seemingly minor issues, such as transportation, parking, and ease of access, are frequently cited as major barriers to participation for elderly persons. The needs of older female coronary patients should be particularly emphasized. They are the most disabled, the most deconditioned, and have the greatest need for exercise rehabilitation, yet they are the least likely of all demographic and gender groups to be referred for exercise rehabilitation [47].

The expansion of programs to include home- or community-based regimes will increase patient participation. In many cases, an intermittent visit to the rehabilitation program can be combined with a home-based or "aging center." Results of studies identifying variables responsible for patient participation in cardiac rehabilitation programs emphasize the importance of physician's strength of recommendation and addressing the demographic, medical, and psychosocial issues involved in patient participation [45–47].

Pulmonary rehabilitation

It is important to discuss the role of pulmonary rehabilitation in the elderly population because chronic obstructive pulmonary disease (COPD) is the fifth leading cause of death in North America and is the only leading cause of death increasing in prevalence [43]. Therefore, it is important to outline its principles and make the practitioner aware of its benefit in conjunction with a cardiac exercise protocol.

Pulmonary rehabilitation teaches a patient how best to manage their chronic disease. In the presence of advanced COPD, particularly for debilitated patients, pulmonary rehabilitation has been proven to be useful in maintaining and in some cases improving health status [48]. A California-based study collected data from 10 established pulmonary rehabilitation programs over 2 years. The mean age of participants was 68 years, and 415 patients completed at least two of four follow-up assessments. The authors concluded that pulmonary rehabilitation was effective in improving symptoms and quality of life and reducing the use of health care resources over 18 months [49]. Most pulmonary rehabilitation programs are inpatient or short-term outpatient programs [43]. Studies shows improvement in quality of life with reduced hospitalization costs over a relatively long treatment period.

Pulmonary function is linked directly to patient's functional capacity [50]. In a cross-sectional study of adult participants in phase 2 of the Third National Health and Nutrition Examination Survey, subjects were classified using spirometric criteria based on the ratio between forced expiratory volumes in one second and forced vital capacity. Subjects were classified as mild, moderate, or severe obstructive, restrictive, or respiratory symptoms alone without evidence of chronic disease. The presence of obstructive or restrictive lung disease or respiratory symptoms in the absence of lung function impairment is associated with increased functional impairment. Functional status, quality of life, distance ambulated, and spirometric measures have been found to improve with a structured pulmonary rehabilitation program [50]. Therefore, it is important for the practitioner to evaluate and treat respiratory symptoms with or without evidence of chronic lung disease. The program should include aerobic training, respiratory muscle strengthening, and breathing exercises and should be prescribed based on the maximal MET level the pulmonary patient is able to perform as noted on initial pulmonary stress testing.

Future trends and research

Future trends and research in cardiopulmonary rehabilitation have emphasized primary prevention. The discussion and data presented in this article emphasize early intervention with the practice of preventative medicine to delay the onset of chronic cardiac and pulmonary disease. The natural physiologic changes that occur with aging can be substantially reduced through early intervention.

Research is continuing to focus on limiting factors for cardiopulmonary rehabilitation participation. Ironically, physician recommendation continues to play a large role. Despite the limitations cited for participation, the potential health benefit with patient adherence to a multidisciplinary program is substantial.

Pharmacologic disease-modifying agents continue to play a large role in treatment. Further research needs to elucidate the benefits of exercise as an exclusive factor in disease modification for all patient groups. Societal dependence on pharmacologic treatment can be reduced substantially with early incorporation of physical activity. Physician recommendation to outpatient cardiac rehabilitation as a preventative treatment to delay the onset of chronic disease may prove to be more cost effective for the long term.

As technology in the field of cardiology continues to advance, it is our duty in rehabilitation medicine to progress accordingly. Recent advances in minimally invasive surgery, left ventricular assistive devices, biologically and chemically treated stents, and robotic cardiac surgeries require the Physiatrist treating these patients to be aware of these technologies. It is important for the physiatrist to create an exercise prescription, set target heart rates, and understand exercise precautions and vital signs limits (min and max) for these patients. Research needs to focus on the creation of a set protocols for patients using these devices and on the efficacy of rehabilitation programs on the function, physiology, and quality of life of these patients.

Medicare reimbursement for long-term outpatient rehabilitation should include a broader range of cardiac and pulmonary patients, including early preventative treatment. Further research focusing on cardiac and pulmonary disease not covered under Medicare guidelines will give a large population access to the health benefits of cardiopulmonary rehabilitation.

References

[1] Ades PA, Savage PD, Tischler MD, Poehlman ET, Dee J, Niggel J. Determinants of disability in older coronary patients. Am Heart J 2002;143(1):151–6.
[2] Pinsky JL, Jette AM, Branch LG, et al. The Framingham Disability Study: relationship of various coronary heart disease manifestations to disability in older patients living in the community. J Public Health 1990;80:1363–8.
[3] O'Connor GT, Buring JE, Yusuf S, Goldhaber SZ, Olmstead EM, Paffenbarger RS Jr, et al. An overview of randomized trials of rehabilitation with exercise after myocardial infarction. Circulation 1989;80:234–44.

[4] Ades PA, Grunvald MH. Cardiopulmonary exercise testing before and after conditioning in older coronary patients. Am Heart J 1990;120:585–9.

[5] Pollock ML, Franklin BA, Balady GJ, Chaitman BL, Fleg JL, Fletcher B, et al. Resistance exerice in individuals with and without cardiovascular disease. Circulation 2000;101:828–33.

[6] Fragnoli-Munn K, Savage P, Ades PA. Combined resistance-aerobic training in older patients with coronary artery disease early after myocardial infarction. J Cardiopulm Rehab 1998;18:416–20.

[7] Aggarwal A, Ades PA. Exercise rehabilitation of older patients with cardiovascular disease. Cardiol Clin 2001;19:525–36.

[8] Lakatta EG. Cardiovascular regulatory mechanisms in advanced age. Physiol Rev 1993;73:413–67.

[9] Vaitkevicius P, Fleg J, Engel J, O'Connor FC, Wright JG, Lakatta LE, et al. Effects of age and aerobic capacity on arterial stiffness in healthy adults. Circulation 1993;88:1456–62.

[10] Superko H, Krauss RM. Coronary artery disease regression: convincing evidence for the benefit of aggressive lipoprotein management. Circulation 1994;90:1056–69.

[11] Celermajer DS, Sornsen KE, Bull C, Robinson J, Deanfield JE. Endothelium-dependent dilation in the systemic arteries of asymptomatic subjects relates to coronary risk factors and their interaction. J Am Coll Cardiol 1994;24:1468–74.

[12] Treasure CB, Klein JL, Weintraub WS, Talley JD, Stillabower ME, Kosinski AS, et al. Beneficial effects of cholesterol-lowering therapy on the coronary endothelium in patients with coronary artery disease. N Engl J Med 1995;332:481–7.

[13] Anderson TJ, Meredith IT, Yeung AC, Frei B, Selwyn AP, Ganz P. The effect of cholesterol-lowering and antioxidant therapy on endothelium dependent coronary vasomotion. N Engl J Med 1995;332:488–93.

[14] Hornig B, Maier V, Drexter H. Physical training improves endothelial function in patients with chronic heart failure. Circulation 1996;93:210–4.

[15] Taddei S, Galetta F, Virdis A, Ghiadoni L, Salvetti G, Franzoni F, et al. Physical activity prevents age related impairment of nitric oxide availability in elderly athletes. Circulation 2000;101:2896–901.

[16] Hambrecht R, Wolf A, Gielen S, Linke A, Hofer J, Erbs S, et al. Effect of exercise on coronary endothelial function in patients with coronary artery disease. N Engl J Med 2000;342:454–60.

[17] Haskell WL, Alderman EL, Fair JM, Maron DJ, Mackey SF, Superko HR, et al. Effects of intensive multiple risk factor reduction on coronary atherosclerosis and clinical cardiac events in men and women with coronary artery disease. The Stanford Coronary Risk Intervention Project (SCRIP). Circulation 1994;89:975–90.

[18] Mount J. Designing exercise programs for the elderly: prevention practice. Strategies for physical therapy and occupational therapy. Philadelphia: WB Saunders; 1992.

[19] Hagberg JM. Effects of raining on the decline of VO2max with aging. Fed Proc 1987;46:1830–3.

[20] Cupples LA, D'Agostino RB. Some risk factors related to the annual incidence of cardiovascular disease and death using pooled repeated biennial measurements: Framingham Heart Study, 30-year follow-up. In: Kannel WB, Wolf PA, Garrison RJ, editors. The Framingham Study: an epidemiological investigation of cardiovascular disease. Bethesda (MD): National Heart, Lung, and Blood Institute; 1987.

[21] MacMahon S, Rodgers A. The effects of blood pressure reduction in older patients: an overview of five randomized controlled trials in elderly hypertensives. Clin Exp Hypertens 1993;15:967–78.

[22] Chobanian AV, Bakris GL, Black HR, Cushman WC, Green LA, Izzo JL Jr, et al. The seventh report of the Joint National Committee on Prevention, Detection, Evaluation, and Treatment of High Blood Pressure: the JNC 7 report. JAMA 2003;289:2560–72.

[23] Aronov WS, Starling L, Etienne F, D'Alba P, et al. Risk factors for coronary artery disease in persons older than 62 years in a long-term health care facility. Am J Cardiol 1986;57: 518–20.

[24] Aronov WS, Herzig AH, Etienne F, D'Alba P, Ronquillo J. 41 month follow-up of risk factors correlated with new coronary events in 708 elderly patients. J Am Geriatr Soc 1989; 37:501–6.

[25] Rossouw JE, Bagdiwala S, Gordon DJ, et al. Plasma lipids as predictors of CHD in older men and women: the LRC Follow-up Study. Circulation 1990;82(Suppl III):346.

[26] Keil JE, Sutherland SE, Knapp RG, Gazes PC. Serum cholesterol: risk factor for coronary heart disease mortality in younger and older blacks and whites. The Charleston Heart Study, 1960–1988. Ann Epidemiol 1992;2:93–9.

[27] Lewis SJ, Moye LA, Sacks FM, Johnstone DE, Timmis G, Mitchell J. Effect of pravastatin on cardiovascular events in older patients with myocardial infarction and cholesterol levels in the average range. CARE trial. Ann Intern Med 1998;129:681–9.

[28] Bang LM, Goa KL. Pravastatin: a review of its use in elderly patients [abstract]. Drugs Aging 2003;20:1061.

[29] Miettinen TA, Pyorala K, Olsson AG, Musliner TA, Cook TJ, Faergeman O. Cholesterol-lowering therapy in women and elderly patients with myocardial infarction or angina pectoris: finding from the (4S). Circulation 1997;96:4211–8.

[30] Vokonas PS, Kannel WB. Epidemiology of coronary heart disease in the elderly. Cardiovasc Dis Elderly Patient 1994;91–123.

[31] Vokonas PS, Kannel WB. Diabetes mellitus and coronary heart disease in the elderly. 1996;12:69–78.

[32] Weslin L, Bresater LE, Eriksson H, Hansson PO, Welin C, Rosengren A. Insulin resistance and other risk factors for coronary heart disease in elderly men: the study of men born in 1913 and 1923. Eur J Cardiovasc Prev Rehabil 2003;10:283–8.

[33] Davidson MB. The effect of aging on carbohydrate metabolism: a review of the English literature and a practical approach to the diagnosis of diabetes mellitus in the elderly. Metabolism 1979;28:688–705.

[34] Lyons TJ. Lipoprotein glycation and its metabolic consequences. Diabetes 1992;41(Suppl 2): 67–73.

[35] Kirwan JP, Kohort WM, Wojta DM, Bourey RE, Holloszy JO. Endurance exercise training reduces glucose-stimulated insulin levels in 60 to 70 year-old men and women. J Gerontol Med Sci 1993;48A:M84–90.

[36] Fried LP, Kronmai RA, Newman AB, Bild DE, Mittelmark MB, Polak JF, et al. Risk factors for 5-year mortality in older adults: the Cardiovascular Health Study. JAMA 1998; 279:585–92.

[37] Banzer JA, Maguire TE, Kennedy CM, O'Malley CJ, Balady GJ. Results of cardiac rehabilitation in patients with diabetes mellitus. Am J Cardiol 2004;93:81–4.

[38] Rozanski A, Blumenthal JA, Kaplan J. Impact of psychological factors on the pathogenesis of cardiovascular disease and implications for therapy. Circulation 1999;99: 2192–217.

[39] Ghiadoni L, Donald AE, Cropley M, Mullen MJ, Oakley G, Taylor M, et al. Mental stress induces transient endothelial dysfunction in humans. Circulation 2000;102:2473–8.

[40] Ziegelstein RC, Fauerbach JA, Stevens SS, Romanelli J, Richter DP, Bush DE. Patients with depression are less likely to follow recommendations to reduce cardiac risk during recovery from a myocardial infarction. Arch Intern Med 2000;160:1818–23.

[41] Krumholz HM, Butler J, Miller J, Vaccarino V, Williams CS, Mendes de Leon CF, et al. Prognostic improtance of emotion support for elderly patients hospitalized with heart failure. Circulation 1998;97:958–64.

[42] Gibbons RJ, Abrams JR, et al. ACC/AHA 2002 guideline update for the management of patients with chronic stable angina. Circulation 2003;107:149–58.

[43] Braddom R. Physical medicine and rehabilitation. 1st edition. Philadelphia: WB Saunders; 1994.

[44] Wegner NK. Cardiac rehabilitation: a guide to practice in the 21st century. New York: Marcel Dekker; 1999.

[45] Ades PA, Waldmann ML, McCann WJ, Weaver SO. Predictors of cardiac rehabilitation participation in older coronary patients. Arch Intern Med 1992;152:1033–5.

[46] Frasure-Smith N, Lesperance F, Gravel G, Masson A, Juneau M, Talajic M, et al. Social support, depression and mortality during the first year after myocardial infarction. Circulation 2000;101:1919–24.

[47] Cooper AF, Jackson G, Weinman J, Horne R. Factors associated with cardiac rehabilitation attendance: a systematic review of the literature [abstract]. Clin Rehabil 2002;16:541–52.

[48] Man SF, McAlister FA, Anthonisen NR, Sin DD. Contemporary management of chronic obstructive pulmonary disease: clinical applications [abstract]. JAMA 2003;290:2313–6.

[49] California Pulmonary Rehabilitation Collaborative Group. Effects of pulmonary rehabilitation on dyspnea, quality of life, and healthcare costs in California [abstract]. J Cardiopulm Rehabil 2004;24.

[50] Mannino DM, Ford ES, Redd SC. Obstructive and restrictive lung disease and functional limitation: data from the Third National Health and Nutrition Examination. J Intern Med 2003;254:540–7.

ELSEVIER
SAUNDERS

Phys Med Rehabil Clin N Am
16 (2005) 267–284

PHYSICAL MEDICINE
AND REHABILITATION
CLINICS OF
NORTH AMERICA

Delivery of rehabilitation services to people aging with a disability

Cathy M. Cruise, MD[a,b,*], Mathew H.M. Lee, MD[a]

[a]Department of Rehabilitation Medicine, Rusk Institute of Rehabilitation, New York
University School of Medicine, 400 East 34th Street, New York, NY 10016, USA
[b]Physical Medicine and Rehabilitation Programs, Veterans Integrated Service Network #3,
130 West Kingsbridge Road, Building #16, Bronx, NY 10468, USA

One often hears discussion about the issues faced by baby boomers as they get older. This group includes individuals who are aging with a disability and those who become disabled as they age. In addition to planning for the resources needed to care for physically fit seniors, we must consider the systems of care required for those who age with a variety of impairments and hope to remain healthy and productive for as long as possible. To this end, systems of care that address preventive strategies and promote a philosophy and lifestyle centered on functional independence offer the greatest opportunity for society to capitalize on the strengths of the elderly population while affording the least economic burden.

It is anticipated that by the year 2030, the population over the age of 65 years will more than double to 70 million people. Within this group we can distinguish between the old (those between 65 and 75 years of age), the old old (those between 75 and 85 years of age), and the oldest old (those 85 years of age and older). The oldest old represents the fastest growing segment of the elderly population and is projected to increase from 4.2 million in 2000 to over 8.9 million in 2030. This is significant because the percentage of individuals with disabilities increases sharply with age, taking a much heavier toll on the oldest old. Almost three fourths (73.6%) of those over 80 years of age report at least one disability. Over half of those ≥80 years of age characterized their disability as being severe, and 35% of those ≥80 years of age reported needing assistance as a result of a disability [1].

The percentages of disabled individuals living in the community and those requiring a nursing home increase dramatically with age. Among persons

---

* Corresponding author. Physical Medicine and Rehabilitation Service/117, Northport Veterans Affairs Medical Center, 79 Middleville Road, Northport, NY 11768.
  E-mail address: cathy.cruise@med.va.gov (C.M. Cruise).

1047-9651/05/$ - see front matter © 2004 Elsevier Inc. All rights reserved.
doi:10.1016/j.pmr.2004.06.007

between the ages of 65 and 69, less than 4% are disabled in the community, and approximately 1% live in nursing homes. Yet, among those over 80 years of age, almost one quarter live in nursing homes, and a little over one fifth of those living in the community report that they are disabled [2].

Individuals with disabilities access health care in a variety of ways. Patients with spinal cord injuries (SCIs) and traumatic brain injuries and patients with multiple sclerosis (MS) and Parkinson's disease are treated through a variety of outpatient clinics and inpatient units throughout the Veterans Health Administration (VHA). Numerous private-sector facilities are establishing interdisciplinary clinics to care for individuals with MS, amyotrophic lateral sclerosis, and Parkinson's disease. One of the benefits of many of these programs is the ability of a disabled individual to age as an integral part of an interdisciplinary health care team providing continuity of care over time. Additionally, nursing homes are supporting rehabilitation units with short- and long-term missions, and subacute rehabilitation programs are gaining in popularity throughout the United States.

As one ages, the systems of care needed may change. In general, individuals tend to require the most care when they are very young and very old. A given individual with a SCI may require infrequent check-ups during young adulthood yet may experience significant clinical changes as he or she grows older, necessitating more frequent and perhaps more specialized medical care. In MS, this is apparent because the effects of immobility and weakness may be complicated by age-related changes in the musculoskeletal system.

Finances often dictate choices in health care, and geography may play an important role. Disabled individuals in farming, mountain, and inner-city communities may share common health care needs, but access to treatment programs may be vastly different. Of significance are differences seen in instrumental activities of daily living (IADL). A trip to the supermarket may mean a 5-minute walk in one area but may entail a 2-hour drive in another. These differences must be appreciated as we consider systems of care. Further, given the cultural diversity within our nation, it is important to be cognizant of the need to convey information in different languages and to recognize and respect different cultural beliefs and customs.

Theoretically achievable goal

The theoretically achievable goal (TAG) is the ultimate attainment in rehabilitation that a disabled person can reach under the most ideal physical, intellectual, mental, physiologic, social, economic, and environmental conditions (Fig. 1). Components of the TAG score include bowel and bladder care, feeding, grooming, dressing, communication, mobility, leisure activity, avocational activity, vocational function, education, and vocational training. Maximum TAG scores are achieved between the ages of 20 and 30 years and gradually decline subsequently with age [3]. We must

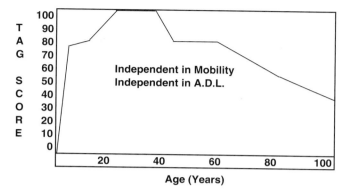

Fig. 1. TAG score according to age. The TAG score sharply increases in early life, reaches maximum at approximately 20 to 35 years of age, and gradually declines as age advances. (*From* Lee M, Itoh M. Geriatric rehabilitation management. In: Joseph Goodgold, editor. Rehabilitation medicine. St. Louis: Mosby; 1988. p. 396; with permission.)

consider all components of the TAG score as we develop rehabilitation programs for the disabled elderly population.

Delivery systems of rehabilitation services: Inpatient systems of care for the disabled elderly population

Rehabilitation provided during inpatient hospital or nursing homes stays has continued to grow in importance over the years. Recent trends reveal that individuals are discharged not only from inpatient medical or surgical units more quickly but also from inpatient rehabilitation units earlier in the course of recovery. This has raised concern regarding access to care for patients with disabilities. There has been a shift in focus from achieving short-term functional goals to setting and achieving long-term goals, including goals addressing quality of life (QOL). Questions have been posed as to whether individuals suffer without the ongoing support of the interdisciplinary team that they would have had on a daily basis as an inpatient. Subacute care is seen as a practical option, and informal support systems have been put into place. Further questions arise as to whether patients get rehospitalized more frequently after a short length of stay and to the extent that the burden on the support system increases. The use of telemedicine aimed at preventing readmission by targeting high-risk patients and following them closely through the use of technology offers alternatives to inpatient rehabilitative care.

Acute medical/surgical hospital units

Admission to an inpatient hospital unit raises concern in disabled and nondisabled individuals. In addition to acute medical-surgical treatment, there is the need to prevent deconditioning and subsequent loss of function. The most significant declines in functional and cognitive capacity often occur during the initial days of hospital care [4]. Research has shown that the muscles of someone on strict bed rest lose 1% to 1.5% of their initial strength per day over a 2-week period, which corresponds to an approximate loss of 10% to 20% strength per week for most persons. The loss is greatest during the first week of inactivity and gradually plateaus at an approximately 25% loss [5]. We must intervene during this early period to prevent future complications.

We often note clinically that it seems easier to prevent loss of strength and function than it is to restore it. It is therefore crucial for rehabilitation staff to intervene early in a patient's hospital stay with the goals of preventing immobility by getting the patient out of bed and moving as much as possible. A simple exercise program should be provided, and the patient should be encouraged to be as active as his medical condition allows. Simple exercises such as ankle pumps may prevent deleterious soft tissue contractures. Proper positioning prevents decubiti. Restorative and rehabilitation nurses are invaluable in the quest to optimize functional status.

Acute Care for the Elderly program

The Acute Care for the Elderly (ACE) program represents a unique approach to providing interdisciplinary, functionally based care for the hospitalized elderly population. Investigators initially identified 651 patients who were ≥ 70 years of age and did not require intensive care upon admission. They randomly assigned half of the patients to the ACE unit and half to traditional ward services. All patients received care from internal medicine physicians who worked on intervention and control units. Care on the control units followed conventional patterns. On the ACE units, a geriatrician and a geriatric nurse practitioner provided supervision, and nurses, aides, rehabilitation therapists, social workers, a pharmacist, and a dietitian functioned as an interdisciplinary team with a rehabilitative orientation. The hospital modified the physical environment of the ACE unit by maintaining uncluttered hallways, displaying large clocks and calendars, and installing carpeting, handrails, door levers, and elevated toilet seats [6]. The study revealed that 21% of patients in the ACE group improved their capacity to perform basic activities of daily living (ADL) by the time of discharge, compared with 13% in the control group. Forty-three percent of ACE patients were discharged to a long-term care facility compared with 60% of the control group. The groups did not differ significantly in mortality or length of stay. The costs of care in the two groups were similar [7]. The ACE philosophy has been used by many medical centers across the United States to address the functional needs of their acutely ill patients.

Acute inpatient rehabilitation

Inpatient rehabilitation programs, within acute rehabilitation units or in rehabilitation hospitals, provide a mechanism for focused interdisciplinary rehabilitative care for the disabled elderly patient. Generally, 2 to 4 hours of therapy is provided per day in acute programs, and outcomes are tracked through the Uniform Data System for Medical Rehabilitation. The Functional Independence Measure is used to obtain functional assessment data on admission, discharge, and 3-month follow-up.

Effective team functioning seems to be a key to the success of the rehabilitation programs [8]. In a recent review, patient-focused rehabilitation team cohesiveness was significantly associated with administrative support, supervisor expectations, attending physician support, and physician involvement. Higher levels of patient-focused team cohesion indicated that patient services were likely delivered with greater interprofessional communication and joint effort [9].

Many inpatient rehabilitation programs have obtained accreditation from CARF, the Rehabilitation Accreditation Commission. CARF standards stipulate that the interdisciplinary team for each individual should be determined based on the patient's assessment, predicted outcomes, and medical and rehabilitative needs. CARF standards further state that team members should include the patient, a rehabilitation physician and nurse, a speech language pathologist, a nutritionist, an occupational therapist, a physical therapist, a psychologist, a social worker, and a therapeutic recreational specialist. Depending on the needs of the patient, formal arrangements may be made for other team members [10].

The literature shows that certain patients with the same diagnosis tend to do better in rehabilitation programs. This is seen most dramatically with stroke. The Stroke Unit Trialists Collaboration concluded that specialized stroke units reduce death, dependency and the need for long term institutionalization compared with general medical care in patients hospitalized with stroke. The success of these units was attributed in part to the high degree of specialized medical and nursing interest in stroke, specialized staff training, interdisciplinary coordination, and involvement of family and caretakers in the rehabilitation process [11]. The setting in which rehabilitative care is provided may also be significant. When comparing community residence, recovery to premorbid levels of function in five ADL skills, Medicare costs and numbers of therapy and physician visits, enhanced outcomes were noted for elderly patients with stroke treated in rehabilitation hospitals in one study. This was not noted in patients with hip fracture [12].

Geriatric Evaluation and Management units

The Geriatric Evaluation and Management (GEM) units within the Veterans Administration provide a comprehensive approach to the care of elderly patients. The GEM unit generally consists of beds within the hospital's intermediate care area in which an interdisciplinary team cares for patients, maintaining direct responsibility for all aspects of patient care. In one program, patients were enrolled into a study on the GEM unit 1 week after admission to the acute areas of the hospital. Veterans in this study were ≥65 years of age and had persistent medical, functional, or psychologic problems that were thought to be likely to interfere with discharge. After discharge, the study patients received follow-up care in the hospital's geriatric clinic, whereas the control group attended the general medical clinics. At discharge, significant differences between the veterans enrolled on the GEM unit and those enrolled on the traditional unit were seen: 73% of the study patients versus 53% of the control subjects were able to return home or to a board-and-care facility. The percentage that died in the hospital was identical. During the following year, the percentage of deaths was significantly lower among the study group (28.3% versus 48.3%). The authors estimated that savings throughout the next year more than recouped the costs of the GEM unit [13]. GEM units continue to be used throughout the VA system.

Geriatric Assessment units

Geriatric Assessment (GA) units parallel GEM units in the private sector. The care on the GA units tends to be similar to that on the GEM unit. In one GA unit, by 6 weeks after discharge, only 8% of patients assigned to the GA unit lived in institutions, compared with 24% of control subjects. By 6 months, these values were 11% and 26%, respectively. Six months after discharge, the intervention group had significantly greater functional improvement than did control subjects, but these differences dissipated over the next 6 months [14]. GEM units and GA units offer an interesting approach to functional care.

Skilled nursing facility

Rehabilitative care may be provided within a skilled nursing facility. Many nursing home residents have multiple and severe impairments. According to the National Nursing Home Survey, the average elderly nursing home resident in 1985 was dependent in 3.9 out of 6 ADLs measured in the survey [15].

Although approximately 5% of persons over 65 years of age reside in a nursing home at any given time, the chance of a given individual entering a nursing home at some point in his or her life is much greater. The vast majority of funds expended on nursing home care are for people who use nursing home care for extended stays. Although 40% to 50% of admissions are for people who stay in a nursing home 6 months or less, only 20% of admissions are for people who reside in nursing homes for 3 or more years [16].

Varying levels of rehabilitation may be provided within skilled nursing facilities. The Minimal Data Set is generally used to determine Resource Use Groups. Patients receive different levels of rehabilitation according to clinical need. An interdisciplinary team approach is used, and appropriate functional goals are set.

Subacute care

Subacute care has become increasingly popular within the Unites States health care system over the last 15 years. Because it is delivered across a continuum, subacute care tends to reduce the focus on discrete episodes of site-specific care. Recent literature defines subacute care as that which is rendered immediately after, or instead of, acute hospitalization. It requires the coordinated services of physicians, nurses, and other professionals in assessing and managing clinical conditions and administering the procedures needed. Subacute care is generally administered for a period of several days to several months or until a condition is stabilized or a predetermined treatment course is completed [17].

Subacute inpatient rehabilitation may be useful to the disabled elderly patient. Short- and long-term restorative goals are set, and individuals generally receive at least 1 hour of therapy per day. Subacute rehabilitation programs before or after an acute rehabilitation program are frequently used. Individuals may participate in a pre-acute rehabilitation program to increase endurance and strength before undergoing a course of acute rehabilitation. Additionally, individuals may participate in a post-rehabilitation program to fine tune self-care and mobility skills before discharge to home. Subacute rehabilitation may also be used as a transitional program before discharge from medical/surgical units and for respite or palliative care.

In one retrospective comparison of acute versus subacute rehabilitation of stroke patients, acute rehabilitation cost twice as much and involved twice as many treatment hours yet achieved greater functional gains. There was no difference in discharge disposition [18].

Respite care

Home care patients may be boarded in an extended care facility for a short period of time to provide temporary relief to the caregiver. Enormous social, psychologic, emotional, and physical stresses are often placed upon a caregiver. Caregivers tend to neglect their own health while caring for a loved one. Additionally, as the population ages, so do the caregivers, many with significant impairments of their own. It is essential to allow caregivers time to rest. While an individual is receiving respite care, it is important to maintain his/her current level of activity and function through rehabilitative intervention using specific physical therapy, occupational therapy, restorative nursing, and other services as needed.

Hospice care

Rehabilitation staff can play an important role in hospice care. Individuals receiving hospice care frequently require assistive devices to remain safely mobile. Patients and caregivers need to be instructed in the proper use of these devices. A physical therapist, an occupational therapist, a rehabilitation nurse, or another rehabilitation professional should be consulted so that proper training may be achieved [19]. Because a holistic approach is often advocated within hospice teams, occupational therapy, operating from a behavioral perspective, can contribute to maximizing the QOL for the terminally ill patient [20]. Information on hospice care and locations can be obtained by calling the National Hospice and Palliative Care Organization at (800) 658-8898 or by visiting their website at www.nhpco.org.

Community systems of care for the disabled elderly population

Program for All Inclusive Care of the Elderly

The Program for All Inclusive Care of the Elderly (PACE) program model is a managed care system that integrates acute and long-term care, inpatient and outpatient care, and Medicare and Medicaid financing to provide cost-effective health care delivery to frail elderly participants [21]. The goal of the program is to maintain participants in their own community for as long as is medically, socially, and economically feasible [22]. Coordination of care and integration of acute and long-term services that characterize the PACE program are developed through effective group processes within interdisciplinary teams at each PACE site [23]. The teams generally consist of a primary care physician and nursing, pharmacy, social work, rehabilitation, nutrition, and recreation therapy and transportation staff [24]. Financing occurs through integration of Medicaid, Medicare, and private funds into a single capitation rate [22].

Adult Day Health Care

Adult Day Health Care programs provide a practical alternative to institutional care in many cases. Adult Day Services are defined by the National Adult Day Services Association as community-based group programs established to meet the needs of functionally or cognitively impaired adults through an individual plan of care [25]. There are generally two models of care, one with a medical focus and the other with a social focus. In each, a variety of health, social, and other related support services is provided for part of a day. Adult Day Services allow increased social interaction in a less isolated setting than traditional home care. They also allow the provider to monitor patients by physically seeing them and enable family caregivers to continue working outside the home [25].

Finding the right Adult Day Health Care Program is an enormous task. Various free brochures that list web sites and resources exist to help the consumer find an appropriate program. Issues of significance when choosing programs include client-to-staff ratios, costs, and services provided.

Geriatric Day Hospital

The Geriatric Day Hospital may offer another alternative to the disabled elderly person. A Geriatric Day Hospital has been described as an outpatient facility where frail older patients can receive subacute or acute medical, nursing, social, or rehabilitative services over any portion of a full day, with return visits as necessary. This definition excludes day hospital programs with more restricted or single purposes, such as rehabilitation, psychiatry, or cancer care and programs with a more social and less medical orientation [26].

Benefits of the Geriatric Day Hospital may include the use of comprehensive functional assessments, interdisciplinary teams, and individualized treatment plans. Geriatric Day Hospitals began in Great Britain. Although the concept spread to the United States, issues with reimbursement may have prevented them from remaining popular within this country.

Outpatient rehabilitation programs

The spectrum of outpatient rehabilitation ranges from comprehensive interdisciplinary programs to single service providers. Comprehensive Outpatient Rehabilitation Facilities (CORFs) are entities established under the federal Medicare program and provide outpatient diagnostic, therapeutic, and restorative services by or under the supervision of a physician. CORFs provide physician services, physical therapy, and social or psychologic services. A visit to the patient's home is generally included to evaluate the home environment in relation to the patient's treatment plan [27]. Comprehensive outpatient medical rehabilitation programs may be accredited by CARF, the Rehabilitation Accreditation Commission. Hospital-based and independent providers may provide physical and occupational therapy and other services.

Systems of care centered in the home

Long-term residential alternatives

A variety of long-term, community-based residential programs exist. Continuing Care Retirement Communities offer housing, residential, and health care services in return for an entrance fee and monthly maintenance fees. Adult foster care provides room, board, and personal care to a small number of elderly residents for a monthly rate. Additionally, the Department of Housing and Urban Development provides a spectrum of subsidized housing programs for low- and moderate-income elderly persons. The Section 202 Housing Program for the Elderly and Handicapped provides below-market interest loans to private nonprofit sponsoring organizations for the development of subsidized housing projects for elderly persons [28].

Home-Based Primary Care

Home-Based Primary Care programs are designed to assist home-bound individuals who do not require ongoing hospitalization yet have significant health care needs that prevent them from remaining independent in the community. Because it is often difficult for these individuals to come to the hospital and clinics for appointments due to their medical conditions, an interdisciplinary team provides care to the person at home. The team generally includes physician, nursing, social work, rehabilitation, pharmacy, and nutrition staff.

The rehabilitative component of Home Based Primary Care is important. Physical and occupational therapists assess patients' homes for safety and provide equipment as needed. Bathroom equipment and kitchen utensils adapted for specific disabilities are commonly provided. Home-Based Primary Care programs are popular within the VHA and many private-sector facilities.

Informal home care

Most long-term care in the United States is provided by informal caregivers, including family members, neighbors, and community groups. Although informal home care is expensive in terms of burden on the caregiver, the financial cost of this care is not often tracked. Expert estimates of expenditures for long-term care generally do not include the costs of informal care. Thus, the total amount of money spent on health care, particularly for the elderly and the disabled populations, is underestimated. Many informal caregivers are elderly. The probability of becoming an informal caregiver increases with age until one reaches 75 years of age [29]. Other caregivers are younger and struggle to balance their loved ones' needs with paid employment and the needs of their own children. The needs of informal caregivers must be addressed to allow them to continue to provide invaluable services.

Formal home care

Data from the 1989 Long Term Care Survey indicates that approximately 20% to 25% of elderly persons in the community have difficulty with ADLs or IADLs. These individuals, numbering approximately 1.6 million, receive formal home care services alone or in combination with informal services [2]. These formal home care services include skilled and nonskilled services.

According to the National Long-Term Care survey, age and disability level are the strongest correlates of formal home care use. Data reveal that 26% of persons with IADL impairments use formal home care services, whereas 40% of persons disabled in three or more ADLs use home care services. Disabled elderly persons living alone are 40% more likely to use formal home care services than are persons who live with others [2].

Telemedicine applications used in the care of disabled elderly persons

Telerehabilitation medicine is an emerging field with great clinical relevance. Telecommunications technology, including video and nonvideo monitors and messaging devices, may be used to access rehabilitative care at remote sites. Data are transmitted over telephone lines, making it easy to use.

Monitors have been used to link patients in rural areas to specialists in main hospitals. Within the VHA, telemedicine has been used to benefit disabled elderly persons through the provision of orthotics and prosthetic clinics, wheelchair clinics, and other specialty clinics, allowing care to be provided to patients in remote locations who might otherwise not be able to receive equipment. Telemonitors may also connect patients in remote sites with specialists in MS, traumatic brain injury, and SCI regional centers.

Tele-home health care applications used with disabled elderly patients

There are significantly different issues regarding access to health care for disabled elderly persons living in different geographic parts of the country and in urban versus rural areas. Although city dwellers who are disabled may have difficulty using public transportation systems, individuals living in rural areas who are disabled, particularly those with failing eye sight or muscular strength and coordination, may not be able to access certain aspects of health care due to distance. Examples of this occur in rural areas of the Midwest where an individual may live 3 hours from a tertiary care facility. Inability to tolerate long car or ambulance rides and financial constraints may combine to preclude certain aspects of health care delivery.

The disabled elderly population will benefit from home messaging devices to assess functional maintenance and rehabilitation needs. Patients may be queried as to changing equipment needs, caregiver roles, transportation needs, fall risk factors and medication management issues. It is hoped that by discovering potential problems before they occur, acute events necessitating emergency room visits can be prevented and that inpatient hospitalizations can be avoided.

In July 2003, the VHA established an Office of Care Coordination to provide the "right care in the right place at the right time." Viewing the place of residence as the optimal place of care, home telehealth technology is being used within the VHA to augment traditional care. Focusing on high-risk populations, a variety of technologic equipment, including text messaging devices, monitors with attached peripheral equipment (eg, blood pressure machines, blood glucose meters, scales, and pulse oximeters) and videophones, is being used.

The Community Care Coordination Service within the Florida/South Georgia Network of the Veterans Health Administration has targeted patients with complex medical/chronic diseases to receive monitoring via home health technology. Data for 1 year showed a 40% reduction in emergency room visits, a 63% reduction in hospital admissions, a 60% reduction in hospital bed days of care, a 64% reduction in VHA nursing home admissions, and an 88% reduction in nursing home bed days of care for veterans enrolled in the program [30].

A unique approach to helping elderly patients remain in the community proposes the use of an Enhanced Activity of Daily Living Index based on a computerized questionnaire form. Additionally, a number of low-cost electronic sensors have been developed that provide electronic measures of functional performance, thus providing a means of continuously and objectively assessing a patient's condition after hospitalization [31].

Delivery systems for the elderly population with specific disabilities

Individuals aging with specific disabilities have specialized needs that must be considered.

Disabled elderly patients with spinal cord injury

There is increasing recognition of the needs of elderly patients with SCI. More older individuals who suffer a SCI are surviving, and those who are injured at a young age are living longer. Significant life expectancies and the potential for functional gains make rehabilitation efforts appropriate for all patients after SCI regardless of age [32].

SCI centers need to adapt to the needs of a population that is more elderly and where the primary caretaker may also be elderly. An innovative approach has been demonstrated within VHA where video monitors have been used to connect veterans in their homes with clinicians in the Medical Center. This has been used with patients with SCI in the New York-New Jersey Veterans Integrated Service Network.

Disabled elderly patients with traumatic brain injury

Post-acute rehabilitation for individuals with traumatic brain injury may be provided in a variety of settings, including day treatment programs, residential treatment programs, and vocational rehabilitation programs. The Brain Injury Association of America provides consumer information, including referrals (www.bia.org).

Disabled elderly patients with post-polio syndrome

Post-polio syndrome can strike a person who has recovered from poliomyelitis between 10 and 40 years after the initial illness. Fatigue, muscle weakness, and pain that may ensue can dramatically affect an individual's access to health care. When post-polio syndrome affects the respiratory system, severe respiratory impairment may occur [33]. There are a number of health care systems with experience in treating post-polio syndrome. One of these is Goldwater Memorial Hospital in New York City, where the staff has expertise in caring for the respiratory complications that may ensue from post-polio syndrome.

Disabled elderly patients with amputation

Specific adaptations to the environment may be needed for an elderly individual after amputation. Changes in the individual's ability to ambulate may affect his or her access to health care services. Amputees may become unable to drive or to use public transportation systems, making systems of care delivery that focus on home services more practical. The National Amputation Foundation provides programs of value to amputees. One of these is the AMP to AMP Program in which a home, hospital, or nursing home visit is available to anyone who has had or will have a major limb amputation. Through these visits, peer counseling and support are provided [34].

Disabled elderly patients with multiple sclerosis

The functional decline experienced by many patients with MS over time may necessitate several changes in the systems of care used. As the patients' needs change, so does the mode of care delivery. The need for home help may increase.

Telerehabilitation offers possibilities in this arena. In one study, data were collected from 27 patients with MS on fatigue, depression, and health-related quality of life (HRQOL) as part of a larger study of the impact of tele-rehabilitation intervention on people with severe mobility impairment. The study consisted of a 9-week intervention with three randomized groups (video, telephone, and standard care) for a 2-year follow-up period. For the video group, HRQOL scores were higher and fatigue and depression scores lower for 24 months. These findings suggest that tele-rehabilitation interventions may be beneficial, although the results need affirmation through larger samples [35].

Financial implications for the disabled elderly population

Changes in the Medicaid and Medicare structures raise many questions for the disabled elderly population. The number of people Medicare serves is expected to nearly double by 2030. In the year 2002, 85% of Medicare beneficiaries were elderly. Nearly 65% of Medicare beneficiaries have annual incomes below $25,000. Among the nearly 30% of beneficiaries who live alone, 56% have an income below $15,000, and 15% are over 85 years of age [36].

Interesting differences exist between elderly Medicare beneficiaries and those younger than age 65 who are disabled. According to the Medicare Health Outcomes Survey Applied Research Center Report on the Health Status of Medicare Disabled Cohort I Baseline data in 1998, when compared with the Medicare beneficiaries over 65 years of age, disabled Medicare beneficiaries under the age of 65 had a higher proportion of ethnic minorities, were more likely to be on Medicaid, were more likely to have a higher number of coexisting chronic conditions, were three times more likely to rate their health as fair or poor and were twice as likely to rate their health as worse than the previous year [37].

Future trends in accessing health care for the disabled elderly population

The future of rehabilitative care for the disabled elderly population is likely to include increased emphasis on preventive programs and case management.

Preventive rehabilitation

The concept of preventive rehabilitation, developed by Lee and Itoh [38], is based on the premise that one should preserve one's health and functional ability so that he/she may die a vertical death, peacefully in one's sleep (Fig. 2). Through a change in emphasis from disease management to health promotion, higher quality, more active, and healthier lives may be obtained, resulting in increased life expectancy. This concept stresses that although genetic make-up is fundamental, environment and lifestyle are equally

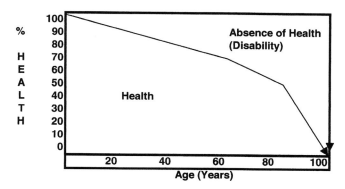

Fig. 2. The objective of Preventive Rehabilitation is to die healthy. Emphasis is shifted from disease management to health promotion. (Courtesy of Mathew Lee, MD and Masayoshi Itoh, MD.).

Box 1. Lee and Itoh Theory on the Concept of Health Status

$$H = g^{(E) + (L)}$$

H = Individual health status
g = Genetic make-up
E = Environmental factors
L = Lifestyle issues

Theory on the Concept of Health Status. Individual Health Status can be viewed as an equation in which health status is equal to genetic make-up raised to the power of the sum of environmental factors and lifestyle issues. (*Courtesy of* Mathew Lee, MD and Masayoshi Itoh, MD.)

---

important, and exercise, diet, and stress management can promote healthy aging. Mental stimulation is also a necessity. Health is equal to genetics raised to the power of the sum of environment and lifestyle (Box 1) [38].

Case management

Case management programs are being implemented throughout the United States. For adults whose loved ones live far from them or who do not have the time or knowledge to provide care themselves, geriatric case managers may be valuable. Functions that may be provided by geriatric case managers include shopping, paying bills, and finding legal help to update estate plans, wills, powers of attorney, and health care directives. Information regarding geriatric case managers can be found on the web site of the National Association of Professional Geriatric Case Managers (www.caremanager.org) [39].

Clinical outcomes and areas of research

Although there is diversity within the systems that exist to care for the disabled elderly population, it is important to obtain quantitative and qualitative data to assess these programs. Factors that need to be considered include medical and mental status, functional status, and QOL. A myriad of measures exist to quantify clinical outcomes, including the Functional Independence Measure, the Katz ADL Scale, the SF-36, and the HRQOL indicator. The challenge is to capture these data in a meaningful way and to share it with others to improve future health care delivery.

The VHA has created a large database known as the Functional Status and Outcomes Database, which assesses functional efficiency over time in veterans with stroke, amputation, and brain injury. Veterans with new onset of stroke and amputation are further subdivided into Function Related Groups (FRGs). Using the FRG system, the VHA is able to compare functional outcomes for different levels of impairment; this can lead to treatment recommendations.

Summary

The disabled elderly population continues to grow. Systems of care for the disabled elderly are vast, ranging from inpatient facilities to outpatient programs and home programs. Recent advances in technology allow us to reach patients in their homes through telemedicine. Support services within the community are growing, and case managers are becoming more necessary as it becomes more difficult to navigate the health care system.

As providers of rehabilitative services, we must help our patients find the most appropriate setting to receive care. As the focus continues to shift from inpatient to outpatient care and to home services, we must approach health care in a dynamic fashion and with flexibility. We must be advocates for our patients and their caretakers.

Significant research questions remain, and health care policy requires development. As the population ages and the disabled elderly population become a focus of fiscal experts, we must look to provide the most cost-effective yet functionally productive health care. We may shift from focusing on functional performance in a therapy gym or inpatient rehabilitation unit to functional performance at home. We must focus on IADL and QOL indicators and must strive to find ways to provide efficient, cost-effective care. Medicaid, Medicare, and third-party insurers offer various options. The VHA offers additional benefit to those who are eligible. Advocacy groups such as the American Association of Retired Persons struggle to meet its members' needs and concerns while generating income to provide education and other resources. We must work to promote the strengths of the elderly population by addressing preventive strategies while maintaining functional independence.

References

[1] Department of Health and Human Services. Administration on Aging. Statistics on the Aging Population. Available at: www.aoa.dhhs.gov/aoa/stats/profile/12.html. Accessed January 20, 2004.

[2] National long term care survey. Washington, DC: United States Department of Health and Human Services; 1989.

[3] Lee M, Itoh M. Geriatric rehabilitation management. In: Goodgold J, editor. Rehabilitation medicine. St. Louis: C.V. Mosby; 1988. p. 394–7.

[4] Hirsch CH, Sommers L, Olsen A, Mullen L, Winograd CH. The natural history of functional mobility in hospitalized older patients. J Am Geriatr Soc 1990;38:1296–303.

[5] Mueller EA. The influence of training and of inactivity on muscle strength. Arch PM&R 1970;51:449–62.

[6] Landefeld CS, Palmer RM, Kresevic DM, Fortinsky RH, Kowal J. A randomized trial of care in a hospital medical unit especially designed to improve the functional outcomes of acutely ill older patients. New Engl J Med 1995;332:1338–44.

[7] Covinski KE, King JT, Quinn LM, Siddique R, Palmer R, Kresevic DM, et al. Do acute care for elders units increase hospital costs? A cost analysis using the hospital perspective. J Am Geriatr Soc 1997;45:729–34.

[8] Stineman MG, Strasser DC. Team process and effectiveness: patients, families, and staff characteristics. Topics Stroke Rehabil 1997;4:21–33.

[9] Smits SJ, Falconer JA, Herrin A, Bowen SE, Strasser DC. Patient focused rehabilitation team cohesiveness in veterans' administration hospitals. Arch PM&R 2003;84:1332–8.

[10] Medical rehabilitation standards manual. Tuscon AZ: The Rehabilitation Commission. The Commission on Accreditation of Rehabilitation Facilities, Inc.; 2003.

[11] Stroke Unit Trialists Collaboration. How do stroke units improve patient outcomes? A collaborative systematic review of the randomized trials. Stroke 1997;28:2139–44.

[12] Kramer AM, Steiner JF, Schlenker RE, Eilertsen TB, Hrincevich CA, Tropea DA, et al. Outcomes and costs after hip fracture and stroke: a comparison of rehabilitation settings. JAMA 1997;277:396–404.

[13] Rubenstein LZ, Josephson KR, Wieland D, English PA, Sayre JA, Kane RL. Effectiveness of a geriatric evaluation unit: a randomized clinical trial. New Engl J Med 1984;311:1664–70.

[14] Applegate WB, Miller ST, Graney MJ, Elan JT, Burns R, Akins DE. A randomized controlled trial in a geriatric assessment unit in a community rehabilitation hospital. New Engl J Med 1990;322:1572–8.

[15] Hing E, Sekscenski E, Strahan G. The National Nursing Home Survey; 1985: summary for the United States. Vital Health Stat 1989;13:1–249.

[16] Spence D, Wiener J. Nursing home length of stay patterns: results from the 1985 National Nursing Home Survey. Gerontologist 1990;30:16–20.

[17] Levenson SL. Subacute care: role and implications for a modernized health care system. In: Katz PR, Kane RL, Mezey MD, editors. Emerging systems in long term care. Springer Series: Adv Long Term Care 1999;4:29–30.

[18] Keith RA, Wilson DB, Gutierrez P. Acute and subacute rehabilitation for stroke: a comparison. Arch PM&R 1995;76:495–500.

[19] Sloan HL, Haslam K, Foret CM. Teaching the use of walkers and canes. Home Healthc Nurse 2001;19:241–6.

[20] Folts D, Tigges K, Weisman T. Occupational therapy in hospice home care: a student tutorial. Am J Occup Ther 1986;40:623–8.

[21] Eleazer P, Fretwell M. The PACE Model (Program for All Inclusive Care of the Elderly): a review. In: Katz PR, Kane RL, Mezey M, editors. Emerging systems in long term care. Springer series: advances in long-term care. New York: Springer Publishing Company; 1999. p. 88–117.

[22] Shen J, Iverson A. PACE: a capitated model towards long-term care. Henry Ford Hosp Med J 1992;40:41–4.

[23] Eleazer GP, Baskins JP, Egbert JR, Johnson CD, Wilson L. Managed care for the frail elderly: the PACE project. J S C Med Assoc 1994;90:586–92.

[24] Eleazer P, Fretwell M. The PACE Model (Program for All Inclusive Care of the Elderly): a review. In: Katz PR, Kane RL, Mezey M, editors. Emerging systems in long term care. Springer series: advances in long-term care. New York: Springer Publishing Company; 1999. p. 96–8.

[25] National Adult Day Services Association. Available at: www.nadsa.org. Accessed January 9, 2004.

[26] Siu AL, Morishita L, Blaustein J. Comprehensive geriatric assessment in a day hospital. J Am Geriatr Soc 1994;42:1094–9.

[27] Comprehensive Outpatient Rehabilitation Facilities. Available at: www.cdphe.state.co.us/hf/static/corf.htm. Accessed January 12, 2004.

[28] Burwell BO, Jackson B. United States Department of Health and Human Services. The disabled elderly and their use of long term care. Cambridge (MA): SysteMetrics; 1994.

[29] Stone R, Cafferta GL, Sangi J. Caregivers of the frail elderly: a national profile. Gerontologist 1987;27:616–26.

[30] Meyer M, Kobb R, Ryan P. Virtually healthy: chronic disease management in the home. Dis Manage 2002;5:1–8.

[31] Doughty K, Costa J. Continuous automated telecare assessment of the elderly. J Telemed Telecare 1997;3(Suppl 1):23–5.

[32] Yarkony GM, Roth EJ, Heinemann AW, Lowell LL. Spinal cord rehabilitation outcome: impact of age. J Clin Epidemiol 1988;41:173–7.

[33] Moss Rehab Resource Net Post Polio Syndrome Homepade. Available at: www.mossresourcenet.org/txtpolio.htm. Accessed March 26, 2004.

[34] National Amputation Foundation. Available at: www.home.comcast.net/~n2fc/natamp/Program. Accessed March 26, 2004.

[35] Egner A, Philips VL, Vora R, et al. Depression, fatigue and health related quality of life among people with advanced multiple sclerosis: results from an exploratory telerehabilitation study. NeuroRehabilitation 2003;18:125–33.

[36] Program information on Medicare, Medicaid, SCHIP and other programs of the Centers for Medicare and Medicaid Services. Baltimore (MD): Centers for Medicare and Medicaid Services, Office of Research, Development and Information. 2002.

[37] Medicare Health Outcomes Survey Applied Research Center. Report on the Health Status of Medicare Disabled. Cohort I Baseline Data, 1998. Prepared by Health Services Advisory Group. November 30, 2000.

[38] Lee M, Itoh M. Healthy aging: preventive rehabilitation. New York: Rusk Institute of Rehabilitation; 2001.

[39] Friedman S. Care managers can help guide the old and alone. Gray Matters Newsday 2004; 28:B5.

ELSEVIER
SAUNDERS

Phys Med Rehabil Clin N Am
16 (2005) 285–305

PHYSICAL MEDICINE
AND REHABILITATION
CLINICS OF
NORTH AMERICA

The role of rehabilitation medicine and palliative care in the treatment of patients with end-stage disease

Ellen Olson[a],*, Adrian Cristian, MD[b]

[a]*Department of Geriatrics and Adult Development, Mount Sinai School of Medicine,
130 West Kingsbridge Road, Routing number 00EX, Bronx, NY 10468, USA*
[b]*Department of Rehabilitation Medicine, Mount Sinai School of Medicine, 130 West
Kingsbridge Road, Bronx, NY 10468, USA*

Advances in medical care are resulting in more and more people surviving, living, and aging with disabilities, including cancer. Due to the progressive nature of some disabilities, practical care issues and ethical dilemmas arise in the care of individuals in the end stages of their diseases.

This article focuses on the issues surrounding the care of patients with end-stage cancer. This model was chosen because it is widely known in the rehabilitation literature, and many of its principles can be used in the care of patients with other end-stage diseases. The goals of the article are (1) to make the reader aware of the principles of palliative care, (2) to describe similarities between palliative care and rehabilitation medicine and highlight the important collaborative efforts of these disciplines in the care of the dying patient, (3) to present a brief history of cancer rehabilitation in the United States, and (4) to discuss some of the ethical and practical issues that arise in the care of patients with end-stage disease, such as cancer. The article concludes with a case study demonstrating how these principles could be incorporated in the care of a patient.

Similarities between palliative care and rehabilitation medicine

Palliative care, as defined by the World Health Organization, is the active and total care of patients whose disease is not responsive to curative treatment [1]. Rehabilitation and palliative care share many characteristics

* Corresponding author.
E-mail address: ellen.olson@med.va.gov (E. Olson).

and goals. The goal of palliative care is to maximize quality of life for patients and their families; the goal of rehabilitation medicine is to help individuals achieve the fullest physical, psychologic, social, vocational, and educational potential, consistent with his or her limitations and goals [2].

Both are multidisciplinary in nature. Disciplines included in the palliative care team model include oncology, neurology, psychiatry, anesthesiology, nursing, social work, pharmacy, clergy, nutrition, and rehabilitation [2,3]. The rehabilitation team is comparable to the palliative care team—it includes nursing, social work, physical therapy, occupational therapy, speech therapy, and physiatry [4]. Medical and surgical specialists are consulted as needed.

Both involve the patient and family in care planning [2]. Both strive to maximize physical function and emotional well-being to the highest extent possible given the nature of the underlying disease process. Both use an array of treatment modalities to address physical and psychologic symptoms. Both aspire to the early identification of persons at risk for pain and disability to minimize suffering and functional loss.

The role of rehabilitation medicine in the care of the dying patient

A recent focus in the field of palliative care medicine has highlighted the contribution of rehabilitation medicine to the care of the dying patient. For many, this is a new blending of complimentary disciplines, both of which focus on maintenance or restoration of function and quality of life in the face of medical or surgical illness. A review of the literature, however, shows that the importance of rehabilitation in terminal cancer is not a new concept.

Rehabilitation and palliative care have a role in the treatment of most advanced chronic diseases, such as amyotrophic lateral sclerosis, multiple sclerosis, spinal cord injury, and end-stage lung and heart disease. Cancer patients commonly face many of the same problems and symptoms faced by patients with other chronic illnesses. Patients with advanced cancer experience a high prevalence of pain, fatigue, generalized weakness, dyspnea, delirium, nausea, vomiting, and depression [5,6]. The same treatments outlined for cancer patients can be applied to patients with other serious illnesses.

Cancer is second to heart disease as the leading cause of death in the United States. It claims the lives of more than 538,000 people each year, usually after months of decline and disability [7,8]. The lifetime risk for men developing cancer is 1 in 2, and for women it is approximately 1 in 3 [9]. As our population ages, cancer incidence rates climb. The incidence rate per 100,000 is 500 for men and women at age 50. By age 80, this number is 2000 for women and 4000 for men [10]. Cancer survival rates have also improved. There is a 5-year survival rate of 58% [11].

For many of these survivors, cancer remains a chronic condition that affects physical and psychosocial functioning [12]. Rehabilitation medicine can maximize function and quality of life for these individuals [13].

A brief history of cancer rehabilitation in the United States

Dietz [14] wrote one of the first and most comprehensive articles on rehabilitation of the cancer patient in 1969. He suggested three categories of goals for rehabilitation, which evolved into the four categories most commonly referred to in current cancer rehabilitation literature. These categories are *prevention* of disability, whenever possible (stage 1); but if not, *restoration* to the premorbid state (stage 2); followed by *support* to reduce cancer-related disabilities (stage 3); then *palliation*, where the goal is reducing complications, maintaining independence, and providing comfort (stage 4) [15].

His article is notable for many insights into cancer care that hold true today. He stated that cancer affects all aspects of the patient's life, including social, economic, vocational, and emotional aspects, thereby requiring a team approach to care that includes psychologists, vocational counselors, and social workers. He advocated early intervention to reduce the degree of disability. This is a goal that palliative care medicine shares with rehabilitation medicine but with reference to reducing symptom burden. He emphasized that disabilities faced by cancer patients were not much different from the disabilities faced by rehabilitation patients in general. The exceptions to this included neuromyopathies secondary to the remote effects of cancer on the nervous system and the focal effects of cancer, such as the pathologic fractures. He noted that most cancer patients are over 55 years of age, and therefore rehabilitation clinicians must deal with age-related disabilities. His article provided a detailed review of problems faced by cancer patients based on the site of the tumor and how to address these problems. The goals that transcended organ systems were maintenance of function and range of motion.

In his article, Dietz reviewed the first 3 years of a collaborative program for the rehabilitation care of the cancer patient that was started at the Institute of Rehabilitation Medicine and Memorial Hospital for Cancer and Allied Diseases in New York (now known as Memorial Sloan-Kettering Cancer Center). Among the 1237 inpatients seen over that time period, the treatment goal into which the largest group fell was the "supportive" category, where progression of disease and disability were kept under at least temporary control. He graded the response to rehabilitation on a scale of 0 to 4, with 0 being no change or improvement and 4 being fully independent with no residual disability. The largest group achieved a response of grade 2, showing moderate improvement and appropriate response to rehabilitative care. He ended the article with the cautionary note that because accurate means for providing estimates of prognosis did not exist for cancer, the provision of rehabilitation services should not be delayed once a need is recognized. Therapy should not be placed on hold pending further determinations of prognosis. He emphasized that there is a need for rehabilitative care even for patients with incurable and terminal disease. These statements hold true today.

The nursing profession was an early advocate of the integral role rehabilitation should play in the care of patients with cancer. The Oncology Nursing Society was the first professional group to offer a practical definition of cancer rehabilitation, which was published in 1989. They defined cancer rehabilitation as a "process by which individuals within their environments are assisted to achieve optimal functioning within the limits imposed by cancer" [16]. Watson [17] provided a history of cancer rehabilitation in an article published in 1992, where she credited the origins of cancer rehabilitation to Drs. J. Herbert Dietz, Harold Rusk, and A.E. Gunn. All three had established rehabilitation programs for cancer survivors with physical disabilities using funding made available 25 years earlier by the National Cancer Institute (NCI). She also credited them with the application of concepts such as the interdisciplinary team and functional assessment to patients with cancer.

Watson stated that cancer rehabilitation continued to receive modest attention and funding support through the 1970s and 1980s but not to the degree anticipated from this early funding initiative. She suggested that this was due to the public and the NCI placing more emphasis on discovering a cure for cancer and early detection and prevention.

Other reasons cited in review article by DeLisa [4] were a subsequent decline in federal funding and emphasis, failure to adequately educate oncologists about the importance of rehabilitation of their patients, failure on the part of the rehabilitation profession to prioritize cancer rehabilitation in physiatry resident education, and the shift in emphasis to outpatient physical medicine. DeLisa reported that a growing body of literature began to appear in the early 1990s that demonstrated the need for cancer rehabilitation and its effectiveness in improving functional status and quality of life.

O'Toole and Golden [18] reported on 70 cancer patients in 1991 who were treated at a rehabilitation hospital. Fourteen percent could walk on admission, and 38% were continent of urine. On discharge, 80% could ambulate independently or with supervision, and 87% were continent. At 90 days post-discharge, 33 patients had died or were lost to follow-up. Of the 37 remaining, 27 had maintained or improved their functional level.

In addition to showing the benefits of rehabilitation services to patients with cancer, O'Toole's other goal in writing this article was to improve the referral rate of cancer patients for rehabilitation by their oncologists. Oncologists were familiar with the Karnofsky Performance scale (KPS) and used it in making treatment decisions but did not use it to determine which patients would benefit from rehabilitation interventions. The Karnofsky Performance scale is a 100-point scale that quantifies cancer patients' ability to function, with 0 being dead and 100 having no functional impairments [19]. His study sought to correlate KPS scores, with which oncologists were familiar, with a Functional Independence Measure (FIM) score, which some feel is a better measure of functional capabilities and rehabilitation potential. His goal was to heighten oncologists' awareness of which patients could benefit from rehabilitation medicine interventions. He devised a table that suggested that even patients with Karnofsky scores as low as 30 (severely disabled, stay in hospital indicated, death not imminent) were candidates for rehabilitation services [18].

The Rehabilitation Institute of Chicago reported in 1996 on 159 patients admitted over a 2-year period for inpatient rehabilitative services for functional impairments from cancer or cancer treatments. They reported significant functional gains in motor function. This study reported that metastatic disease did not affect functional outcome and that radiation therapy was associated with greater functional improvement than when it was not provided or completed before starting rehabilitation [20].

In an article published in 2001, Cheville [21] felt that the most compelling reason to provide comprehensive care, including rehabilitation, to advanced cancer patients is that it enhances and maintains physical function. The threats of disability and becoming a "burden" to caregivers are among the most distressing concerns to cancer patients. Concerns over caregiver burden have been cited as a reason for requests for physician-assisted suicide and euthanasia [22]. The kinds of symptoms and conditions Cheville describes as treatable with comprehensive rehabilitation programs include motor deficits, sensory deficits, cerebellar dysfunction, cranial and oromotor deficits, cognitive dysfunction, deconditioning, and osseous mets. Cheville cautions that treatment goals in these situations must be reviewed frequently, specifically with respect to whether they are consistent with patient wishes.

Problems commonly encountered in the care of the dying patient with cancer

Patients who are in the end stages of their disease, including terminal cancer, have a variety of potentially treatable problems including fatigue, weakness, pain, dyspnea, and delirium. Even modest attempts to address them can help improve the patient's quality of life and functionality. This section addresses these issues and offers suggestions on how to ameliorate them.

Asthenia

A significant problem that faces cancer patients that is not related to any type of tumor or location of disease is cancer asthenia. Asthenia is characterized by physical fatigue, poor endurance, inability to initiate activity, and impaired memory and concentration [23]. It is usually seen in advanced cancer among patients who have been actively treated for cancer, who may have had adverse side effects from treatment, and for whom palliative and hospice care is being considered.

Other etiologies of fatigue that are seen in advanced cancer patients include cachexia, infection, anemia, and metabolic and endocrine disorders. These must be considered in any advanced cancer patient presenting with asthenia. The above conditions may be partially reversible with treatment if the patient with advanced illness requests treatment of underlying disorders [2].

Because previous studies had not addressed the response of cancer asthenia to rehabilitative techniques, Scialla et al [23] documented the effects of comprehensive inpatient rehabilitation on elderly patients who showed signs and symptoms of cancer asthenia. All patients studied had a Karnofsky Performance Status score of 60 or less and a FIM total score of <80. All patients received comprehensive multidisciplinary rehabilitation from an oncologist, a physiatrist, oncology nurses, physical therapists, recreational therapists, social workers, psychologists, nutritionists, speech pathologists, and cancer support groups. The FIM was used to measure functional improvement.

The FIM rates independence in 18 individual areas including cognitive function on a 7-point scale. A score of 18 implies complete dependence. A score of 126 represents complete independence. A total of 110 patients were reviewed [24–26]. Sixteen had blood-related neoplasms. The rest had a variety of solid tumors. The mean age was 75.3 years. All were Dietz stage III or IV with regard to goals of care. The mean hemoglobin level was 10.7. The median Karnofsky Performance Score was 50.0. The median total FIM score was 71. Patients were taken from a retrospective review of all inpatient rehabilitation admissions 60 years and older over a 30-month period if the record showed signs of cancer asthenia. The mean discharge FIM score was 88, which was a statistically significant improvement in physical and cognitive functioning. However, it only changed the description of the patients' functional status from "in need of significant assistance in all activities of daily living" to "requiring moderate assistance with self-care." This improvement was felt potentially to have a significant effect on caregiver burden once the patient returned home. Each one-point gain in a FIM score is felt to decrease caregiver time by 3 to 4 minutes [27,28]. Although the study provided evidence that a diverse group of cancer patients could experience functional improvement after a rehabilitation program, the authors concluded that more work needs to be done to accurately predict which patients will achieve the greatest benefit [23].

Winningham [29] addressed the same problem in 2001. She cited more recent articles that identify what she labels as "cancer-related fatigue syndrome (CRFS)" as the most distressing experience among cancer patients, affecting their daily lives more than pain [30,31]. Although she would agree with Scialla in that CRFS is amenable to rehabilitation efforts, she suggested that those efforts should be directed to the root of the cause of CRFS, which is impaired oxygen delivery to cells due to disease and treatment effects on oxygen availability. This results in anaerobic metabolism that leads to lactic acid formation and associated symptoms of dyspnea and fatigue. Although in the past rest was recommended to address fatigue, it is now recognized that physical inactivity induces further muscle wasting and deconditioning and that the treatment for cancer-related fatigue may be endurance exercise training.

Winningham [29] cites numerous studies on the effects exercise protocols have had on various cancer populations. She states that exercise has been shown to improve muscle mass and plasma volume, improve pulmonary ventilation and perfusion, increase cardiac reserve, and result in higher concentrations of oxidative muscle enzymes. This is important to cancer patients because physical performance and lean mass are important predictors of survival. Anorexia, weight loss, and dyspnea place cancer patients at high risk for morbidity and mortality [32,33]. Winningham also makes the case that improved physical function can enhance feelings of control, self-esteem, and independence, thereby improving social interaction and reducing anxiety and fear. The benefits of exercise on muscle function may in part be mediated through the immune system, whereby interleukin-1 and other myotoxic cytokines are downregulated [34]. Resistance exercise has also been shown to reduce steroid-induced loss of muscle mass. She cautions, however, that patients must be adequately evaluated for risk factors before pursuing an exercise program.

Pain

Pain is a symptom common to palliative care and rehabilitation. Seventy to ninety percent of patients with advanced disease have significant pain [2]. Pain can interfere with the progress made in physical therapy. It is incumbent upon clinicians in both areas of practice to become knowledgeable in the use of analgesics, including the various opioid medications, and in nonpharmacologic techniques to treat pain. Pain management in people aging with disabilities is covered in another article in this issue.

Dyspnea

Dyspnea is defined as a subjective experience of breathing discomfort, which can be characterized only by the person who is experiencing it [35,36]. Dyspnea is a common symptom in older adults, even in the absence of cardiac or pulmonary disease [37]. It is a common symptom in all forms of advanced lung disease, including lung cancer and chronic obstructive pulmonary disease (COPD) [38]. It is also a common symptom in patients with advanced malignancy of any kind, occurring in 70% of terminal cancer patients [39]. The differential diagnosis of dyspnea includes an obstructive airway process (asthma, COPD), parenchymal or pleural disease (cancer, pneumonia), vascular disease (pulmonary embolus), cardiac disease (congestive heart failure, ischemic heart disease), primary neurologic disease (amyotrophic lateral sclerosis [ALS]), metabolic disease (anemia, renal failure), or generalized weakness. Generalized weakness can be seen in advanced disease of any etiology but especially advanced cancer.

Dyspnea is almost always associated with some degree of anxiety and a negative impact on quality of life [36]. Given the diverse etiologies of dyspnea, the treatments may vary. The first approach is to reverse the underlying cause consistent with the patient's goals for care. The patient with advanced cancer or ALS whose course is further complicated by pneumonia may choose to receive oxygen therapy, bronchodilators, and morphine for dyspnea as opposed to more aggressive treatment with antibiotics and tracheal intubation. The goal of treatment should be to reduce the symptom burden and improve the patient's quality of life given the circumstances of their disease process and their wishes for care.

Bronchodilator therapy with drugs such as albuterol and ipratropium bromide can play a role in malignant and nonmalignant lung diseases. Corticosteroids are also useful in exacerbations of COPD and in several cancer-related conditions, including superior vena cava obstruction and tumors causing airway obstruction. Morphine is a mainstay of treatment for dyspnea in cancer patients. It has been shown to be more effective in relieving dyspnea among cancer patients than patients with COPD [40,41]. Detailed dosing of the pharmacologic agents used to treat dyspnea is beyond the scope of this article but can be found in two reference texts on palliative care [36,42]. Supplemental oxygen therapy has been used with mixed results for dyspnea at rest associated with advanced lung disease and advanced cancer [43,44]. A fan at the bedside of the dyspneic patient may be more effective than supplemental oxygen [45].

Nonpharmacologic approaches to dyspnea include pulmonary rehabilitation, relaxation techniques, noninvasive positive pressure ventilation, positioning, humidified air, acupuncture, cognitive-behavioral therapy, and simple reassurance [36]. Noninvasive positive pressure ventilation has become an accepted therapy for patients with chronic respiratory failure from neuromuscular disorders when $Paco_2$ is >45 mm Hg or when there is significant nocturnal desaturation [46].

Delirium

Delirium is a common symptom at the end of life, occurring in as many as 85% of patients in the days before death [47]. Delirium, as defined in the Diagnostic and Statistical Manual of the American Psychiatric Association, is (1) a disturbance of consciousness, with associated disturbances in attention; (2) a change in cognition or the development of a perceptual disturbance that cannot be explained by a pre-existing dementia; (3) the disturbance develops over a short period of time and may fluctuate over the course of the day; and (4) there is evidence of a change in the general medical condition that could result in direct physiologic consequences to the patient who is exhibiting the above symptoms [48].

Dementia renders patients more susceptible to delirium of any cause and to side effects from anticholinergic and opioid medications. Constipation and urinary retention can contribute to delirium, especially in the older patient with dementia.

Other risk factors include multiple severe or unstable medical problems, polypharmacy, dehydration, infection, fractures, visual impairment, psychoactive drug use, male gender, and alcohol abuse [49,50]. Old age is also felt to be a risk factor, possibly because of age-related brain changes leading to reduced cholinergic activity or because other risk factors, such as dementia and polypharmacy, are more prevalent in old age [51]. Because delirium is often multifactorial, the relative risk of developing delirium increases with the number of risk factors [52]. Delirium in the palliative care setting is characterized by declining function, behavioral difficulties, caregiver burden, and loss of ability to direct one's care and communicate with loved ones. Patients with delirium also experience more falls [49,50].

Delirium should be anticipated, and the underlying causes should be treated as early as possible. Some early signs of delirium include disordered sleep, social withdrawal (refusing to speak with staff or family), irritability or forgetfulness that is new, or the new onset of incontinence. Later signs can approach those of an acute psychosis, with hostile outbursts, refusal to cooperate, agitation, and illusions, delusions, and hallucinations with paranoid features [53]. Delirium may also be associated with a depressed motor state. This "hypoactive delirium" is associated with more severe medical illness, longer hospital stays, the development of pressure ulcers, and a worse prognosis [54]. Hypoactive delirium in elderly patients is often misdiagnosed as depression or not recognized as a problem [55]. Reversible causes of delirium in advanced cancer patients include psychoactive medications (especially opioids) and dehydration. Delirium associated with hypoxia and metabolic disturbances in advanced cancer is less likely to be reversible [56]. Rehydration in the setting of terminal illness can present other concerns, however. This is further discussed later.

Pharmacologic treatment is indicated when patients are a danger to themselves or seem to be frightened or distressed by their symptoms [57]. Neuroleptics are the drugs of choice in treating the agitation, fearfulness, hallucinations, paranoia, and aggression associated with delirium. They are less effective in treating confusion, wandering, and restlessness and may be associated with the development of akathisia or motor restlessness.

Haloperidol is the neuroleptic of choice for short-term use. It has a lower incidence of hypotension and cardiovascular side effects and can be given via many routes. Although short-term use of haloperidol is not likely to cause extrapyramidal side effects, it is recommended that the atypical neuroleptics, such as risperidone, be used for longer-term treatment. They are, however, associated with more side effects, including more anticholinergic activity, which may worsen delirium. Withdrawal from alcohol or sedative hypnotic medications is also associated with delirium, in which case benzodiazepines are the recommended treatment.

When opioid medication is felt to be associated with delirium, opioid rotation can be helpful if the patient needs this category of drug for symptom management.

Any medication with anticholinergic effects can contribute to delirium, including H2-blockers and scopolamine, which are commonly used in the palliative care setting. These drugs should be discontinued in the setting of delirium, especially in elderly patients [58].

Nonpharmacologic measures are important in the treatment of delirium. A supportive environment that avoids overstimulation and isolation is important. The patient should be surrounded by familiar items even if they are in a hospital or nursing home. Having family and friends spend time with the patient and keeping the patient involved in meaningful activity to the extent allowed by their behavioral symptoms can be helpful [59,60]. Physical restraints should be avoided because they are associated with increased agitation, discomfort, increased falls, and death [61–63].

Rehabilitation medicine program

Although this article does not cover the topic of cancer rehabilitation in detail, certain basic principles need to be emphasized. The role of rehabilitation medicine is to help the patient achieve his/her highest possible level of function and independence, given the diagnosis and prognosis. Rehabilitation medicine uses prescribed exercises to maximize range of motion, muscle strength and endurance, with the ultimate goal of improved functionality and independence. Whenever possible, appropriate orthotics, prosthetics, and adaptive equipment are used to help achieve these goals.

A crucial component of the rehabilitation prescription is the use of appropriate precautions while providing treatment. For example, using an appropriate assistive device and close supervision in an individual with an unsteady gait and impaired balance helps minimize the risk of falls and fractures. Cardiac and pulmonary precautions can also provide safe parameters for exercise.

Patients with end-stage disease may not tolerate long periods of exertion, and therefore the treating team should incorporate frequent rest periods during the exercise sessions. Therapies should not be scheduled back-to-back so the patient has time to rest between sessions.

Adaptive equipment can be used to compensate for lost range of motion, strength, and endurance. Occupational therapists can perform an evaluation of the patient's activities of daily living or perform a home visit to make recommendations on the use of various devices, such as reachers, sock-aids, raised toilet seats, and grab bars.

Physical therapists and occupational therapists can educate the caregivers on techniques of transfers, hygiene, grooming, and dressing that will make it easier for them to care for the patient.

Orthotics can be used to protect and support an injured extremity and substitute for lost function. For example, an ankle foot orthosis can make it easier for foot clearance during the gait cycle of a cancer patient with absent ankle dorsiflexion due to metastatic brain disease.

Ethical dilemmas in patients with end-stage disease receiving rehabilitation medicine and palliative care

End-of-life care raises issues regarding resuscitation, advance directives, decision-making capacity, resource allocation, and medical futility. The Hastings Center, an organization committed to the study of ethical issues in medicine, the life sciences, and the professions, convened a task force in 1985 to explore the ethical concerns associated with rehabilitation and chronic care. The issues they identified included the role of the family in decision-making and caregiving, confidentiality issues in a health care team delivering rehabilitative services, goal setting, decision-making in the context of changes in functional abilities, paternalism, and access to rehabilitative services [64,65].

To further elaborate the ethical concerns of rehabilitation professionals, Kirschner et al [66] undertook a survey in an urban specialty rehabilitation hospital. They used a questionnaire developed by the research team that addressed everyday ethical issues and educational approaches to ethics education. Two hundred seventeen clinicians out of 411 (53%) responded to the survey. Among the issues identified were health care reimbursement for rehabilitative services; setting rehabilitation goals; decision-making capacity; confidentiality issues (especially as they pertain to billing practices); decisions to withdraw life-sustaining treatments; adequacy of discharge plans; advance directives and DNR status; and patient, family, or caregiver refusal to follow through with a care plan.

The team approach to setting goals of care and how conflicts are resolved among team members and with patients and families with unrealistic wishes for care was a prominent concern. This is of relevance to the practice of palliative care and to rehabilitation where the team approach to care is the accepted model. The investigators of this study used the information gathered to develop an educational curriculum that would assist the rehabilitation clinicians in their daily clinical experience [66].

Appropriate goal-setting

The issue of appropriate goal-setting is a major challenge faced by the teams that provide palliative and rehabilitative care. Patients with advanced disease often have a desire for continued or renewed independence, but the ravages of disease leave the success of rehabilitation in question. Balancing hope for continued function with the realization of the toll that the disease is extracting is a challenge. Purtilo and Meier [67] characterize this as "helping a person become accustomed to living in an altered situation." Conversely, it might be the palliative care or rehabilitation team that expects the patient to want to function at the highest level possible when the patient is more interested in assuming an accepting role of their progressive physical decline and focusing on psychosocial goals. The ethical principle that should guide these decisions is patient autonomy. As Purtilo and Meier [63] describe, honoring patient autonomy shows respect for the patient, their goals, values, fears, and hopes.

Purtilo and Meier [68] describe six factors that impair the team's ability to let patient preference guide the care plan. These include (1) the "can't turn back now factor," whereby the patient feels too invested to change the course of action; (2) the "fatigue" factor, whereby the patient is too engaged with multiple team members and activities to seek alternatives; (3) the "anxiety" factor, whereby the patient is too anxious to risk new approaches; (4) the "gratitude" factor, whereby the patient feels thankful to the team and does not want to hurt anyone's feelings even though the recommended course of action no longer suits the patient's goals for care; (5) the "reasonable expectation" factor, whereby the team seems to demand patient cooperation; and (6) the patient feels outnumbered by the team members. Team members need to be aware of these dynamics and the threat they pose to patient-centered goals of care.

Informed consent and decision-making capacity

Another ethical principle operative in goal setting is that of informed consent. The conditions of informed consent are closely aligned to decision-making capacity. To give informed consent, a patient must (1) be capable of making and communicating a decision; (2) be presented with and understand the information relevant to the decision at hand, including the risks and benefits of the proposed treatments and alternative treatments; (3) understand that the treatment decision at hand applies to them and make a decision based on their particular values system; and (4) the decision should be free from coercion of any kind [69,70].

Another criterion often mentioned is that of "durability" of the decision. Is this decision consistent with previous health care decisions and with the patient's values? If not, has the patient changed his mind, or does the patient not fully understand what is being asked of him? An example of this is the tetraplegic spinal cord injury patient who has refused to be placed on a ventilator over a period of years and then presents to the emergency room consenting to tracheal intubation for respiratory difficulty. Such a decision warrants further discussion. However, this may not be possible in a moment of crisis when the patient is in distress. If in doubt about what decision to make in such a situation, the rule is to treat and then try to ascertain patient wishes after the patient is stabilized or a surrogate decision-maker can be identified.

Decision-making capacity is variable, especially in older patients. Medications, illness, dehydration, and time of day can influence the patient's understanding of the decision at hand. Decision-making capacity is also not "all or nothing." The rule of thumb is that the greater the potential burden a treatment decision imposes on a patient, the greater the capacity to make decisions must be. If time allows, the patient with compromised capacity should be assessed over a period of hours or days before decisions are turned over to a surrogate decision maker.

Family members with unrealistic goals of care can influence decision-making in such a way that the patient's wishes become secondary. Every opportunity should be made to speak with patient alone when discussing care issues unless the patients requests that family or friends be present. If the patient is not alone, those present during conversations should be encouraged to listen to what the patient is saying and let patient's wishes guide the decisions at hand.

If the patient is not capable of informed consent for the treatment decision at hand, the team must turn to a surrogate decision-maker who represents the patient's wishes if the patient could speak for himself/herself. This is the principle of "substituted judgment." Identification of this person varies from state to state but can include the person chosen by the patient to speak for them if they can no longer speak for themselves (known as a Health Care Proxy or Durable Power of Attorney for Health Care), a family member or friend (depending on local state law), or a court-appointed guardian.

If the surrogate decision-maker cannot exercise substituted judgment, the ethical principle invoked would be the "best interest" standard. This is the decision that would be in the best interests of the patient under the existing circumstances [70]. Another description of this standard is the "reasonable person" standard-the decision that most reasonable persons in the same situation would choose [71].

The goals of care provided by the rehabilitative and palliative care team should be based on the expressed wishes of the patient with decision-making capacity, following the principle of patient autonomy. In the event the patient does not have decision-making capacity, the goals of care should be determined by a surrogate who represents the patient, following the guidelines outlined above, and the treating team. This collaboration should result in a treatment plan by which the patient, his or her family, and the treating team can abide [69–71].

The use of cardiac resuscitation, mechanical ventilation, antibiotics, artificial nutrition/hydration, and hospitalization in the end stages of disease

The use of mechanical ventilation, antibiotics, artificial nutrition, and hydration are dependent on the patient's wishes and to a lesser degree on their prognosis. If life-prolongation is desired, these modalities and hospitalization may be tried. If the primary goal is comfort, the goal may be attained without the use of these interventions.

The discussions with the family and patient should include all the information needed to make the decision, keeping in mind the above-mentioned criteria for informed consent. The issues of cardiac resuscitation, mechanical ventilation, antibiotics, artificial nutrition, hydration, and hospitalization should be discussed as early as possible in the course of advanced disease. This is done in an effort of identify the health-care wishes of the patient, thereby reducing the burden of decision-making for the surrogate [72].

Cardiopulmonary resuscitation is an example of where there is disagreement among health care providers and patients as to the appropriateness of providing this treatment to terminally ill patients. When originally conceived in the 1960s, CPR was felt to be indicated only in situations of unexpected death. In 1974, the American Medical Association endorsed a policy that included the statement that "Cardiopulmonary resuscitation is not indicated in cases of terminal irreversible illness where death is not unexpected" [73]. This was in response to what had become the standard of care in the medical community that everyone would prefer to be resuscitated. Although subsequent studies showed that terminal illness was a strong predictor of poor outcomes with CPR, others have shown an initial response rate equal if not better than those of nonterminally ill patients. Survival to discharge remains poor, however. Nevertheless, resuscitation remains a choice available to patients with advanced disease, and there is no consensus that it should be withheld from patients based on their diagnosis [74].

Artificial nutrition and hydration is another area where consensus has not been reached with regard to terminally ill patients. Two review articles found no evidence of benefit in terms of survival or comfort when advanced dementia is the underlying cause of failure to take in adequate nourishment [75,76]. However, with cancer patients, extent of disease, functional status, and patient goals of care must be considered when making this treatment decision.

Before a decision is made regarding artificial nutrition or hydration in a terminally ill patient, good palliative care dictates that all reversible causes of poor oral intake be adequately addressed to. Decreased appetite can be due many factors associated with terminal illness, including constipation and fecal impaction, nausea, urinary retention, untreated pain, infection, medications, depression, changing food preferences, dysphagia, and poor oral hygiene. Terminal illness is associated with loss of appetite that may respond to appetite stimulants such as megestrol acetate, corticosteroids, and dronabinol.

Cachexia syndrome is a condition in which loss of appetite is associated with marked weight loss, weakness, and muscle wasting. It is most common in cancer patients but can be seen in advanced heart failure, COPD, liver and renal failure, and AIDS. It is a catabolic process that breaks down skeletal muscle, fat, and carbohydrates in the setting of reduced nutritional intake. It usually cannot be reversed with short-term nutritional supplementation [77]. Studies of enteral and parenteral feeding in advanced cancer patients with cachexia show no benefit in terms of improved nutritional status or survival [78–81]. Therefore, a request from a patient with advanced disease of any type for artificial nutrition or hydration must be carefully considered because parenteral and enteral feeding carry risks and most likely little to no benefit.

Artificial nutrition and hydration should not be started out of concern that the terminally ill patient who is not eating will otherwise suffer. A study of dying cancer patients who were no longer eating or drinking showed that the only discomfort they experienced was that of a dry mouth. This symptom was successfully treated with ice chips, sips of fluid, and artificial saliva [82]. Other studies on dehydration at the end of life show that patients are felt to be more comfortable if not provided with excess fluid beyond that needed to keep the mouth moist. This is best achieved with local mouth care, not artificially provided food and fluids [83,84].

When patients cannot decide what to do with regard to treatments such as feeding tubes, or the surrogate decision-maker is unsure of how to proceed, a time-limited trial of the treatment or treatments in question is an acceptable alternative. If the treatment proves ineffective or the burdens too great, then the treatment may be withdrawn. Withdrawing some treatments, especially feeding tubes and ventilators, is difficult for many clinicians and families. There is legal and ethical consensus, however, that withdrawing ineffective treatments is the preferred alternative to not starting potentially beneficial treatments at all [85]. Artificial nutrition and hydration are treatments that a patient can refuse or ask to be discontinued if they are not helping to achieve his or her goals for care [86,87]. How such decisions are made for patients who no longer have the capacity to do so varies from state to state but usually involves a surrogate decision-maker and explicit documentation of what the patient's wishes for care would be under the circumstances (eg, an advance directive) [77].

A case study is presented to help illustrate some of the principles outlined above.

Case study

History

Mr. S is a 77-year-old man with a history of stage IIIB lung cancer with bilateral pleural effusions and diabetes mellitus. He was admitted to an inpatient palliative care unit because of progressive weakness, anorexia, dizzy spells, and falls at home. He had received several courses of chemotherapy, but the lung cancer had continued to progress, and he was felt to be too weak to try new treatments. His primary caretaker was his wife, who could no longer manage his care needs. She reported that he could no longer walk up and down the flight of stairs in the home. However, he was able to ambulate with a rolling walker and one-person assist for a few feet.

Physical examination

The patient was thin, had a depressed affect, and was dyspneic with speech and minimal exertion. He had a blood pressure of 85–95/50–60 without orthostatic changes, a heart rate of 80, decreased breath sounds at the left lung base on chest examination, and 2 to 3+ lower extremity edema. His upper extremity strength was 3/5, hip flexors were 3/5, knee extension and flexion was 4/5, and dorsiflexion was 5/5. He had fair sitting balance and poor standing balance. Functionally, he needed assistance to transfer from bed to wheelchair and was able to walk only 4 feet with a rolling walker and contact guarding. His endurance was rated as poor, and he was noted to be dyspneic with the slightest exertion.

Functionality

The patient had a score of 40 on the Karnofsky performance status scale, which translates into an inability to care for himself and requiring institutional care.

Laboratory tests

Laboratory tests were significant for a hemoglobin level of 10 and an albumin level of 1.9.

Patient's goal

The patient's goal was to regain enough function to be able to assist in his care at home. His wife confided in the palliative care team that she did not think he could regain enough function to return home because she knew his cancer was progressing and that she was finding his care emotionally draining. However, she supported his wishes.

Assessment

The patient was reviewed at a joint meeting of the palliative care unit team and the rehabilitation team. His poor appetite was attributed to his cancer process and to dyspnea. His progressive weakness was attributed to his advancing cancer, exacerbated by poor nutritional intake, mild anemia, low blood pressure, and deconditioned state. It was felt that the edema in his legs was secondary to his poor nutritional status and low albumin. He was also felt to be depressed.

Treatment plan

These findings were shared with the patient and his wife. Although the physical therapist was not hopeful that the patient could regain meaningful function, a trial of an active rehabilitation program was suggested that included training in transfers, ambulation, balance, strength, and functional mobility. To this, occupational therapy added range-of-motion exercises and strengthening to the upper extremities, training in activities of daily living, bed mobility, and wheelchair training.

The patient's diuretic was discontinued, and he was instructed to liberalize the salt intake in his diet. It was also recommended that he take an appetite stimulant and to begin taking antidepressant medication. Erythropoietin was recommended for his anemia.

Advance directives were discussed with the patient. He appointed his wife as his health care proxy, with his son as an alternate. He requested an attempt at resuscitation but stated that he would not want to be kept alive on a ventilator if he was not awake and could not communicate with his family and if there was no expectation that he would ever do so. He said he did not want artificial nutrition and hydration under any circumstance. He would agree to any other treatments for the sole purpose of making him more comfortable, not for prolonging his life. The patient agreed to the treatment plan as outlined.

Course

Early on, the patient required supplemental oxygen to participate in the rehabilitation program. In approximately 1 month, his appetite and mood were much improved. He could ambulate without supplemental oxygen with a rolling walker for 150 to 300 feet per session, with occasional rest periods, and could negotiate 13 stairs two to four times per session. He was independent in bed mobility and transfers. He was discharged home in the care of his wife and remains there 1 year later, his disease held in check with a new chemotherapy regimen.

This case illustrates many of the principles outlined in the article. The patient was felt to have advanced untreatable disease, but with a comprehensive and multidisciplinary approach, he was able to regain physical and emotional function and improve his quality of life despite the initial expectation that this could not happen.

The challenges ahead

Despite renewed recognition regarding the importance of cancer rehabilitation, barriers exist. Watson [17] comments on a changing health care system where there is more focus on outpatient care and therefore less time to evaluate and plan for rehabilitative services. There is also less contact with facilities where the rehabilitation can be provided.

DeLisa [4] adds that although the number of physiatrists has increased by sixfold since 1975, many are engaged in outpatient musculoskeletal and sports medicine. There is a need for physiatrists to address the rehabilitative problems faced by patients with cancer. Additionally, identification of the rehabilitation needs of patients with advanced disease by their treating practitioners remains a major barrier to the provision of appropriate rehabilitation services [11].

Continuing educational activities need to be developed for oncologists, primary care physicians, and others taking care of patients with end-stage diseases to make them more aware of the benefits that palliative care and rehabilitation medicine can provide.

References

[1] Cancer pain relief and palliative care. Geneva: WHO; 1990.
[2] Santiago-Palma J, Payne R. Palliative care and rehabilitation. Cancer 2001;92:1049–52.
[3] Billings J, Pantilat S. Survey of palliative care programs in United States teaching hospitals. J Palliat Med 2001;4:309–14.
[4] DeLisa JA. A history of cancer rehabilitation. Cancer 2001;92:970–4.
[5] Curtis EB, Krech R, Walsh TD. Common symptoms in patients with advanced cancer. J Palliat Care 1991;7:25–9.
[6] Donelly S, Walsh D. The symptoms of advanced cancer. Semin Oncol 1995;22:67–72.
[7] Ries LAG, Kosary CL, Hankey BF, Miller BA, Harras A, Edwards BK, editors. SEER cancer statistics review, 1973-1994: tables and graphs. Bethesda (MD): National Cancer Institute; 1997.
[8] McCarthy EP, Phillips RS, Zhong Z, Drews RE, Lynn J. Dying with cancer: patients' function, symptoms, and care preferences as death approaches. J Am Geriatr Soc 2000; 48(Suppl):S110–21.
[9] Cancer facts and figures. Atlanta: American Cancer Society; 1993.
[10] Cancer rates and risk. 4th edition. Bethesda (MD): National Institutes of Health; 1996.
[11] Landis SH, Murray T, Bolden S, Wingo PA. Cancer statistics, 1998. CA Cancer J Clin 1998; 48:6–31.
[12] Stafford RS, Cyr PL. The impact of cancer on the physical function of the elderly and their utilization of health care. Cancer 1997;80:1973–80.
[13] Movsas SB, Chang VT, Tunkel RS, Shah VV, Ryan LS, Millis SR. Rehabilitation needs of an inpatient medical oncology unit. Arch Phys Med Rehabil 2003;84:1642–6.
[14] Dietz JH. Rehabilitation of the cancer patient. Med Clin North Am 1969;53:607–24.

[15] Dietz JH. Rehabilitation oncology. New York: Wiley Medical; 1981.

[16] Mayer D, O'Connor L. Rehabilitation of persons with cancer: an ONS position statement. Oncol Nurs Forum 1989;16:433.

[17] Watson PG. Cancer rehabilitation: an overview. Semin Oncol Nurs 1992;8:167–73.

[18] O'Toole DM, Golden AM. Evaluating cancer patients for rehabilitation potential. West J Med 1991;155:384–7.

[19] Mor V, Laliberate L, Morris J, Weimann M. The Karnofsky performance status scale. Cancer 1984;53:2002–7.

[20] Marciniak CM, James JA, Spill G, Heinemann AW, Semick PE. Functional outcome following rehabilitation of the cancer patient. Arch Phys Med Rehabil 1996;77:54–7.

[21] Cheville A. Rehabilitation of patients with advanced cancer. Cancer 2001;92:1039–48.

[22] Breitbart W, Rosenfeld B. Physician-assisted suicide: the influence of psychosocial issues. Cancer Control 1999;6:146–61.

[23] Scialla S, Cole R, Scialla T, Bednarz L, Scheerer J. Rehabilitation for elderly patients with cancer asthenia: making a transition to palliative care. Palliat Med 2000;14:121–7.

[24] Granger CV, Hamilton BB, Sherwin FS. Guide for the use of uniform data set for medical rehabilitation. Buffalo (NY): Uniform Data System Medical Rehabilitation; 1986.

[25] Heineman AW, Linacre JM, Wright BD, Hamilton BB, Granger CV. Relationship between impairment and physical disability as measured by the functional independence measure. Arch Phys Med Rehabil 1993;74:566–73.

[26] Dodds TA, Martin DP, Stolov WC, Deyo RA. A validation of the functional independence measure and its performance among rehabilitation inpatients. Arch Phys Med Rehabil 1993; 74:531–6.

[27] Granger CV, Cotter AC, Hamilton BB, Fielder RC, Hens MM. Functional assessment scales: a study of persons with multiple sclerosis. Arch Phys Med Rehabil 1990;71:870–6.

[28] Granger CV, Cotter AC, Hamilton BB, Fielder RC. Functional assessment scales: study of persons after stroke. Arch Phys Med Rehabil 1993;74:133–8.

[29] Winningham ML. Strategies for managing cancer-related fatigue syndrome: a rehabilitation approach. Cancer 2001;92:988–97.

[30] Vogelzang NJ, Breitbart W, Cella D, Curt GA, Groopman JE, Horning SJ, et al. Patient, caregiver, and oncologist perceptions of cancer-related fatigue: results of a tripart assessment survey. Semin Hematol 1997;34:4–12.

[31] Winningham ML, Nail LM, Burke MB, Brophy L, Cimprich B, Jones LS, et al. Fatigue and the cancer experience: the state of the knowledge. Oncol Nurs Forum 1994;23:23–36.

[32] Gerber LH. Cancer rehabilitation into the future. Cancer 2001;92:975–9.

[33] Reuben DB, Mors V, Hiris J. Clinical symptoms and length of survival in patients with terminal cancer. Arch Intern Med 1988;148:1586–91.

[34] Deuster PA, Curale AM. Exercise-induced changes in populations of peripheral blood mononuclear cells. Med Sci Sports Exerc 1987;20:276–80.

[35] American Thoracic Society. Dyspnea: mechanisms, assessment, and management: a consensus statement. Am J Respir Crit Care Med 1999;159:321–40.

[36] Pan CX. Dyspnea. In: Morrison RS, Meier DE, editors. Geriatric palliative care. New York: Oxford University Press; 2003. p. 230–55.

[37] Landahl S, Steen B, Svanborg A. Dyspnea in 70-year-old people. Acta Med Scand 1980;207: 225–30.

[38] Claessens MT, Lynn J, Zhong Z, Desbiens NA, Phillips RS, Wu AW, et al. Dying with lung cancer or chronic obstructive pulmonary disease: insights from SUPPORT. Study to understand prognoses and preferences for outcomes and risks of treatments. J Am Geriatr Soc 2000;48(Suppl 5):S146–53.

[39] Reuben DB, Mor V. Dyspnea in terminally ill cancer patients. Chest 1986;89:234–6.

[40] Poole PJ, Veale AG, Black PN. The effect of sustained-release morphine on breathlessness and quality of life in severe chronic obstructive pulmonary disease. Am J Respir Crit Care Med 1998;157:1877–80.

[41] Bruera E, Macmillan K, Pither J, MacDonald RN. Effects of morphine on the dyspnea of terminal cancer patients. J Pain Symptom Manage 1990;5:341–4.

[42] Waller A, Caroline NL. Dyspnea. In:Handbook of palliative care in cancer. 2nd edition. Boston: Butterworth-Heinemann; 2000. p. 239–244.

[43] Liss H, Grant B. The effect of nasal flow on breathlessness in patients with chronic obstructive pulmonary disease. Am Rev Respir Dis 1988;137:1285–8.

[44] Booth S, Kelly MJ, Cox NP, Adams L, Guz A. Does oxygen help dyspnea in patients with cancer? Am J Respir Crit Care Med 1996;153:1515–8.

[45] Schwartzstein RM, Lahive K, Pope A, Weinberger SE, Weiss JW. Cold facial stimulation reduces breathlessness induced in normal subjects. Am Rev Respir Dis 1987;136:58–61.

[46] Robert D, Willig TN, Leger P. Long-term nasal ventilation in neuromuscular disorders: report of a consensus conference. Eur Respir J 1993;6:599–606.

[47] Shuster JL. Palliative care for advanced dementia. Clin Geriatr Med 2000;16:373–86.

[48] American Psychiatric Association. Diagnostic and statistical manual of mental disorders, vol. IV. Washington, DC: American Psychiatric Press; 1994.

[49] Inouye SK. Predisposing and precipitating factors for delirium in hospitalized older patients. Dement Geriatr Cogn Disord 1999;10:393–400.

[50] Fann JR. The epidemiology of delirium: a review of studies and methodological issues. Semin Clin Neuropsychiatry 2000;5:64–74.

[51] Trzepacz PT. Delirium: advances in diagnosis, pathophysiology, and treatment. Psychiatr Clin North Am 1996;19:429–48.

[52] Inouye SK, Bogardus ST Jr, Charpentier PA, et al. A multicomponent intervention to prevent delirium in hospitalized older patients. N Engl J Med 1999;340:669–76.

[53] Fleishman SB, Lesko LM. Delirium and dementia. In: Holland J, Rowland J, editors. Handbook of psychooncology. New York: Oxford University Press; 1990. p. 342–55.

[54] O'Keefe ST, Lavan JN. Clinical significance of delirium subtypes in older people. Age Aging 1999;28:115–9.

[55] Farrell K, Ganzini L. Misdiagnosing delirium as depression in medically ill elderly patients. Arch Intern Med 1995;155:2459–64.

[56] Lawlor PG, Gagnon B, Mancini IL, Pereira MB, Hanson J, Suarez-Almazor, et al. Occurrences, causes, and outcomes of delirium in patients with advanced cancer: a prospective study. Arch Intern Med 2000;160:786–94.

[57] Goy E, Ganzini L. Delirium, anxiety, and depression. In: Morrison RS, Meier DE, editors. Geriatric palliative care. New York: Oxford University Press; 2003. p. 286–303.

[58] Tune LE. Serum anticholinergic activity levels and delirium in the elderly. Semin Clin Neuropsychiatry 2000;5:140–53.

[59] Shuster JL. Palliative care for advanced dementia. Clin Geriatr Med 2000;16:373–86.

[60] Volicer L, McKee A, Hewitt S. Dementia. Neurol Clin 2001;19:867–85.

[61] Morrison RS. Pain and discomfort associated with common hospital procedures and experiences. J Pain Symptom Manage 1998;15:91–101.

[62] Tinetti ME, Liu WL, Ginter SF. Mechanical restraints use and fall-related injuries among residents of skilled nursing facilities. Ann Intern Med 1992;116:369–74.

[63] Miles SH, Irvine P. Deaths caused by physical restraints. Gerontologist 2001;32:762–6.

[64] Haas JF, Mackenzie CA. The role of ethics in rehabilitation medicine: introduction to a series. Am J Phys Med Rehabil 1993;72:228–32.

[65] Caplan AL, Callahan D, Haas J. Ethical and policy issues in rehabilitation. Hastings Cent Rep 1987;17:S1–S20.

[66] Kirschner KL, Stocking C, Wagner LB, Foye SJ, Siegler M. Ethical issues identified by rehabilitation physicians. Arch Phys Med Rehabil 2001;82:S2–8.

[67] Purtilo RB, Meier RH 3rd. Team challenges: regulatory constraints and patient empowerment. Am J Phys Med Rehabil 1988;72:327–30.

[68] Purtilo RB. Ethical issues in teamwork: the context of rehabilitation. Arch Phys Med Rehabil 1988;69:318–22.

[69] Beauchamp TL, Childress JF. Principles of biomedical ethics. New York: Oxford University Press; 1989.

[70] Sliwa JA, McPeak L, Gittler M, Bodenheimer C, King J, Bowen J, and the AAP Medical Education Committee. Clinical ethics in rehabilitation medicine: core objectives and algorithm for resident education. Am J Phys Med Rehabil 2002;81:708–17.

[71] Jonsen AR, Siegler M, Winslade WJ. Clinical ethics: a practical approach to ethical decisions in clinical medicine. 4th edition. New York: McGraw-Hill; 1998.

[72] Teno JM. Advance care planning for frail, older persons. In: Morrison RS, Meier DE, editors. Geriatric palliative care. New York: Oxford University Press; 2003. p. 307–13.

[73] Standards for cardiopulmonary resuscitation (CPR) and emergency cardiac care (ECC). JAMA 1974;227(Suppl):833–68.

[74] Waisel DB, Truog RD. The cardiopulmonary resuscitation-not-indicated order: futility revisited. Ann Intern Med 1995;122:304–8.

[75] Finucane TE, Christmas C, Travis K. Tube feeding in patients with advanced dementia: a review of the evidence. JAMA 1999;282:1365–70.

[76] Gillick MR. Rethinking the role of tube feeding in patients with advanced dementia. N Engl J Med 2000;342:206–10.

[77] Easson AM, Hinshaw DB, Johnson DL. The role of tube feeding and total parenteral nutrition in advanced illness. J Am Coll Surg 2002;194:225–8.

[78] Evans WK, Nixon DW, Daly JM, Ellenberg SS, Gardner L, Wolfe E, et al. A randomized study of oral nutritional support versus ad lib nutritional intake during chemotherapy for advanced colorectal and non-small-cell lung cancer. J Clin Oncol 1987;5:113–24.

[79] Ovesen L, Allingstrup L, Hannibal J, Mortensen EL, Hanson OP. Effect of dietary counseling on food intake, body weight, response rate, survival, and quality of life in cancer patients undergoing chemotherapy: a prospective, randomized study. J Clin Oncol 1993;11: 2043–9.

[80] Koretz R. Parenteral nutrition: is it oncologically logical? J Clin Oncol 1984;2:534–8.

[81] Lipman TO. Clinical trials of nutritional support in cancer: parenteral and enteral therapy. Hematol Oncol Clin North Am 1991;5:91–102.

[82] McCann RM, Hall WJ, Broth-Juncker A. Comfort care for terminally ill patients: the appropriate use of nutrition and hydration. JAMA 1994;272:1263–6.

[83] Huffman JL, Dunn GP. The paradox of hydration in advanced terminal illness. J Am Coll Surg 2002;194:835–9.

[84] Byock IR. Patient refusal of nutrition and hydration: walking the ever-finer line. Am J Hosp Palliat Care 1995;12:8–13.

[85] Council on Ethical and Judicial Affairs. American Medical Association: decisions near the end of life. JAMA 1992;267:2229–33.

[86] Boisaubin EV. Legal decisions affecting the limitation of nutritional support. Hosp J 1993;9: 131–47.

[87] Groher ME. Ethical dilemmas in providing nutrition. Dysphagia 1990;5:102–9.

ELSEVIER
SAUNDERS

Phys Med Rehabil Clin N Am
16 (2005) 307–316

PHYSICAL MEDICINE
AND REHABILITATION
CLINICS OF
NORTH AMERICA

Basics of elder law and legal liabilities of negligence and malpractice for physicians as they apply to individuals with disabilities

David Ullman, Esq[a,b,*], Michael E. Zuller, Esq[c]

[a]New York State Bar Association, Section on Trustees & Estates,
1 Elk Street, Albany, NY 12207
[b]American Trial Lawyers Association, 1050 31st Street NW, Washington, DC 20007
[c]Private Practice, New York, NY 10018

In the normal course of treating patients, there are legal issues that require that the physician have an overview of what is beyond the charts and lab results. The physician is often the first to confirm that someone needs greater assistance than expected or anticipated. Although it is sometimes obvious that a person has difficulties making decisions for themselves, more often this is a subtle observation. A slowly progressing disease process can gradually diminish an individual's ability to formulate adequate responses to situations.

Patients choose their course of treatment provided that they are competent to do so. If they are not competent, then the legal issue of competence takes center stage because the physician (outside of emergency care) may not know what to do in relation to the patient's wishes. If the patient lacks capacity, it is important for the treating physician to know that there are provisions in place for someone to make decisions over treatment, discontinuance of treatment, etc. Some questions arise: Is the family unified in their view of the patient's course of treatment? Are there legal documents in place? What legal steps can be taken to protect the affected individual? Is there a Guardian? What is the role of the physician? When should a physician speak out or intervene? What are the ramifications for malpractice? The importance of these interactions to the physician becomes obvious in regard to treatment, ethical concerns, billing, and legal liability.

* Corresponding author. 600 Old Country Road, Suite 314 Garden City, NY 11530.
E-mail address: UllmanEsq@aol.com (D. Ullman).

Health care proxies

It is vital for the physician to know who is legally responsible for making health care decisions for the patient. All states have laws that enable individuals to identify others to act as their agents in making medical decisions for them when they can no longer direct their own treatment. This is generically called a health care proxy (HCP) (also known as a "power of attorney for health care directives").

In its simplest form, the HCP is a statement in which an individual designates one or more people to make medical decisions for them when they are no longer competent to do so. Most commonly, these documents are presented to or requested by a treating facility. The medical facility needs to see and know that the HCP is properly executed, contains the necessary language, and contains the names of the agent (if there is more than one agent, all should be listed, and the medical facility needs to know the order of priority).

Another document sometimes incorporated into the body of the HCP is a "living will." This is a declaration made while the person is competent that they do not seek extraordinary care in the end stage of their illness. The living will contains the patient's wishes regarding the use of heroic measures to resuscitate or treat and calls for specific direction, such as the withholding of food, water, or medicine, while allowing maximum palliative treatment. The living will information should be kept in the medical chart for all staff to see.

These documents assist the physician in directing conversations regarding treatment to the appropriate person. Difficulties can arise if there is more than one person named as the HCP proxy agent. Many attorneys do not like more than one person named but prefer to keep an order based on discussions with the family or caregivers. For example, it is common for a husband and wife to appoint each other, with the children named as successors, one at a time. This way potential confusion is minimized. It is a good idea for the physician to review the document with the patient and family in advance before a crisis arises and emotions cloud judgment.

The document's ability to determine the degree of competency can sometimes become an issue. For example, does the document specify at what point the HCP kicks in if a patient is not fully incompetent? Often, a committee or the treating physician (alone or with another doctor) is asked to provide a statement in writing that the patient has essentially lost the ability to participate in a meaningful way in their health care. At that point, the agent named in the HCP has the authority to act.

Historically, the family has been responsible for making decisions once it was determined that the patient could not. Typically it is the spouse who makes the decisions; if there is no spouse, the children make the decisions. Problems can arise when there is disagreement between the spouse and the children. In this case, the physician has a dilemma as to who is making the decisions for the patient. In such a case, a hospital board may have to convene a special meeting to resolve the matter.

Advances in medical technology have created additional problems with respect to questions surrounding life support. Who has the authority to disconnect the life support equipment? There were a number of cases in the late 1980s and early 1990s across the nation in which hospitals (some with obvious religious affiliations) did not accept a statement from the family regarding the patient's wishes when there was no written document.

In other cases, the family was split: The spouse wanted one course of treatment, and the children wanted another. These led to costly and excruciating court battles where judges had to step in and render a decision. In part, as a result of these cases, all states have since allowed for HCPs to be used to eliminate this problem.

When there is no HCP or living will, a family has to go to court to obtain the right to remove life support equipment (usually under a Guardianship petition). These are expensive and often traumatic events where they are contested. There have been reports of outside interested groups unrelated to any of the parties who had sought to impose their own religious or political agendas on the family.

The fact that there may already be a HCP on file does not assure that the family members will be able to effectively deal with the issues. Depending on its content, it can create more problems than it solves. For instance, if more than one person is named as the agent, are they all present and willing to undertake their designated role? Do they all agree? What happens if they disagree?

Additionally, hospital admissions personnel may be more interested in knowing that a patient has a HCP than seeing it and having the physician review it. Often the document is not produced until it is needed, which is the wrong time to discover its limitations.

Physicians should openly discuss the importance of the HCP with their patients and encourage them to obtain it. If they do not have a HCP, then a referral to a lawyer that specializes in "Elderlaw" or estate planning can be helpful in drafting such a document. Over the past decade, Elderlaw has become a legal specialty (differing from Trusts and Estates lawyers). Elderlaw attorneys deal with issues such as HCP, Powers of Attorney, health directives, Medicare, Medicaid, and guardianships.

Once the HCP is obtained, it is good practice to have a copy of it as part of the patient's medical chart in case the family cannot locate it in a time of crisis. Almost always, the attorney who drafted it will have a signed copy in his/her file.

Case study 1

MC is a 75-year-old woman who had a stroke that left her with cognitive impairments and left-sided weakness. During her hospitalization, she demanded to be discharged home, although the opinion of the treating physician was that she was not ready. Going home would have placed her at a great risk of falling and possible fracture. He had recommended a transfer to an inpatient rehabilitation facility. This could have been a difficult situation were it not for the fact that she had a HCP that gave her husband the authority to make decisions for her. The husband, following the directions in the HCP, and in cooperation with the treating physician, was able to certify that she could not make decisions for herself, and she was transferred to a rehabilitation facility.

There are times when the lack of a HCP could be a devastating situation for the patient's family. In a case where an elderly disabled individual is on life support without a clear HCP and Living Will, there is the potential of pitting the surviving spouse against the children if they disagree on whether or not to discontinue the life support. If there is no surviving spouse, the children may be pitted against each other. The HCP is even more critical when there are family members of equal stature, such as only children, where there is no natural decision-maker, such as a surviving spouse.

Case study 2

In a recent case originating in Florida, Theresa Shiavo, age 27, lost consciousness due to a cardiac episode and was in a vegetative state for many years. After 8 years of seeing his wife in that chronic vegetatice state, dependant upon full life support, the husband petitioned the lower court for guardianship rights so as to withdraw life support (he did not have a HCP). Theresa Shiavo's parents objected and fought the petition. The husband prevailed in the lower court battles each time. The case became a national cause and ultimately Governor Jeb Bush obtained a legislative change in the law to stop the discontinuance of life support. The Florida Supreme Court overruled the Governor, indicating that the legislation passed was unconstitutional and that the trial court that allowed the husband to be guardian had processed the case correctly. While the final outcome at the time of this writing is not known, the animosity between two parties who loved Theresa Shiavo caused untold grief, massive expenses, and embroiled nationwide debate over the rights of a vegetative patient, and the issue of who has the authority to direct, or discontinue treatment [1].

Power of attorney

Different from the HCP is the power of attorney (POA) (known as "health power of attorney" in some jurisdictions). Whereas the HCP covers medical treatment, the POA covers legal and financial issues. It allows an agent limited or full legal authority to act on behalf of the impaired individual.

The value of the POA to physicians is that is assures a means to "get things done" that might otherwise be significantly delayed. These include having the family to do things in preparation for events likely to occur, such as completing the necessary forms and procedures for obtaining financing for a long-term care facility, or acting on plans to hire people or preserve assets because she had those documents in place.

Case study

EF is a 70-year-old man with a long-standing spinal cord injury who was exhibiting symptoms of paranoia. His wife was advised to apply for Medicaid to offset the costs associated with nursing home placement. During the application process, it was noted that there were about $40,000 worth of bonds in his name, which had to be transferred to his wife for him to obtain Medicaid benefits. He was able to handle the distribution of several hundred thousand dollars of assets to the wife, including his interest in the house, but for some reason he was unreasonably attached to the bonds. His wife used the POA to transfer the bonds, as this was in his long-term benefit. She was then able to obtain the Medicaid benefits for him.

The role of the physician

What does a physician do when he suspects or knows that the patient is no longer fully competent? The first answer is to discuss this with the relevant family members, hence the importance of the HCP. Due to the sensitive nature of this issue, it is important that this discussion be performed with the appropriate individual identified in the HCP.

It is equally important that the patient's family or caregivers be aware of the various day-to-day issues that the patient will have to deal with. Here the physician's discussion with the family or caregivers can be crucial in the long-term planning for the patient. The physician should be prepared to answer questions about the nature of the disability, possible progression of the disease, and the eventual loss of some or all of the patient's abilities to handle their household and financial affairs. The physician may be asked about any increased need for attendants, medical equipment, or long-term institutionalization. The earlier that the family knows about such issues, the better the planning will be.

The physician should be aware of his/her hospital's policies with respect to incompetence because the facility may have their own internal standards and methods of determining it.

Guardianship

There are cases when it is evident that no one has the legal authority to act on behalf of the patient. In such circumstances, a guardianship may be sought. A guardianship (available in all states) is a legal proceeding that can be brought by any interested party. It does not need to be brought by a relative.

In a guardianship proceeding, a court looks for the least intrusive way to assist an "allegedly incompetent person." For example, this could mean help with finances or assistance in making health decisions. The court hears testimony in this regard and appoints someone, usually a family member, who is empowered to make these decisions. In effect, the family has to go through a full legal procedure costing thousands of dollars for what could have been done in advance for a tiny fraction of the cost.

Case study

AN is a 63-year-old man who suffered a stroke while undergoing brain surgery. This left him with some cognitive deficits, such as short-term memory loss and an inability to deal with financial matters. He is articulate, alert, and otherwise in good health. His wife recently died, but he has several children from his previous marriage and one stepdaughter.

After the surgery and the stroke, the stepdaughter noticed significant problems in AN's behavior. He could no longer handle money and needed supervision for basic care, such as cooking and bathing. He exhibited dangerous behavior, such as burning things on the stove.

The stepdaughter sought a guardianship because his children refused to deal with the situation and could not see the serious nature of their father's illness. The court was requested to make a determination on whether he was in need of a guardian and if so to what extent and to appoint a person if warranted. The fact that a nonblood relation brought the petition did not mean she would or should be appointed, and in this man's case, the stepdaughter did not seek the position for herself and did not oppose the court in naming one of the other children. The court allowed the appointed child full HCP powers and access to assets with the requirement of periodic reporting to the court.

What to do if there is no family

Most hospitals and nursing homes have patient advocates who have connections to the local legal community and who know of the local options available. Most of these institutions can assign a social worker to assist the patient. If the patient is no longer able to dictate their own course of treatment, it goes back to the guardianship provisions discussed above. These same options are used where there is family but no one is willing to assist.

Liability for accidental versus intentional actions

Any discussion of medical malpractice law must initially draw a distinction between professional and lay liability. A "simple negligence" case involves a question of carelessness determined by a jury (or other finder of fact) based upon common knowledge. The "medical malpractice case" generally concerns issues of whether the treatment rendered was proper and in keeping with the general standards of care practiced by other doctors under similar circumstances. Because specialized knowledge is required, such a determination, as made by the jury, is based on predictably conflicting expert testimony. An example of a simple negligence claim might be a fall due to failure by a nurse or orderly to engage bedside guardrails. Not timely diagnosing a treatable disease, such as a pressure ulcer, would be one of medical malpractice, proof of which would require an expert's opinion. As in every liability case, even imposing defense evidence does not guarantee a favorable verdict to the defendant doctor/hospital/nursing home. Overwhelming probability is not the same as certainty. Juries are famous for disregarding the proof and allowing feelings of sympathy for an injured victim (termed "plaintiff") to decide a case. There are safeguards—notably the appeals process—built into the legal system to reverse such plaintiffs' verdicts, but that discussion is beyond the scope of this article.

A third type of claim in a hospital or nursing home setting is termed "intentional tort," as in the nature of physical assault, detention, or deliberate deprivation. Whereas the previous types of claims stem from neglect, the intentional tort is deliberate in nature. Factual patterns can be easily envisioned involving all manner of intentional mistreatment of patients, such as sexual assault, denial of food or medication, locking patients into rooms, or denying patients access to outsiders, visitors, or the premises and grounds of the facility. Even the less serious examples can give rise to civil actions against the institution and individual employees grounded in battery (eg, unlawful physical contact, touching, striking, or hitting) or false imprisonment (eg, denying a patient freedoms of movement, choice, activity, etc.) and result in awards of significant monetary damages. More serious situations could result in criminal prosecution.

Nursing home liability and the doctrine of respondeat superior

In civil actions targeting the hospital or nursing home institution, the liability theories center on negligent hiring, retention, or supervision. In New York State, the broadly worded Public Health Law Section 2801(1) places a nursing home, a free-standing rehabilitation facility, and many other kinds of health care centers within the definition of "hospital." All are subject to a large number of regulations in the Article 28 of that body of statutes. There are similar statues in all other states. In the context of nursing home (or free-standing health care center) liability, the doctrine of respondeat superior applies, making an institution responsible and legally liable for the negligent acts of its employees [2]. Determining whether an employee's careless act was performed within the scope of employment is critical. When an employee's careless action falls outside the scope of employment, a defense may arise for the nursing home, permitting it to sever its ties to the negligent employee. Its insurance carrier might not provide a defense [3]. If, for example, a surgical resident sexually assaults a patient in a recovery room, the hospital may successfully argue the resident's actions were outside the scope of employment, relieving it of all legal responsibility for the attack, even in its obligation to supervise or safeguard patients from harm inflicted by third persons [4].

In the case of a doctor working at the nursing home, it is crucial to determine whether his relationship with the facility was that of employee or affiliation. Once it is determined that a person is an employee, the master (nursing home) becomes subject to "vicarious liability" for his/her negligent or tortuous conduct. Thus, if he/she is employed by the nursing home or acting as its agent, the doctor is treated as any other employee whose negligence could cast the institution in vicarious liability (under respondeat superior) [5].

Generally, the nursing home is not be liable for the actions of the privately affiliated doctor so long as the staff properly carries out that doctor's orders [6]. Such a doctor would likely be termed an "independent contractor" and would be legally responsible for his own actions. Many nursing homes require such independent contractor physicians to carry their own medical malpractice insurance for just such contingencies, but a nursing home could face liability if its staff knows or should know that a private doctor's orders are so contraindicated by normal practice that inquiry would be expected [7].

In the context of nursing home liability for the actions of employees, claims can stem from negligent hiring, negligent retention of a troublesome employee, or negligent supervision. The latter three theories can be integrated into the following factual scenario: Mr. D, a nursing home worker, applies a hot pack to the insensate skin of a patient's leg. Instead of checking back in the prescribed 20 minutes, Mr. D. forgets and does not return for an hour. By that point the patient has suffered severe second-degree burns. Follow-up investigation yields important background information on Mr. D. Claims of a master's degree on the job application turn out to be false. Previous complaints by doctors and patients about the worker were never thoroughly explored, and supervision by doctor-employees or department heads or periodic job performance evaluations was virtually non-existent. Here, the actions of several employees may combine to make a successful plaintiff's case against the nursing home facility and can involve claims of ordinary negligence and medical malpractice if Mr. D is a professional.

Medical malpractice claims go toward the professional care rendered by professional nursing home staff, with an emphasis on whether the person causing injury was a nursing home employee, administrator, or professional and, if so, whether he was acting within the scope of employment. If both criteria are met, the nursing home is liable for the negligent acts of its employees. A mere affiliation is insufficient to impute the doctor's negligence to the nursing home and hold it liable, even where staff members rendered minimal assistance and did not stray from the doctor's orders. As with almost all malpractice cases, the final decision rests with the jury and turns on the credibility and reliability of the evidence [8].

What of the liability of the independent contractor or private physician who must decide whether to refer a patient to a health care facility? A physician who fails to timely transfer a patient to a hospital or nursing home may face personal liability consequences because this decision is not always considered an exercise of professional judgment. Once more, the evidence takes the form of expert opinions. Ordinarily, the referral of the patient to a nursing home does not impose liability on the referring physician for malpractice/negligence on the part of the nursing home physicians or staff. A question of fact would arise when a referring physician who periodically visited the patient knew or should have known of mistreatment or neglect and was in a position to exert some general authority and control and did or said nothing on the patient's behalf. In such cases, the physician might find himself held liable as an independent contractor for injury to the patient, together with the nursing home [9].

Because the movement of law in recent years has been in the direction of broadening liability and stretching the boundaries of responsibility to include anyone within the patient's circle of medical care, retention by the referring doctor of any control or authority over the patient in a nursing home setting should be presumed to confer potential liability if things go awry.

Defenses to liability claims

Classic defenses to medical malpractice claims are professional judgment and "bad result." As with any claim of professional malpractice, the practitioner may assert his decision-making and consequent action or inaction based upon the fairly wide judgment latitude accorded to doctors. If a doctor's decision is conceded to be a matter of judgment, liability does not attach for any unfortunate outcome. It is only when the doctor's judgment and action (or inaction) go beyond the parameters established by the large majority of practitioners that a malpractice finding can be obtained [10]. If a jury believes the doctor defendant acted on a reasonable professional judgment call, the case will likely fail for plaintiff, even when the end results of the doctor's decision have proven disastrous. A physician's duty is therefore to provide the level of care acceptable in the medical community in which he practices and to have the skills of an average member of his profession and specialty.

Resources

Cites that can be of assistance include the various state and county bar associations, the National Academy of Elder Law Attorneys (www.naela. com), and the National Network of Estate Planning Attorneys (www. nnepa.com).

References

[1] Bush v Schiavo, Florida Supreme Court, No. SC04-925 (2004).
[2] Morris v Lenox Hill Hospital, 232 A.D.2d 184, 647 NYS2d 753 (1996).
[3] Judith M. v Sisters of Charity Hospital, 93 NY2d, 932, 693 NYS2d 67 (1999).
[4] N.X. v Cabrini Medical Center, 280 AD2d 34, 719 NYS2d 60 (2001).
[5] Shafran v St. Vincent's Hospital and Medical Center, 264 AD2d 553, 694 NYS2d 642 (1999).
[6] Hicks v Ronald Fraser Clinic, 169 AD2d 558, 565 NYS2d 484 (1991).
[7] Somoza v St. Vincent's Hospital, 192 AD2d 429, 596 NYS2d 789 (1993).
[8] Tuzeo v Hedge, 172 AD2d 747, 569 NYS2d 134 (1991).
[9] Einaugler v Supreme Court, 109 F.3d 836 (1997).
[10] Ibguy v State of New York, 261 AD2d 510, 690 NYS2d 604 (1999).

ELSEVIER
SAUNDERS

Phys Med Rehabil Clin N Am
16 (2005) 317–326

PHYSICAL MEDICINE
AND REHABILITATION
CLINICS OF
NORTH AMERICA

Index

Note: Page numbers of article titles are in **boldface** type.

A

Acetaminophen, for pain, in disabled
adults, 70

Acupuncture, for pain, in disabled adults,
75–76

Alzheimer's disease, with traumatic brain
injury, 170–171

Amantadine, for post-polio syndrome, 210

Amputation, aging with, **179–195**
    and physical activity, 47–48
    diagnostic tests before, 184
    energy expenditure in, 181–182
    epidemiology of, 179–180
    future research on, 190
    heel ulcers and, 188
    impact of, 188–189
    level of function before, 182
    pain management in, 58, 63, 80
    pre- and postoperative care for,
      181–184
    predicting further limb loss in,
      187–188
    prevention of, 188
    prosthetic phase in, 184–187
      complications of, 186–187
      K-modifiers scale in, 186
      predicting outcome of,
        186
      socket designs in, 185
    rehabilitation for, 277
    risk factors for, 184
    versus revascularization and limb
      salvage, 181

Anesthetics, local, for pain, in disabled
adults, 73

Anthracycline analogs, for multiple
sclerosis, 229

Anticonvulsants, for spinal cord injury, 81

Antidepressants, for pain, in disabled
adults, 72

Antiepileptics, for pain, in disabled adults,
72

Antioxidant activity, age-related changes in,
20

Aquatic exercise, for post-polio syndrome,
212–213

Arthritis, cerebral palsy and, 238

Articular cartilage, age-related changes in,
27–29

Artificial nutrition and hydration, for
end-stage cancer, 296–297

Asthenia, and rehabilitation and palliative
care, for end-stage cancer, 287–288

Atherosclerosis, and amputation.
    See Amputation.

Avonex, for multiple sclerosis, 229

Azathioprine, for multiple sclerosis, 229

B

Baclofen, for pain, in disabled adults, 73

Behavioral dyscontrol, with traumatic brain
injury, 171–172

Betaseron, for multiple sclerosis, 229

Bladder complications, of cerebral palsy,
241
    of multiple sclerosis, 225–226

Bones, age-related changes in.
    See Musculoskeletal system.

Botulinum toxin injections, for pain, in
disabled adults, 78

Bowel complications, of multiple sclerosis,
226

Brief Fatigue Inventory, to measure fatigue,
in elderly, 97–98

C

Cachexia syndrome, and rehabilitation and
palliative care, for end-stage cancer,
297

doi:10.1016/S1047-9651(04)00101-9